Your Vegetarian Pregnancy

A Month-by-Month Guide to Health and Nutrition

DR. HOLLY ROBERTS

Board-Certified Obstetrician-Gynecologist

A FIRESIDE BOOK

Published by Simon & Schuster

New York London Toronto Sydney

FIRESIDE
Rockefeller Center
1230 Avenue of the Americas
New York, NY 10020

FIRESIDE and colophon are registered trademarks
of Simon & Schuster, Inc.

For information regarding special discounts for bulk purchases,
please contact Simon & Schuster Special Sales at
1-800-456-6798 or business@simonandschuster.com

Designed by Jill Weber

Manufactured in the United States of America

3   5   7   9   10   8   6   4

Library of Congress Cataloging-in-Publication Data

Roberts, Holly, date.
Your vegetarian pregnancy : a month-by-month guide to
health and nutrition / Holly Roberts.
p.   cm.
"A Fireside book."
Includes bibliographical references and index.
1. Pregnancy—Nutritional aspects.   2. Vegetarianism.   I. Title.
RG559.R635   2003
618.2'4—dc21   2002042701
ISBN 0-7432-2452-3

This publication contains the opinions and ideas of its author. It is intended to provide helpful and informative material on the subjects addressed in the publication. It is sold with the understanding that the author and publisher are not engaged in rendering medical, health, or any other kind of personal professional services in the book. The reader should consult his or her medical, health, or other competent professional before adopting any of the suggestions in this book or drawing inferences from it.

The author and publisher specifically disclaim all responsibility for any liability, loss, or risk, personal or otherwise, that is incurred as a consequence, directly or indirectly, of the use and application of any of the contents of this book.

This book is dedicated to my husband, Patrick,

who encourages me to live my dreams,

and our daughters, Brigette, Rose, and Heather,

who give me inspiration.

ACKNOWLEDGMENTS

I extend my deepest thanks to Sister Maureen Conroy

for her faith in my medical/humanitarian book for

pregnant vegetarian women, to my dedicated young

editor, Anne Bartholomew, for guiding me along my

literary path, and to all my patients who permitted me to

share their joy during their creation of life.

In gratitude to

Divine Intervention.

Contents

Part III: NOW THAT YOU ARE A MOTHER   307

Preface

Your deepest female instincts
have led you and compelled you
toward this dedicated path of creation.

These guiding instincts are not part of your knowledge,
not part of your education,
nor are they part of your job.

They are part of a universal force.
A force that drew
every inch of your body
and every millimeter of your essence
to long for a child.

A longing that could be realized only
in the conception, the nurturing, and the birthing of
a human life.

As you begin your journey
you will find yourself guided by the needs of your body,
by the advice of concerned healers,
and by the wisdom of your instincts.

Each of you who has chosen to read this book,
a guide to your health and nutrition
and a source of
questioning, contemplation, and compassion,
will follow your own path to motherhood.
That path will be strewn
with wisdom and dignity.

I have faith in you,
as I know you each have the strength in your character,
and the belief in your own convictions,
to find the true answers to all your questions.

Introduction

For as long as I can remember, I never liked to eat meat. It was at the age of thirteen that I became inspired to be a physician and to cease eating the flesh of other animals. Both concepts occurred to me when I awoke after having my appendix removed. I recognized that the doctor looking over my bed had saved my life, and I decided that someday, I too would save lives. I also truly appreciated the sanctity of life and resolved that I would seek to live my life without taking the life of any other creature.

I did not realize how circuitous my journey to become a physician would be. The journey took me from Brooklyn College in New York City to Kirksville College of Osteopathic Medicine in Missouri. It was within this altruistic and holistic medical school environment that I was taught that doctors do not heal patients, but are facilitators in their healing process. The power to heal lies within each individual. I was taught that all are blessed with the natural abilities to cure most diseases themselves but must make wise health choices throughout life, lest their natural healing modalities become depleted.

After I graduated from medical school, my quest for knowledge and training took me to Pennsylvania, New Jersey, New York, Maryland, and Tennessee. I left residency to work at a Cuban refugee clinic and then to become a medical missionary in Honduras, Mexico, and Peru. Three days after returning from Peru, I met my husband-to-be. We were soon blessed with three daughters. I completed obstetrics residency and trained in advanced gynecologic cancer surgery in New York and Maryland. I opened a medical practice in New Jersey, in which I delivered more than five thousand babies and cared for several thousand other pregnant women.

My ability to witness so many births was a spiritual blessing. Through those many years and many births, I always knew that I was on a mission to reach an even greater number of women, to share my experience and knowledge with them.

This book is for every woman contemplating pregnancy while striving for the best of health and showing the greatest mercy to others. The information it contains will help you safely, authoritatively, and wisely fulfill your dreams of giving birth to a strong, healthy child while adhering to a compassionate and healthy lifestyle. Whether you are decreasing your intake of red meat, limiting your intake of dairy products, or fully committed to a vegetarian or vegan lifestyle, there is an abundance of valuable information within this book that will help you optimize your baby's and your health during your pregnancy.

Having been a vegetarian, a physician, and a mother, each for over twenty-five years, I've thought about most of the questions you are now facing. When I was carrying my own children I asked these questions, but there were no answers. After years of studying nutrition, studying medicine, and gaining obstetric experience, I have learned how to guide and educate young women who share the same quest for answers about diet and health that engaged me.

The answers to many of your questions do not lie conveniently in medical journals. Although the basis for the knowledge is there, the complete answers can be found only at a deeper level of consciousness. You will obtain this knowledge as you learn about creation, birth, health, and nutrition. By striving to achieve a peaceful and wise lifestyle and being open-minded to new concepts, you will increase your chances of finding that humane and healthy life you so desire. By combining the medical knowledge you find here with your own maternal intuition, you will be able to answer each and every question about your health during pregnancy. I know that our journey together will benefit you and your baby. My best wishes are with you both.

IS THIS BOOK RIGHT FOR ME?

If you are browsing through this book, you will probably think about how your diet affects your health and might affect your tiny fetus. You may have recognized already that the typical American meat-based diet may not truly be the best diet for your baby or yourself. Because you have strayed from the dietary norm, I know you make your own choices. I hope to share my medical knowledge with you so you can continue to make your own choices—but make them at a higher level of medical and nutritional expertise.

You may already be among the peripheral group termed "vegetarians," and although you may or may not be among the strictest of the group, you are a thinker, a humanitarian, and a person with purpose. As you begin to prepare for your vegetarian pregnancy, it is important that you know which type of vegetarian lifestyle best suits your health needs and ethical choices. I will review the basic types of vegetarian lifestyles to help you discern which group applies to you.

An individual decreasing meat in her diet: You may be among the large and growing percentage of people moving toward a semi-vegetarian diet. You may be limiting your meat intake to fewer portions, may still eat fish or poultry or both, or may have completely eliminated red meat. Although yours is not a totally vegetarian diet, it warrants serious consideration during pregnancy. You definitely need the same nutritional knowledge for yourself and your unborn baby as does any other type of vegetarian. Also, you may be approaching a full vegetarian diet, and the completion of that path might occur before the end of your pregnancy.

Lacto-ovo-vegetarian: If you are a lacto-ovo-vegetarian, you do not eat beef, pork, fish, or poultry. Basically, you do not believe in eating the body of any animal or in taking the life of any animal. You may, however, eat products derived from animals, including eggs and dairy products—milk, butter, cheese, and yogurt. You are among a varied group of individuals. Some lacto-ovo-vegetarians believe in eating animal-derived products as long as the animal has not lost its life. Other lacto-ovo-vegetarians do not wish to eat the actual animal-derived food for specific health reasons, such as decreasing cholesterol or avoiding the pesticides, antibiotics, and synthetic hormones stored in animal fat. Because most eggs are not fertilized and would never have become chickens, lacto-ovo-vegetarians may not find the eating of eggs morally offensive, although most would prefer eggs from noncaged or free-roaming chickens. Most people who are lacto-ovo-vegetarians usually choose this diet for a combination of philosophical, humanitarian, and health reasons.

Vegan: Vegans are the purest vegetarians. If you are vegan, you avoid consumption of all animal-derived products. You will not eat any meat, fish, fowl, eggs, or dairy products. Your healthy diet consists of vegetables, fruits, nuts, legumes, grains, and seeds and is low in fats but high in protein, vitamins, minerals, and fiber. Because present-day farming techniques have depleted the soil of nutrients, you may need to pay closer attention to your diet to obtain sufficient quantities of vitamin D, vitamin B_{12}, and omega-3 fatty acids. These nutrients are not abundantly available in foods of plant origin. However, it is actually quite simple for you as a vegan to obtain adequate amounts of these nutrients. Many vegans have adopted a lifestyle in which their clothing, shoes, and cosmetics do not contribute to animal cruelty.

Macrobiotic vegetarian: If you follow a macrobiotic diet, you believe that eating a diet consisting of whole grains is superior physically and philosophically. You may also believe that the grains and plants you eat should vary with the seasons of the year and with the place in which you reside and should be indigenous to the area in which you live. Macrobiotics is not just a diet; it is a philosophy and a lifestyle based on principles of balance and harmony between nature and the universe. There is a strong Asian influence in the macrobiotic lifestyle, reflecting the principles of yin and yang. Because a macrobiotic diet is low in fats and animal products and high in nuts, grains, and seeds, you may have chosen this diet to attain a healthier lifestyle.

Part I
Preparing for Pregnancy

CHAPTER 1

Before You Become Pregnant

As you begin to plan for pregnancy,
many people will offer you advice.

Your doctor, midwife, friends,
and family
will all want to share the wisdom of their experiences
with you.

At first, you may feel overwhelmed.
But you will find yourself listening closely
to what they say.
And with their love and wisdom
you will become educated, inspired, and enlightened.

As you look forward to motherhood,
You will learn anew
how to eat, to sleep, to work, and to play.

Others will guide you,
but mostly,
your guiding force
will be your own inner wisdom.
You are the one who knows
how best to support that new life within you.

You will be the one to make all the final choices.
And they will be wise choices.
They will be carefully considered, intuitive,
and humane.

The inner wisdom of your soul,
the wisdom that is guiding you
as the educated and compassionate woman
you are,
will give you all the knowledge you need
on your journey toward motherhood.

PREGNANCY IS NATURAL

During pregnancy, there is so much medical information to absorb. I do not want to think of my pregnancy as purely scientific. How can I strike a balance between what I'm learning and what I'm feeling?

When you think about having a baby, so many visions will come to your mind. You will imagine the joy of finding out you are pregnant; you will visualize your pregnancy and birth as being an entirely natural phenomenon, as natural as life itself; and you will feel female instincts consuming your body, filled with the instinctive wisdom women have felt through all generations. These will be sustaining you during your creative journey to motherhood. Need you plan for the work of nature?

Nothing in your life will be closer to nature than your creation of life. We as vegetarians respect the power of nature in its primitive, earthy, and spiritual process called birth. I have been awed thousands of times by the instinctive strength of a woman's body and the fortitude of her mind throughout pregnancy and in birth.

However, having witnessed thousands of births, I know that many aspects of our complicated society give women conflicting messages about what is "natural" and what is "medical." In our present culture, we have tamed nature in numerous aspects of our lives, and we have come to be-

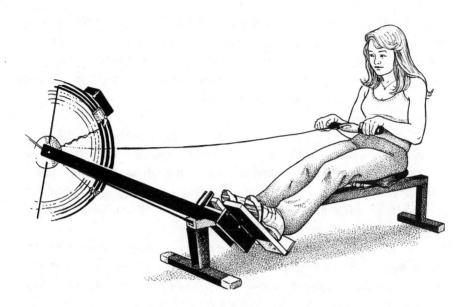

lieve that we can tame it in all aspects. But in actuality, we cannot and should not. Pregnancy and birth are times during which nature rules. Nature is perfect, but we might not like her perfect plan. Not all that is given us in nature is what we would have wished for, and that is what frightens us.

Following your instincts and increasing your medical knowledge will help you to strike a healthy balance. You will be informed and prepared without having to compromise what you know is best for your baby. I have seen pregnant women ignore their instincts and make poor health choices, such as working in an environment laden with toxic chemicals, discontinuing healthy exercise, or eating meat simply because the misinformed have told them it is healthier. Please listen to your instincts.

It is difficult for a woman to differentiate between prenatal information that is intuitive and factual and that which is born of ignorance and popular opinion. I hope that the following chapters will answer your questions and help you to bring your new life into this world with both wisdom and peace.

I am forty-five years old. Am I too old to have a baby? I married late in life, and I would love to have one, but only if it is safe for the child.

I believe that no woman is ever too old to have a baby, as long as she will love it. And obviously you will. There are risks to everything in life, but if you do not take chances, you will gain nothing. You do have an increased risk of having a miscarriage, however, due to your age. The rate of miscarriage when you were twenty-two years of age was 9 percent. At forty-five, your risk is 75 percent. On the positive side, you have a one in four chance of not having a miscarriage and of having the greatest blessing in your life.

Your chance of having a child with a chromosomal disorder is also higher. Every woman of every age has a chance of having a normal or an abnormal baby, so your age should not stop you any more than it should stop any other woman. There are no guarantees at any age, except the guarantee that if you try, your dreams might be fulfilled. Your chance of having a child with a chromosomal disorder at age forty-five is one in twenty. Reversing those statistics, you have a 95 percent chance of having a baby without a chromosomal problem. If you have an amniocentesis, you can further improve your chances of delivering a healthy baby. Hopefully, this testing will serve to alleviate your fears.

As an older pregnant woman, you will have a higher chance of developing either gestational diabetes or toxemia of pregnancy. At delivery, you will also have a statistically higher chance of needing a cesarean delivery. Studies indicate that your probability of requiring a cesarean section will be between 22 and 32 percent. One main reason contributing to this higher rate is that your cervix may not dilate well during labor. It may have become firm and rigid from years of never having dilated and may not be able to budge open, even during labor. A cesarean may be necessary as a result, but when it is over, you will have your baby for the rest of your life.

My husband is quite a few years older than I am. I am thirty-two years of age and he is fifty-five. Does that mean we are at risk?

The risk that you will have a child with a genetic disorder is increased because your husband is older. The traits for these specific disorders are carried on tiny genes within a large chromosome, so it isn't possible to detect these with an amniocentesis.

The disorders that occur more often when a baby's father is older include neurofibromatosis (elephant man disease), achondroplasia (dwarfism), Alpert syndrome (in which a baby is born with a misshaped head and fused fingers), and Marfan syndrome (a disorder in which the individual's hands and feet will become elongated with age). Although these diseases can become hereditary in future generations, they can occur for the first time in a family when the father is older.

There is also an increase in the incidence of specific disorders in the grandsons of men who were older when they fathered these boys' mothers. The fathers pass on a defective mutated gene to their daughters, who then become unsuspecting carriers of these diseases. The daughters will have no symptoms, but their sons or the grandsons of the older father will have the disease—this is called the "grandfather effect." These diseases can be serious—they include hemophilia and muscular dystrophy—and more often than not they will become hereditary for future generations.

ADVICE, ADVICE, ADVICE

I believe strongly in being vegetarian, yet now I am second-guessing myself because everyone wants me to eat meat during my pregnancy. I'm so torn.

It's natural for you to feel confused—you want to do what's best for your baby, but you also need to know that you cannot compromise your ideals. Talk to people about vegetarianism and tell them that the number of vegetarians in our country is increasing in leaps and bounds—15 percent of all Americans now consider themselves vegetarian to some extent. Ask these people if they know that those leaning more toward vegetarian lifestyles today are educated young students, older adults, individuals studying Asian philosophies and religions, and people who have medical disorders. Many of the latter individuals had been misled during their entire lives as to their dietary choices, and now, many are beginning to regain their health by following vegetarian diets. Teaching people about what it means to be vegetarian will help you gain the confidence you need, especially when you teach them that vegetarians choose their lifestyle for combinations of philosophical, health-related, religious, humanitarian, and ecological reasons. In turn, you'll find that your friends and family will understand more about your ideals and be more willing to support your choices.

HELPING OTHERS SUPPORT YOUR
VEGETARIAN CHOICE

My family insists that I start eating animal products so my baby will be healthy. What can I do to relieve their fears so they will support me as I continue my vegetarian diet during pregnancy?

This book will be a factual and reliable aid for you. Although there are many vegetarian books on the market, they were not written by board-certified obstetricians who were also vegetarian. I will share my obstetric experience, medical and nutritional knowledge, and understanding of recommended dietary guidelines to ensure that your vegetarian diet will be safe, healthy, and optimal for your baby and you.

The facts within this book will give you all the support you will need to teach your concerned family members about your vegetarian diet, to document that your diet is in no way inferior to a meat-based one, and to show them that in numerous instances your diet is superior. Be patient with them. Your family members are a product of a culture based on a carnivorous diet, and it's difficult for them to stray from the norm. They love you. When you will be able to teach them about your vegetarian lifestyle, they will respect you and support you.

I am vegetarian, but my husband is not. He is concerned that during my pregnancy, I will not be giving enough nourishment to our baby. What can I tell him to convince him that our baby will be healthy?

First, you must be patient with him. It is very difficult for non-vegetarians to accept this way of life. Everything he has read, has been taught, and has been shown has convinced him that the only diet that is safe and healthy includes animal flesh. Also, his opinion is the majority within our country, so he may find it hard to accept that your nontraditional opinions and views are valid. You will need to convince him that your diet contains a full variety of nutrients, in both quality and quantity, and that it is not the *source* from which you obtain these nutrients that is significant, but their presence and the quantity in which they are present.

Let him know that humans have existed for thousands of years on vegetarian-based diets and that vegetarians in our country have lower rates of heart disease, stroke, cancer, diabetes, kidney disease, obesity, hypertension, and osteoporosis. Inform him that vegetarians in our country live an average of eight years longer than their meat-eating counterparts. He will be less worried when he learns that all the nutrients recommended and required for pregnant women can be found in a healthy vegetarian diet. Also, he will gain renewed respect for your dietary choices when he learns of the improved health bestowed upon those individuals raised on and practicing vegetarian lifestyles.

As your pregnancy progresses, so too will all of your complaints. With each pregnancy-related complaint, your husband might be quick to assume that the underlying problem is your diet. Show him the American College of Obstetricians and Gynecologists guidelines I have included in chapter 2. He'll see how vegetarian foods fulfill each and every requirement. He will know that you are obtaining all the essential nutrients that both your baby and you need from a vegetarian diet.

You will have to accept his non-vegetarian lifestyle, so that he will reciprocally accept your vegetarian one. By your example, you will show him that as a vegetarian, you are not here to change him, only to live by your own principles. Feel free to mention that the woman physician who wrote this book had three healthy, bright vegetarian children, two of whom played varsity ice hockey in college for four years (he may like that).

A HEALTHY PREPREGNANCY LIFESTYLE

I do not know if some aspects of my life would be considered unhealthy during pregnancy. Can you review what a healthy pregnancy lifestyle should be like?

There are many aspects of your life that contribute to your total health during pregnancy. All aspects are of equal importance, because one unhealthy act can negate numerous healthy ones. During your pregnancy, think of your life as an interrelated chain, with every link as important as every other. If your weakest link is not healthy and breaks, the others cannot compensate. This is why you need to foster good health in every aspect of your life.

Look at your own health, as well as your family's genetic history. If you have a chronic illness, you should make sure you are at an optimum state of health and that your medications are safe for your unborn child. Next, ask your family and your partner's family if there have ever been any genetic diseases in family members of either side. It is beneficial for you to learn your full ethnic heritage. By knowing this, you can avail yourself of screening for a whole variety of ethnic-related diseases.

It is important that you not expose your body to unnecessary toxins, such as cigarettes, passive cigarette smoke, marijuana, street drugs, or alcohol. Further, you need to think about toxic substances present in your work environment. You should also recognize that your work environment may be a source of infection, particularly if you work in a school, day care center, hospital, health care clinic, prison, laboratory, pet store, or veterinary clinic.

Your food supply is another major area that should be checked for harmful bacteria or toxins. You should look at your diet to confirm that you have sufficient vitamins, minerals, and protein and limited amounts of fats, cholesterol, and empty calories.

If you have a weight problem, devise a realistic plan as to how much weight you can attempt to lose prior to becoming pregnant and how little weight you can afford to gain during your pregnancy. You should attempt this control of your weight only if it does not compromise your basic nutrition. This is also an important time for you to consider starting an exercise program. You can reasonably maintain one that will keep you strong and fit throughout your pregnancy.

Chronic Diseases

I have asthma and need to take several medications daily to prevent attacks. Should I inform my allergist that I am trying to conceive?

Most definitely. Whatever medications and inhalers you need to take a deep breath, you should take. It is critical that you supply sufficient oxygen to both your baby and yourself during pregnancy. Your pulmonary specialist might modify some of your asthma medications and switch you to safer ones; he also may try to decrease doses of other medications. You will still be permitted to take your beta-agonists, your bronchodilators, and your steroids as needed.

You should not try to decrease your medication dosages yourself, as in your enthusiasm you may lower them to such a level that you end up in the emergency room with a full-blown asthma attack. If that occurs, you might not only deplete your baby of needed oxygen, but you may also require more medication than you were taking initially. Take care of your condition just as you would normally. Inform your doctor of your plans to conceive, and you will be fine.

Why does my endocrinologist consider my being diabetic so significant during pregnancy?

If you are diabetic and dependent on insulin to control your diabetes, your chances of having a child with a congenital malformation may be increased if you do not keep your blood glucose in excellent control. When you visit your endocrinologist, she will check your daily glucose levels, and she may also check your blood for hemoglobin A1c. Your hemoglobin A1c level indicates your average blood glucose levels over the past three months. If your blood glucose levels have been normal, that will decrease the probability that your baby will develop "caudal regression syndrome," an abnormality that occurs in children of diabetic mothers whose glucose levels have not been in good control. Caudal regression syndrome affects the developing internal and external organs within the lower region of a fetus's body.

You will need to observe and control your diet and your blood sugar levels very closely, and you will most likely need to meet with your doctor regularly to make sure your levels remain normal. Before pregnancy, if your blood sugars are elevated minimally, there is no immediate harm to you. When you become pregnant, if your blood sugar elevates because you cannot produce sufficient insulin to metabolize all of your ingested glucose, this excess blood sugar will pass through your placenta to your baby. Your baby's tiny pancreas is not diabetic, so it will start to work overtime to metabolize the excess sugar coming to it from your body. Its pancreas will be working like a Trojan, but it will not be able to metabolize all of the sugar that it is receiving. This serious condition may have significant detrimental effects on your baby's health, including both developmental abnormalities and loss of life.

I am on seizure medication for epilepsy. Should I see my neurologist prior to becoming pregnant?

Yes, you should. It might be necessary for him to switch you to a safer anti-seizure medication. Initially, he will need to confirm that you are under perfect seizure control, and then he will place you on very high levels of folic acid to prevent possible congenital abnormalities from developing in your baby. This is because many seizure medications interfere with the body's absorption of folic acid, one of the B vitamins. This decreased level of folic acid within your body places you at higher risk for having a child with spina bifida (see chapter 2). Although the average woman planning to become pregnant should take 400 micrograms to 1 gram of folic acid daily, women taking seizure medication should take 4 grams of folic acid daily. Even though you will be taking 4 grams of folic acid daily, the amount absorbed into your system might be equivalent only to the 1-gram dosage a woman not on seizure medication is taking. You will be started on this dose prior to conceiving because the most important time to prevent birth defects in your baby is immediately after you conceive.

Unfortunately, the fact that you have epilepsy means you have a 6 to 8 percent chance of having a child with an epilepsy-related birth defect. This is based solely on the fact that you have epilepsy and has nothing to do with the medications you do or do not take. This rate of abnormalities is three times that of women within the general population. Each and every seizure medication has some potential side effects when given during pregnancy, so it is best to let your doctor decide which one is both the safest choice for your baby and the most effective in controlling your seizures. It is important that you discuss all these issues with your neurologist.

I have a heart condition. Will it be safe for me to conceive, carry a pregnancy, and deliver vaginally?

It will be very important for you to discuss your plans with your cardiologist. You may be in good health from a cardiovascular perspective and as healthy as any other woman who never had heart problems or heart surgery, but your cardiac function will need to be evaluated prior to your becoming pregnant. Pregnancy places an excess burden on the heart. This burden is created not just because of the size of your baby and your enlarged uterus, but also because of an increase in the circulating blood volume within your bloodstream. You will most likely be placed on anticoagulants to decrease the chance that your blood will develop clots. In general, your chances are approximately 56 percent that you will successfully complete your pregnancy in perfect health and leave the hospital with a healthy baby. There still exists, however, a relatively large chance that you may have a miscarriage or may lose your baby later in pregnancy as a direct consequence of having a heart condition.

Whether you decide on a vaginal delivery or a cesarean section may depend on how you are feeling toward the completion of your pregnancy. Contrary to what many people might believe, a calm vaginal delivery in a mother who has had an epidural for pain relief may present less of a strain on the heart than a cesarean section. Many factors come into play when you're trying to decide on the safest mode of delivery for you; only time and careful observation will answer this question.

I have been told that I might have more complications during my pregnancy because I have lupus. What problems might I expect?

Lupus is a chronic disease in the category of illnesses termed "autoimmune disorders." This category includes all diseases that manifest themselves by producing antibodies to tissues within an individual's own body. Lupus is the prototype for these illnesses, and as its name implies, lupus ("wolf") ravages many organs of an individual's body, just as an attacking hungry wolf might. Lupus is a disease that affects predominantly women—often young women. Women afflicted with this disease experience flare-ups and remissions. Studies have shown that if you postpone your entire pregnancy until you have been in a remission phase for six months, the final outcome of pregnancy will be positive for both your baby and yourself. When your immunologist learns that you have become pregnant, she might place you on medications beginning in the earliest phases of your pregnancy. You might be given medication, including steroids, to prevent a flare-up of your illness. You might also be advised to take baby aspirin to prevent blood clots from forming within your placenta.

The benefits of being in remission at the inception of your pregnancy will be significant. This will markedly lower your chances of developing lupus-related kidney disease, lung disease, hypertension, and toxemia of pregnancy. If you already have kidney disease and hypertension due to your lupus, this adds another layer of complexity to your risk status, but not an insurmountable one. Having lupus does not place you at increased risk for having a miscarriage, having a baby with a congenital problem, or having a stillbirth. However, if your lupus is not under control, you will be more likely to experience a premature delivery. Studies have shown that if your illness is not in remission, your chance of delivering prematurely may be as high as 30 percent.

I have had colitis since I was a teenager. I have heard that this can affect my pregnancy, but I do not know how.

Ulcerative colitis is common among young adults and affects many women, giving them cramps and diarrhea during pregnancy. The most significant indicator of your health during this pregnancy will be your health at the time you conceived. If your colitis was not active when you conceived, the rest of your pregnancy should be healthy. Women who develop ulcerative colitis for the first time during their pregnancy have an increased number of pregnancy complications, the main one being premature delivery. Pregnant women with colitis have been shown to fare better if they begin their pregnancies when the disease is in an inactive phase.

Although studies have shown that women with ulcerative colitis have no higher rate of infertility, miscarriage, having babies with lower birth weights, or having babies with intrauterine growth retardation, please discuss your colitis with your physician. Treatments for colitis include prolonged courses of sulfasalazine, 5-aminosalicylic acid, and corticosteroids. None of these has had a negative effect on the newborns of women treated for their colitis during pregnancy.

I have been diagnosed with Crohn's disease. How will this affect my pregnancy? Is my vegetarian diet safe to follow?

Crohn's disease is a serious inflammatory disease of the intestines that can create ulcers, scarring, and even total blockage of the bowels. When it is acting up, you will suffer from diarrhea and abdominal cramping and find blood, mucus, and pus in your stool. The disease process may affect your small intestine, your large intestine, or both. Genetic predisposition may have increased your chance of developing Crohn's disease; it is more prevalent in Caucasian women and in women of Jewish heritage.

Pregnancy will not trigger your Crohn's disease; whether or not you are pregnant, your risk of relapse is always 26 percent. Your risk of delivering prematurely, however, will be increased if you have Crohn's disease. This is particularly true if you had your first attack of Crohn's disease or if you had a reactivation of it during your pregnancy. Fortunately, your Crohn's disease does not increase your chances of having a miscarriage.

Your vegetarian diet may be advantageous during the times you are in remission, but it can be problematic when your Crohn's disease is active. A high-roughage vegetarian diet is considered the healthiest diet during times of remission because it may help to prevent recurrences. When your disease is active, however, a low-roughage diet is necessary. Your gastrointestinal specialist will guide you during your pregnancy to help you choose low-roughage nutritious foods. You may also need to increase your bed rest and take prescription steroids and sulfa medications when the disease is active. Some low-fiber vegetarian foods that will be less irritating for you include pasta, rice, bananas, peanut butter, molasses, white breads, eggs, and dairy products. The sulfa medications you're taking to stop the intestinal inflammation will decrease the quantity of folic acid that your body will absorb. It is best for you to take a folic acid supplement to counteract this effect.

Cigarette Addiction

I would like to stop smoking before I become pregnant. Are patches, gums, and pills that help people quit smoking as dangerous as cigarettes?

These products are almost as unhealthy as cigarettes, but they have been proven effective in helping smokers quit. It is so important for you to stop smoking before you become pregnant. If you feel you need one of these aids to help you quit, don't hesitate to ask your doctor which one would be best for you. Please do not feel ashamed to tell your physician that you smoke and you need help. Twenty-nine percent of all women of childbearing age smoke. Your doctor will not judge you; in fact, she will be very anxious to help you.

Over 2,500 different chemicals are present in fumes released when you smoke. Nicotine and carbon monoxide are the chemicals that cause the most detrimental side effects. The carbon monoxide in your cigarettes places you at particularly serious risk because it decreases the oxygen supply to your baby and placenta.

The following summary includes some of the side effects cigarette smoking causes during pregnancy. The list is here not to frighten you, but to motivate you.

◆ If you smoke, you have a higher chance of having a miscarriage. Forty-two percent of smokers miscarry, compared with only 19 percent of nonsmokers.

◆ As a smoker, you have a higher chance of premature separation of your placenta, premature rupture of the membranes, and premature delivery. If a woman stops smoking before she becomes pregnant, she decreases by 50 percent the chances of losing her baby due to premature separation of her placenta.

◆ If you smoke, your chance of having a baby of low birth weight is three to four times higher than that of a nonsmoker.

◆ When all other factors are considered, it is estimated that 30 percent of all infant deaths from SIDS (sudden infant death syndrome) can be directly attributed to a baby's being exposed to cigarette smoke within its mother's uterus.

◆ If all women in our country were to stop smoking, there would be a 10 percent total decrease in the deaths of fetuses and newborns.

◆ There is evidence that attention deficit hyperactivity disorder in a child may be linked to his exposure to cigarette smoke while in his mother's uterus.

What are some medical aids I can use to help me stop smoking?

If you elect to use any of these medical treatments to achieve your goal of becoming a nonsmoker, please use them in combination with the non-medical aids—you will have greater success. Both nicotine gum and the nicotine patches release nicotine into your body to provide relief from cravings for and withdrawal from nicotine. Nicotine gums are designed to gradually decrease the addiction to nicotine. However, when you use them, you create surges in nicotine levels (when you chew) and decreases (when you do not chew). These gums do not decrease your desire for nicotine; they simply give you less nicotine than cigarettes. For many smokers, nicotine gum is not strong enough to be fully successful. Nicotine patches, the next step, have been a great improvement over gums, because they supply a continuous level of nicotine. Most of the patches (Nicoderm, Habitrol, Prostep, and Nicotrol) can be used for eight weeks. To use them, apply a patch as soon as you get up in the morning and do not smoke at any time while you are using it. The amount of nicotine in the starting patch is equivalent to the amount of nicotine inhaled from twenty cigarettes. If you smoked only ten cigarettes a day, you must start with the midlevel patch rather than the strongest one. Your doctor and pharmacist will inform you of the dose of nicotine in each commercial patch. The gums and patches are not without risk in pregnancy, as your baby is still exposed to nicotine with each of these—another excellent reason to eliminate your smoking habit *before* you become pregnant.

There are currently two oral antidepressants, Wellbutrin and Zyban, that are prescribed to help individuals combat their urge to smoke. They should not be used together, as they contain the same components and people have had seizures when they have taken both simultaneously. These medications are placed within category B safety levels in pregnancy, which means that if you accidentally become pregnant while taking one of these medications, you do not need to worry. Nevertheless, if you can free your system of cigarettes, gums, patches, and medications before you become pregnant, that will certainly be a wonderful achievement for you.

What will your success rate be? That depends upon your prior addiction and your motivation, and we know you are very motivated now. This is not the time to be concerned about the twelve-pound weight gain that typically occurs when women stop smoking. Those twelve pounds will not hurt your baby, but 20 cigarettes daily for 266 days or 9 months—a total of 5,320 cigarettes—will.

What are some nonmedical aids I can use to help me stop smoking?

Hypnosis can be a wonderful tool to help you stop smoking. A professional hypnotist will teach you that all hypnosis is really self-hypnosis. The hypnotist will teach you how to place yourself in your own hypnotic state—your own special place away from the stress of this world—so that you can bring yourself into a nonsmoker state of being whenever you feel the urge to smoke. If you truly let yourself ascend to this state, you may be surprised at the success you achieve.

SmokeStoppers is a self-help group that has helped many people quit smoking. Whether or not joining this group will help you might be influenced by the degree to which the environment outside of your class is supportive. Your motivation to have a strong and healthy baby will be the most significant factor in your ability to quit.

You may also consider receiving acupuncture and acupressure treatments, joining a stress management group or meditation group, or seeing a private counselor. Establish your plan of action and the date by which you will achieve your goal, and aim toward it.

I've tried to stop smoking before, without much success. If I am still smoking after I conceive, is it safe to use nicotine gum, the patch, or pills like Wellbutrin or Zyban now to help me quit?

Before you use any of these products, remember that it is always best to live naturally while pregnant before you think of placing another substance in or on your body. The true effects of medications are often unknown until many years after their use. On the other hand, the true effects of nicotine use during pregnancy are known, and they are serious.

When you smoke, your baby does, too. That is why smokers have a higher incidence of miscarriage, smaller newborns (less than five pounds at birth), and newborns with a range of birth defects, including deformed arms and legs, attention disorders, and growth retardation. Smoke filters through your placenta and causes scarring in the placental tissue. These scars prevent blood, oxygen, and nutrients from getting through to the baby, all of which lead to poor health and development. Studies show that if you stop smoking before you are twenty weeks pregnant, your baby's growth will not be restricted. Even if you stop smoking by your thirtieth week, your baby will be larger than that of a woman who has continued to smoke all the way through her pregnancy.

If you are a heavy smoker, you can use nicotine gum or a nicotine patch to help you stop smoking. Both of these are considered safe, because although they contain nicotine, they do not contain carbon monoxide, cyanide, or the other toxins present in cigarettes. You cannot smoke at all while you are on either of these medications, or you and your baby will receive even higher doses of nicotine than you would have were you just smoking. The U.S. Food and Drug Administration (FDA) places both these drugs in category D status for use during pregnancy. This means that there is positive evidence of human risk from both the nicotine gum and patch, and their use can be justified only by the end result. If these help you to stop smoking, they are worth the risk. If you do not truly want to stop smoking, it is best not to use them.

The FDA places both Wellbutrin and Zyban in category B for safety during pregnancy, meaning no risks have been found in animal studies and no risks have been found in humans. You will need to speak with your physician about your use of these medications during pregnancy. There are always some risks with any medical preparation used for any purpose, so if you can stop smoking by going to a hypnotist, an acupuncturist, or a self-help group, try that first. If your husband smokes, his passive smoke will also be going to your baby. He had best stop smoking, too, or at least step outside to smoke. Please continue to decrease the number of cigarettes you smoke. Even if you wean yourself down to five cigarettes a day, you have done a great job. This will certainly be better for your baby than for you to continue smoking two packs a day.

Alcohol

I drank alcohol before I knew I was pregnant, and now I am worried. Have I hurt my baby?

No one knows exactly how much alcohol may cause fetal alcohol syndrome in an infant. It might be as small a quantity as two alcoholic drinks in one day, or it might be much larger quantities on a daily basis. That is why it is important that you not drink any alcohol. You cannot turn back the clock, you can only move forward and do what is best for your baby. Your doctor will be familiar with the concerns and fears you have about how alcohol may affect your baby's health, so don't hesitate to tell her. Some effects of fetal alcohol syndrome can be detected with ultrasound before the baby's delivery. If she thinks it is necessary, your doctor will do an ultrasound to check for anything out of the ordinary.

Caffeine

I like to drink coffee. Should I stop now that I am pregnant?

Yes. Coffee affects both your baby and you adversely. Although coffee is the most widely used herbal beverage in our country, if it were a newly developed drug, it might not pass FDA guidelines. The word *coffee* comes from Caffa, the region in Ethiopia where it was first discovered. Prehistoric East Africans ate the red unroasted beans before tribal wars for their stimulant properties. Coffee may increase your anxiety, raise your blood pressure and heart rate, cause an increase in your secretion of gastric acid, and contribute to insomnia, irritability, and nervousness. Do you need to be stressed any more while you are pregnant?

It is known that caffeine crosses the placenta. Women who drink large quantities of caffeine have had a higher level of birth defects and a higher rate of spontaneous miscarriages. Caffeine enters breast milk, so if you have not broken your coffee habit during pregnancy, you will need to if you plan to breast-feed. Caffeine causes your kidneys to lose many important minerals (such as potassium, magnesium, and zinc) and vitamins (such as vitamin C and vitamin B_1). A cup of coffee contains 120 to 150 milligrams of caffeine. Even if you have only two or three cups of coffee daily, your caffeine intake is high.

CAFFEINE LEVELS IN COMMON BEVERAGES AND FOODS

◆ Coffee	1 cup	120–150 mg
◆ Cola soda	1 cup	30–65 mg
◆ Instant coffee	1 cup	65 mg
◆ Black tea	1 cup	50 mg
◆ Green tea	1 cup	30 mg
◆ Milk chocolate	1 oz	10 mg
◆ Decaf coffee	1 cup	5 mg

To decrease your craving for caffeine, follow a diet that creates an alkaline residue; good choices are fruits, greens, corn, and whole-grain and soy products. To decrease your caffeine habit, avoid foods that give you an acid residue, such as meats and sugar. Most people who stop drinking coffee have withdrawal symptoms. These include headaches beginning eighteen to twenty-four hours after they stop the caffeine and continuing off and on for several days. They also usually experience constipation for one to two days.

Aside from decaf coffee, there are several beverages that are good substitutes for coffee and do not contain any caffeine. These include Postum, a blend of richly roasted bran and wheat, and Roma, a blend of roasted malt, barley, and chicory. The taste of Roma is stronger and closer to that of coffee. Both of these contain a minimal amount of calories.

I have been told that consuming caffeine will increase my chances of having a miscarriage. Is this true?

Unfortunately, it is. Recent studies have shown that among women who miscarry between their sixth and twelfth weeks of pregnancy, more have been consuming large quantities of caffeine. If a healthy woman consumes 500 milligrams or more of caffeine daily, her miscarriage rate will increase to almost 50 percent, compared to the 25 to 30 percent rate of a woman who consumes less than 100 milligrams of caffeine on a daily basis. It takes only three to four typical 8-ounce cups of coffee to reach 500 milligrams. No one can be certain if there is a direct cause-and-effect relationship between caffeine and miscarriages, but in this case, it is better to be safe than sorry.

Can I drink tea while I'm pregnant, since it has less caffeine than coffee?

Yes, tea is a better choice for you than coffee because it contains less caffeine, but water-decaffeinated tea is an even better choice. Commercial teas contain tannin, which, like caffeine, is a stimulant. It can also irritate your stomach lining and your kidneys. One benefit of drinking tea is its high fluoride content, but the drawback of drinking tea is that tannin can decrease your absorption of iron by 80 percent. This is quite important for a vegetarian.

Are herbal teas safe to drink during pregnancy?

That depends. Teas are made from various leaves, roots, or flowers. Some teas are safe and actually beneficial for use during pregnancy, while others create problems. Most teas that are sold in the supermarket, such as Celestial Seasonings teas, are safe. Following is a reference list you can use when shopping for herbal teas during your pregnancy.

SAFE TEAS

◆ Chamomile tea: Chamomile is safe during pregnancy and has a soothing effect to aid digestion. Do not drink chamomile if you are allergic to ragweed.

◆ Peppermint and spearmint tea: Mint tea is safe during pregnancy. It aids digestion and has been used for centuries to relieve nausea.

◆ Ginger tea: Ginger tea is safe and may help you combat morning sickness. Grate 1 tsp of ginger, then add sugar, lemon juice, and boiling water.

◆ Raspberry tea: Raspberry tea has been used as a uterine relaxant in the last month of pregnancy, but it is difficult to determine if it helps women to have an easier labor, since each labor is so individual.

UNSAFE TEAS

◆ Black haw tea: Black haw is very similar to aspirin and may cause bleeding.

◆ Licorice tea: This may cause high blood pressure, headache, and swelling.

◆ Celery tea: This kind of tea can deplete potassium from your body.

◆ Senna tea: Senna tea may cause severe intestinal cramping and diarrhea.

◆ Black cohosh: Indian women used to use black cohosh for menstrual cramps and childbirth. Pregnant women should never use it because it contains estrogen, and hormone preparations should not be given during pregnancy.

◆ Any teas containing angelica, goldenseal, juniper, lavender, motherwort, myrrh, passionflower, rhubarb, sage, thyme, or vervain may be harmful. Although herbs may be safe for you as an adult, it is difficult to know how they may affect your unborn baby.

I drink green tea regularly and just found out that I am pregnant. Have I harmed my baby?

There is no specific component in green tea that is harmful to a baby. Green tea and black tea are quite similar. Black tea is dried and then fermented, while green tea is only dried. Green tea itself does not have a high level of caffeine, usually 30 to 40 milligrams per cup. That is certainly less than a cup of percolated coffee, but still significant. You would be safer switching to decaffeinated green tea.

Street Drugs

Are all common street drugs dangerous?

Every illegal drug can be associated with either miscarriage, death of your baby, or abnormalities in your baby. They are much more harmful to a tiny fetus than they are to an adult, and the effect of using them in pregnancy is frequently tragic. If you have been using any street drugs, please tell your doctor. She will help you get treatment so that you will be able to remain drug-free when you are ready to create that vulnerable life within your body. I've listed the most common illegal drugs and how their use during pregnancy can affect your baby.

Cocaine and Crack

Pregnancies during which mothers have been taking crack have a greater chance of resulting in miscarriage, birth defects, the unexplained death of a baby during the last three months of pregnancy, separation of the placenta from the uterine wall, a decrease in oxygen given to the fetus, and sudden infant death syndrome.

Heroin

Heroin use in pregnancy is associated with intrauterine fetal death, growth retardation of babies, and premature labor and delivery.

Glue Sniffing

Glue sniffing creates many of the same effects in a baby as alcohol does. An exposed baby may have a small body, a defective heart, abnormal facial features, and abnormalities of the arms, legs, and joints. The baby may also have attention deficit disorders.

LSD

LSD crosses the placenta and has been shown to cause a variety of birth defects, including malformations of some of the fetal organs.

Marijuana

Marijuana use in pregnancy has been shown to have effects on a baby later in its life. The affected child may have difficulty with memory and reasoning skills, and a variety of learning disabilities. Studies show that compared with nonusers, women who use marijuana during their pregnancies have two and a half times the risk of delivering a baby of low birth weight and double the risk of delivering prematurely. Marijuana definitely crosses the placenta.

Amphetamine (Speed)

A speed baby may have retarded growth, shaking, fussiness, and an inability to bond and to relate to its mother.

Safety of Medications

There are so many medications available. How can I know which medications are safe for me to take while I am trying to conceive and, then, when I become pregnant?

Fortunately, the United States Food and Drug Administration has classified all medications to inform us how safe or how dangerous they are. Each medication is listed in a book called the *Physicians' Desk Reference* (PDR), with a code letter next to it to indicate its safety. This book is reprinted and updated yearly.

All medications are listed as A, B, C, D, or X:

Category A: Controlled studies in humans have never shown any risk to an unborn baby.

   Example: Vitamin C.

   B: Studies in animals have shown no risk to their fetuses, but no studies have been done in humans.

   Example: Ampicillin.

   C: Studies in animals have shown dangerous effects to their fetuses, but no studies in humans have been reported.

These medications can be used if their benefit justifies any risk to a baby.

Example: Some medications for treatment of HIV.

D: Risk to a human fetus has been demonstrated, but the medication can be used if there are no other options.

Example: Dilantin for seizures.

X: Studies in animals and in humans have shown serious abnormalities in newborns. These medications should never be used by pregnant women.

Example: Accutane for acne.

If you need medication, your doctor will always try to place you on the preparation with the greatest safety. There are very few medications in the A group except vitamins. Most of the medications doctors strive to give pregnant women are in category B, such as penicillin or erythromycin. Your doctor may also give you medications in the C and D categories but will absolutely never give you a preparation in the X category during your pregnancy.

The decision as to whether or not your doctor gives you medication in the C or D category will depend greatly upon the information you supply him. For example, if you have pain in your leg and a category B medication is not giving you relief, you may tell the doctor that you desperately need pain relief. Your doctor may seek to ease your pain, and the only available options may be category C or D medications. The relief is for you, not for your doctor. If you can bear the pain, however, and tell your doctor that you will stay with the milder medication and use a heating pad or bed rest to ease the pain, your baby will benefit from your resourceful actions.

Which medications should I avoid while trying to conceive and once I become pregnant?

The following list contains common medications you should never take while trying to conceive and when you become pregnant. If you have taken any, please tell your doctor. All of these medications may have serious side effects on a developing baby. If you need to take any of them, postpone becoming pregnant until you do not require the medication.

Accutane: This medication is used for cystic acne. Twenty-five percent of fetuses that have been exposed to Accutane will be born with abnormalities, including malformations of the brain, spinal cord, heart, thymus gland, and facial bones. After Accutane is taken, it will remain in a woman's system for at least four months. Even subsequent to that time, it may be metabolized into another dangerous chemical called etretinate, which remains in the body for many months. It is best to wait two years following your last course of Accutane before trying to conceive.

ACE inhibitors: These medications are used for the treatment of high blood pressure. They can cause kidney and bone damage in 30 percent of newborns.

Aspirin: Aspirin was initially derived from the bark of the white willow tree, which is considered a symbol of joy. Chinese physicians have been using willow bark to relieve pain since 500 B.C.E., but it took five hundred years for the European world to recognize its value. It is considered safer for you not to take aspirin during pregnancy. If you've taken it once or twice since conceiving, don't worry—just switch to a pain reliever in the acetaminophen family for the duration of your pregnancy. There are two reasons you should not use aspirin while you are pregnant. One is that in animal studies, aspirin increased the risks of birth defects. But no similar defects, thank goodness, have ever been shown to occur in humans. The second reason is that aspirin will increase your tendency to bleed. If you experience trauma in your uterus while you are pregnant, your ingestion of aspirin might increase the chance that your placenta will bleed.

Chemotherapy, such as methotrexate and aminopterin: These medications, which help to fight cancer, cause miscarriages. They also use the body's folic acid. This medication-induced deficiency in folic acid increases the incidence of newborns with spina bifida.

Coumadin, Warfarin: These medications used to prevent blood clots may cause abnormalities of the hands, bones, eye, and brain in 20 percent of fetuses.

Depakote, Depakene (valproic acid): These seizure medications can cause spina bifida in a baby.

Dilantin: This seizure medication can cause mental retardation and growth disorders in 30 percent of affected newborns.

Lithium: This medication used for treatment of manic-depression can cause heart abnormalities in a baby.

Male hormones: These hormones may cause gender malformations in the development of a male or female fetus.

Streptomycin: This antibiotic is rarely used, but it can cause loss of hearing in a baby.

Tetracycline: This antibiotic, taken during pregnancy, can ultimately cause poor growth of the enamel of the child's teeth and also cause the teeth to appear gray in color.

Thalidomide: This drug had been used as a sleeping pill to treat insomnia during pregnancy. It caused severe deformities of the arms and legs in 20 percent of affected newborns. It was taken off the market but has recently appeared because it has proven effective in the treatment of HIV/AIDS and rheumatoid arthritis. It is never prescribed for pregnant women.

Thyroid-suppressing medications: PTU and iodide can suppress the baby's thyroid gland and cause its thyroid gland to swell, creating a goiter.

Trimethadione and paramethadione: These medications used to prevent seizures cause miscarriages and abnormalities of the face, defects of the heart, retardation, and other serious effects in 60 to 70 percent of newborns.

Vitamin A and products derived from it: Excess synthetic vitamin A from animal-derived sources, also called retinol, can cause miscarriages, facial abnormalities, heart defects, nervous system anomalies, cleft lip, and palate abnormalities in fetuses. It is also advisable to stop using skin care products that contain retinol, such as Retin-A for acne and wrinkles, as these preparations contain vitamin A (see chapter 2).

Your Hair, Skin, and Nails
Electrolysis and Waxing

I usually have electrolysis on my bikini region. Can I continue electrolysis during my pregnancy?

You should not continue electrolysis on your bikini region. The electric current from electrolysis does not stop at the surface of your skin. Your uterus is just under your pubic bone, and the electric current can be transmitted there. For a similar reason, you will have to stop waxing your bikini area during pregnancy. The heat from the hot wax penetrates to your deeper body tissues and can be dangerous for your baby. However, you can continue waxing other parts of your body, including your face.

So how can you remove the hair? Using a razor is your safest bet. Before you apply soap or shaving cream to your pubic area, clean the region with rubbing alcohol or peroxide to kill the bacteria there. Many bacteria live in this location, and if one hair follicle is infected, as you nick the other hair follicles you will spread the infection to the whole area. Using an antiseptic will prevent this from happening.

Dyeing Your Hair

I have gray hair that I have been dyeing for several years. Is it safe to dye during pregnancy?

Previously, studies had shown no detrimental effect to a fetus if a mother dyed her hair during pregnancy. One recent study, however, did show a relationship between women who used hair dye and heart defects in their newborns. This medical study may someday be disproved—only time will tell—but for the present it is best not to dye your hair until you have completed your first trimester. Your baby's heart and other internal organs are forming during this period; after that time, most of your baby's organs have formed and are just growing. If it is very important for you to dye your hair, you can do so with vegetable dyes. These will not give quite the same effect as commercial dyes, and they will wash out after a few shampoos, so you will need to reapply fairly often. The good thing is that using the natural dye will leave you with the peace of mind that you have not caused any harm to your baby. I always highlighted my hair in pregnancy, but I waited until after the first three months. Pregnancy has a drabbing effect on hair, and women want to color their hair more than ever.

Hair Straightening and Perms

Can I straighten or perm my hair while I'm pregnant, and will these hold?

There is no known medical reason why you cannot perm or straighten your hair during pregnancy, but as with most chemicals that you might apply on, or absorb into, your body, it is always wiser to wait until you have completed the first three months of pregnancy. There is a better chance that your hair straightening will hold during pregnancy than your hair permanent will. Within a week after having a perm, your hair may become limp and you may lose both the body and curl as well as the money you paid for it. If you straighten your hair, it should hold and maintain its straightening for several months. Several medical studies suggest that the chemicals used both to curl and to straighten hair can penetrate the scalp, but it is not known if these chemicals can pass through the placenta. That is why it is best to wait until after your first three months of pregnancy before attempting either a permanent or a straightening.

Hair Changes

Most women notice that their hair becomes thicker during pregnancy but will start to thin out three to six months after delivery. Under normal nonpregnant conditions, a percentage of a woman's hair falls out each month, so that a constant amount of hair is on her head. While you are pregnant, this hair does not fall out, so you have more hairs during these months. For example, if each strand of your hair normally grows for three years before falling out, then one thirty-sixth of your hair falls out every month, since there are thirty-six months in three years. Normally new hair grows in, so you have a steady loss and gain of hair. Over the nine months of your pregnancy, however, one-fourth of your hair does not fall out, so your hair is 25 percent thicker.

Hair length also increases noticeably during pregnancy. Normally your hair grows half an inch each month. Because your hair is not falling out during the nine months of your pregnancy, it can grow four more inches in length before it falls out. For example, if each strand of your hair grows for two years before falling out and being replaced, normally you will be able to grow your hair almost twelve inches in length (one-half inch for every twenty-four months of your hair's life span). When you are pregnant and you do not shed your hair each month, you will have nine more months of length in your hair, which works out to almost four inches. You will enjoy this extra length until your baby is three to six months old.

Skin Changes

In my last pregnancy, I developed little white dots on my face. Can I do something to prevent these?

These white dots have no formal name but are commonly known as "acid spots." They develop temporarily when pregnant women eat an abundance of acidic foods, like tomatoes, grapefruits, oranges, strawberries, and other citrus fruits. Women often get these earlier in pregnancy, when they crave acidic foods, and then later, when they stop craving such large amounts of these foods, their spots disappear. You don't need to stop eating the acidic foods that cause the rash, as most of the foods are healthy for you and the rash resolves itself anyway.

Why does a pregnant woman's skin become discolored under her earrings, rings, and watch?

Almost all jewelry, except twenty-four-karat gold, is a mixture of two or more metals. Often one of them is copper. When you are pregnant, your body tissues react differently to chemicals. In moist areas, such as under a ring, the copper precipitates a green layer called a "patina" that prevents the copper from corroding. As your tissues naturally will become warm and moist during pregnancy, they react with the copper easily. You would do best to take off your metal jewelry and use nonmetal accessories if this reaction occurs on your skin. After pregnancy, your body chemistry will return to normal and you will be able to wear all of your jewelry without any problem.

Travel as a Vegetarian

My job requires that I travel. What can I do to keep my baby and myself healthy while I'm traveling?

When planning your trip, try to make your reservations for an aisle seat so that it will be easier for you to get up and move around the aircraft. If you'll be having a meal on the plane, discuss the vegetarian options with the airline beforehand to make sure it is something that will appeal to you. I have received meals on planes with no sugar, no salt, no shortening, and no spices. Some commercial carriers have the impression that the word *vegetarian* is synonymous with the word *sacrifice*. The people who prepare these bland meals apparently never tasted foods from predominantly vegetarian countries like India! If the vegetarian meal option sounds too bland, bring your own food as a supplement. For example, if you know that they will give you vegetables with no flavoring, bring a small plastic bag with grated nuts or Parmesan cheese to sprinkle. You may also want to bring a container of mixed nuts and fruit. Keep drinking water or other liquids on the airplane to prevent dehydration. Instead of drinking soda, please ask for orange juice and club soda and mix the two together.

When going through security, you do not have to worry about the luggage scanner, as this is an ultrasound unit and does not emit radiation. The security poles you walk through are only metal detectors, so those will not harm you, either. Also, pack an extra pair of wider shoes in your carry-on, as your feet may swell on the plane.

If you are going to a third world country, follow the same safe food precautions that you would follow were you not pregnant. Do not drink water that is not bottled or sterilized; do not drink liquids that have ice cubes in them; eat only fruits or vegetables from which you are able to peel an outer protective surface, such as bananas and oranges. You may want to bring your own individual water-boiling unit to boil each cup of water and to use this water in your room and when you brush your teeth. If you will be traveling to regions that are high risk for certain infections, make sure you inform your doctor and receive whatever vaccinations are necessary.

After your twentieth week of pregnancy, it is best not to fly to a third world country. The health care available to you were you to go into premature labor and to deliver might not give your baby the same chances of survival as would the care in the United States.

PREPARING YOUR HOME
FOR YOUR PREGNANCY

Should I worry about using cleaning solutions while I am trying to become pregnant?

If you are using solvents as cleaning solutions (and most commercial cleaning solutions are solvents), then you should definitely be aware of the potential risks. You should learn the characteristics of the solutions you currently have, so that you use as few as possible. Solvents are chemicals that dissolve other substances and are found in a wide range of home and commercial cleaning products. Many medical studies have shown that women who use cleaning solvents during pregnancy have a higher incidence of newborns with cleft lips and cleft palates. Some typical solvents are glycol ethers, aliphatic solvents, biocides, and trichloroethylene. The Consumer Product Safety Commission has determined that over 150 chemicals in ordinary household products cause birth defects.

The children of women employed as housecleaners, hairdressers, leather workers, and shoe factory workers all have a higher incidence of cleft lips and cleft palates. In the case of the women working with leather and in shoe manufacturing, these defects result from solvents used to clean and soften the leather product.

Should I start drinking bottled water?

Not necessarily. In general, there is nothing wrong with tap water. Each municipality filters tap water to remove impurities. Your local water comes either from a surface reservoir (such as a lake) or, if you live in a rural area, from deep groundwater. There are several situations under which you might wish to have your tap water checked. If you live in a home that is over thirty years old, you should have your water checked for lead. Years back, lead was used to solder the joins of pipes, and this can precipitate into your water. If you live in an agricultural area, you might want to check your water for pesticides, herbicides, and nitrates present as a residue of fertilizers. These chemicals may have seeped into your water supply after having been sprayed on crops.

If your source of drinking water is well water, you might consider switching to bottled water. You should definitely have your well water checked for bacteria, minerals, herbicides, and pesticides. Well water should be tested yearly to make sure that bacteria and fertilizer nitrates have not contaminated your water supply. You can call the EPA Safe Drinking Water Hotline at 800-426-4791, or visit www.epa.gov/safewater/pwells1.html for more information.

Is mineral water safer and healthier for my baby and myself?

If your water at home is safe, you may not be gaining much, excluding a difference in taste, by bringing home mineral water. Bottled mineral waters must meet a standard mineral content, but your water at home must also meet similar standards. The process of injecting carbon dioxide into bottled water adds most of the carbonation in "sparkling water." Although this might add zest to your water, your body does not need more carbon dioxide absorbed into your tissues; actually, the body is always trying to get rid of it. Carbon dioxide obtained from drinking carbonated beverages is not necessarily beneficial to your baby or yourself. Mineral water is usually free of microorganisms but may contain the same amount of minerals and pesticides as your tap water, or an even greater amount.

Is it dangerous to use computers, cell phones, microwaves, or any kind of home technology while I'm pregnant?

Most technical devices emit electromagnetic radiation. The radiation does not stop when it leaves the device: it travels outside the device in waves. So far, there have been no conclusive studies showing a correlation between the use of technical devices and pregnancy-related problems, nor have there been any studies conclusively proving these devices are safe. Researchers studying the effects of electromagnetic fields on pregnant women admit there are limitations that prevent them from drawing clear conclusions. The primary limitation is that our present-day exposure to electromagnetic radiation is so pervasive, it is virtually impossible to obtain control subjects who have not been similarly exposed.

Some individuals, such as military personnel and air traffic controllers, have been exposed to very large quantities of electromagnetic radiation. They may be at risk for a higher rate of malignancy due to this exposure. There are no indications that you should leave your computer job or leave your cooking job. However, you should try to avoid any unnecessary exposure to electromagnetic radiation, such as sleeping all night on a heated waterbed or under an electric blanket.

EATING FOR PREGNANCY: YOUR VEGETARIAN DIET, YOUR BABY, AND YOU

Will my baby be as healthy as one whose mother eats meat during her pregnancy?

Without a doubt! As a vegetarian, your baby will be as strong and healthy as that of any woman on a meat-based diet and will certainly be large enough. Maintaining a vegetarian diet will not cause any kind of disease in infants born to well-informed and well-motivated vegetarian mothers.

Like any pregnant woman, vegetarian women need to build a strong nutritional foundation to ensure their baby's health. One health issue unique to vegan women is the possibility of vitamin B_{12} deficiency. Long-standing vegans who exclusively breast-fed their babies have had children with vitamin B_{12} deficiency, though these cases are very rare. The mothers in these studies had not attempted to obtain vitamin B_{12} from plant sources, nor had they taken vitamin supplements. Vegans can prevent vitamin B_{12} deficiency in their newborns by taking standard vitamin supplements containing vitamin B_{12}.

Contrary to what many people imagine, there is not a higher incidence of calcium deficiency in children of vegans as compared to children born to meat-eating mothers. Vegetarians and vegans do not excrete calcium from their bodies as rapidly as do meat-eaters, so they maintain high calcium levels within their blood. They are then able to pass on to their baby the calcium they maintain within their system. As older adults, vegetarians actually have a lower incidence of osteoporosis than do meat-eaters, and for exactly the same reason, they do not excrete their calcium.

Any diet, vegetarian or carnivorous, can be healthy or unhealthy, depending upon the knowledge and judgment of the individual making the dietary choices. A woman consuming only candy and french fried potatoes cannot expect her baby to achieve optimum nutrition, whether or not she is vegetarian!

So many people tell me I do not ingest enough protein to support a growing baby. What can I say to convince them that my vegetarian diet is healthy?

Many people think of meat as equivalent to protein. They simply don't know that plants are just as protein-rich as meat (and in some cases even more so). If you share with them these statistics about the protein content of vegetarian diets, they will recognize how protein-rich and nutritionally sound your vegetarian diet is.

- ◆ Beans contain approximately 25 percent protein.
- ◆ Soybeans contain 40 percent protein.
- ◆ Soybeans have twice as much protein as cheese.
- ◆ Soybeans have twice as much protein as red meat.
- ◆ Soybeans have ten times as much protein as whole milk.
- ◆ Soybeans actually contain all eight of the essential amino acids and, weight for weight, have a higher quantity of all eight essential amino acids than meat or eggs.
- ◆ Soybeans contain calcium, phosphorus, iron, and more B vitamins than eggs.
- ◆ As a vegetarian, if you eat soy protein at one meal, grains at another, and beans at a third meal, you will easily obtain your full complement of amino acids.
- ◆ The United States government recommends 65 grams of protein daily for men and 60 grams of protein daily for pregnant women. These are generous amounts, leaving a large room for margin.
- ◆ Following a balanced vegetarian diet, you can consume at least 60 grams of protein daily without any difficulty.

If I become nauseated and cannot eat protein-rich foods at every meal, will that affect my baby's growth?

The protein you eat does not go directly, like a funnel, into your baby's little body. The protein you ingest, whether of plant origin or animal origin, is broken down in your intestines into its amino acid components. These amino acids are then carried to your liver, where they are broken down into their basic components and recombined. After that, these new compounds are distributed to their final organ destination for use, either in your baby's body or in your own. At these final sites, the amino acids will be joined to form the specific protein necessary for that part of the body to use. Any excess protein that is not used, by either your baby or yourself, will be stored in your body as fat tissue for potential use at a later date. Your body has many stores of protein. If you cannot eat protein at every meal, don't be concerned. Soon your nausea will dissipate and you'll be able to start eating more protein again.

Your Prepregnancy Diet and Fitness

I would like to lose weight before I become pregnant. Can you explain how I can do this and remain healthy?

First, there are some basic concepts you should know (if you don't already) concerning weight gain and weight loss. When you gain weight, it is because you have taken in more calories than you have used, so your body stores these calories in the form of fat. From a practical perspective, each pound of fat you have is equal to 3,500 extra calories. All the foods you eat give you energy, and you need this energy to move, think, breathe—to carry out all of life's functions. Calorie counts vary with each food—for instance, one piece of candy may contain many more calories than a salad. In general, vegetarian foods are low in calories; that is why fewer vegetarians have problems watching their weight. Even as a vegetarian, however, you can gain excess weight from foods like oil, salad dressing, fried foods, milk shakes, protein shakes, or peanut butter—basically any food with a high fat content.

The number of calories you need to maintain your present weight, as well as the number of calories you must decrease in your diet to lose one pound of weight, varies with your age, your current weight, your height, your muscle mass, and your activity level. However, there are some general guidelines you can use to help determine to what extent you should decrease your caloric intake to lose weight. Most women need only 2,000 calories a day, but women who exercise a great deal may *burn* 4,000 calories a day (double the number of calories!). To lose one pound a week, you need to burn up to 3,500 calories. For example: To lose one pound a week if you don't exercise, you will need to decrease your daily intake of calories from 2,000 to 1,500 (or 500 calories less a day for seven days). If you exercise, you will need to decrease your daily intake of calories from 4,000 to 3,500 (still 500 calories less a day). It is much easier to remain hunger-free on 3,500 calories a day and work out than it is to deprive yourself on 1,500 calories daily. That's why combining exercise with a full, healthy diet is the best way to lose extra pounds.

If I want to become pregnant in six months, how much weight can I realistically lose during that time frame and still begin my pregnancy as a healthy vegetarian woman?

The only way to determine how much you will be able to lose will be to begin your diet now and evaluate your weight loss after two months. Many women can lose ten pounds or more during their first month of a weight-reduction and exercise-enhanced diet. Much of that, however, is due to fluid loss, as they are often limiting chips, cheeses, sodas, and other salt-retaining foods. During your second month, you will have a more realistic idea of the amount you can anticipate losing during the months to come. The fact that your diet is restricted in calories and fat content in no way means that it should be deficient in vitamins, minerals, fiber, and protein—please make sure you are getting enough of these nutrients in your diet.

Start now to evaluate the healthy foods listed in chapter 2 to supply you with all the nutrients required for you to have a healthy baby. Most of these foods are low in calories, and there will be no conflict in your consuming them while on your calorie-restricted diet. You should also take a multivitamin to ensure that you maintain high levels of B vitamins, particularly folic acid. Please call your obstetrician and tell her that you are trying to lose weight before you conceive. She will probably place you on prenatal vitamins now: certainly one of the main reasons prenatal vitamins were first designed was to ensure optimum nutrition.

Is there a way I can determine if I need more or less than the average 2,000 calories that an inactive women needs daily?

One way to determine your caloric need is to chart the number of calories you consume in an average week and divide that by seven. You may find that you consume much more, or much less, than that amount. To determine how many calories you can burn if you exercise and do not increase your caloric intake, you can estimate by using the following rule:

- At rest, you burn about 10 calories for each pound you weigh daily. This is called your basal metabolic rate (BMR).

- Sedentary people burn an average of 13 calories per pound daily.

- Moderately active people burn an average of 15 calories per pound daily.

- Active people burn an average of 18 calories per pound daily.

Low levels of activity include walking or playing golf; medium levels include swimming, jogging, or walking briskly; strenuous levels include aerobic exercises, cycling, or lifting weights.

When I increase my exercise, what matters more, the activity I choose or the time I spend working out in general?

Given the time constraints all of us face day-to-day, it is the quality, not the quantity, of exercise that sets the foundation for the number of calories you will be able to burn. That is because most of us have only a limited number of hours in which to work out. Therefore, if you walk three miles in one hour or jog six miles in that hour, obviously you will be burning more calories if you jog. If you are able to exercise for only a particular length of time, the more strenuous the exercise, naturally the greater the number of calories you will burn. In general, if you do aerobic exercises, such as walking, for thirty to forty-five minutes three times a week, and do not increase your intake of calories, you should be able to lose weight.

I am forty years old and just can't seem to lose weight. Why?

You will be able to lose weight on a carefully controlled healthy diet and an exercise schedule, but it will be harder because you are older. One reason is that our metabolism slows down as we age, and another reason is that we generally have a lower percentage of body muscle mass as we age. As increased muscle mass helps us to burn calories, the decreased mass makes the process of weight loss more difficult.

Why does everyone say that exercise is so important if I want to lose weight?

In order to lose weight, you will need to decrease your caloric intake relative to the number of calories you burn. When you don't exercise, the basic rate at which you burn calories, your "basal metabolic rate," is at a standard level "specific" for you. When you exercise, you can increase that rate by 10 percent, and this metabolic rate may remain at that increased level for up to forty-eight hours. So if you exercise in the morning and spend the rest of your day sitting at a computer, you will still be burning more calories during the rest of the day.

The number of calories of fat that you will burn depends upon the duration and the intensity of the exercise you do; this amount is specific for you. If you do not lose weight easily, you should not despair and give up. By increasing your exercise, you will definitely reach a level of "decreased calories in and excess energy out" at which you will lose weight. You may wonder why it is more difficult for you to lose weight than it is for your husband. If a man weighs 250 pounds, with much of this weight in muscle mass, he will expend many more calories per hour than you will if you weigh 145 pounds and have minimal muscle mass. You may actually need to exercise twice as long to burn the same number of calories that your husband is able to lose in half that time.

How often should I exercise to help me lose weight?

If you cannot exercise every day, it is recommended that you exercise every other day (rather than exercising three days in a row and not exercising for four days in a row). By exercising every other day, you will be able to achieve a sustained increase in your basal metabolic rate for the entire week.

Can I just lose weight by dieting, rather than by combining dieting and exercising?

You can, but weight loss by dieting alone is much less effective, takes much longer, and creates a greater chance that you will gain back the weight than if you combine dieting and exercise. If you lose weight just by dieting, 25 percent of your loss will be from your lean body mass (muscles) and only 75 percent will be from your body fat. If you lose weight by dieting and exercising together, 98 percent of your weight loss will come directly from your body fat.

The compounding problem with weight loss from dieting alone is that when you gain some weight back after dieting (an almost universal phenomenon), the weight that you initially lost as 25 percent muscle and 75 percent fat will be gained back totally as fat, and you may look broader and actually need to wear a larger size than you did before your initial weight loss.

Can all kinds of foods create fat in my body, or will just "fatty foods" make me fat?

If you consume an excess number of calories from any food group, your body will store this as fat. For every extra 3,500 calories you have consumed from any food group—be it from fats, proteins, or carbohydrates—your body will store this as a pound of fat. The picture, however, is much more complicated. That is because an equal volume of food rich in fat or protein contains approximately twice the number of calories as a meal of natural carbohydrates, such as starches or natural sugars. Another complicating factor is that sugars and refined carbohydrates may increase your appetite, so although each portion contains fewer calories, you might be tempted to eat more than you would have had you eaten a meal of fats and protein.

This is a problem that some people face when they first become vegetarian. Because a vegetarian diet is often lower in fats and proteins than is a meat-based diet, a newly converted vegetarian may feel hungry all the time. The solution to combat this hunger is quite simple: just snack on foods higher in fat and protein—such as avocado salad, nuts with fruits, and banana with peanut butter—in between meals.

Is it true that if I develop larger muscles, I will burn more calories?

Yes, it is. Besides the fact that weight lifting and muscle training are great exercises themselves, once you have developed muscles from these exercises, the muscles themselves actually burn calories more efficiently than fat and other body tissues. That is one reason muscular people will find it easier to remain in shape than will someone with minimal muscle mass. A common misconception among non-vegetarians is that vegetarians cannot gain a large amount of muscle mass. Vegetarians can obtain as much muscle mass as any other body builder. Everyone can develop muscles by lifting weights, doing strenuous exercises, and eating a well-rounded nutritious diet.

When I try to evaluate whether or not I am at my ideal body weight, I cannot tell if my frame is small, medium, or large. Is there an easy method I can use to determine my body type?

An easy method is to compare your weight to your height. As a rule of thumb, women should weigh one hundred pounds for their first five feet of height and then add an additional five pounds for each additional inch. If you have a small frame, you can deduct 10 percent of that total weight, and if you have a large frame, you can add 10 percent to that amount.

To determine if you have a large frame or a small frame, you can use this key, comparing your wrist size to your body type:

If your height is under five feet two inches:
- Small = wrist size less than 5.5 inches
- Medium = wrist size 5.5 to 5.75 inches
- Large = wrist size over 5.75 inches

If your height is five feet two to five feet five:
- Small = wrist size less than 6 inches
- Medium = wrist size 6 to 6.25 inches
- Large = wrist size over 6.25 inches

If your height is over five feet five:
- Small = wrist size less than 6.5 inches
- Medium = wrist size 6.5 to 7.5 inches
- Large = wrist size over 7.5 inches

Why is it that I have such a difficult time losing weight, even when I eat less and exercise?

There are different theories about how people experience weight loss. One is called the "set point theory." This theory conjectures that our bodies try to maintain a certain amount of fat within them. How much fat we retain is determined by the number of fat cells we have, which may in turn be determined by our genetics and our early eating patterns.

According to this theory, when you start to lose weight below the level of your set point, your metabolic rate will slow down as your body tries to conserve every calorie. If you try to lose weight on a severely calorie-restricted diet, your metabolism will come to such a screeching halt that you may actually gain weight. You can conquer this problem if you maintain a regular exercise regimen and follow a long-term healthy eating pattern—steady in content and only slightly lower in calories—instead of committing to a calorie-restricted diet.

I'm aware that my eating habits are poor. How can I plan a consistent healthy vegetarian diet for my pregnancy?

The following list of techniques may help you maintain a healthy vegetarian diet prior to pregnancy, while still helping you to follow a weight-loss program if that is your goal:

- Learn about the fats, calories, and nutrients in your vegetarian foods.
- If you are hypoglycemic, do not eat fruits without nuts or cheese.
- Minimize salad dressing and oils, as well as fried coatings on your vegetables.
- Avoid fatty desserts such as cakes, cookies, or ice cream.
- Limit your intake of refined foods, such as soda and ice pops.
- Eat fruits and raw vegetables as your snacks.
- Exercise, exercise, exercise!
- Avoid alcohol and caffeine and minimize salt.
- During meals, fill up first on low-calorie foods such as soup and salad.

- Drink eight glasses of water daily.

- Drink freshly squeezed vegetable or fruit drinks instead of prepared ones.

- Plan your meals ahead of time, so you have healthy foods to reach for when you are hungry.

- Don't shop when you are hungry.

- While shopping, buy finger foods, such as cut fruits and vegetables, for snacks.

- If you fall off your healthy diet, don't give up—just get back on it.

- Weigh yourself only once every one or two weeks.

- If you feel hungry when you should not be, try working out instead.

- Use smaller plates and portions.

- Remember the big picture; your plan is not to diet, but to develop a lifetime of healthy eating habits.

Can you give an example of a healthy meal plan I can follow to lose weight and still begin my pregnancy in optimum health?

The basic components of a healthy prepregnancy vegetarian diet include adequate vitamins, minerals, protein, fiber, and liquids. Here is a general plan of food groups you can follow—it will be easy for you to choose the foods you want within these categories:

EARLY MORNING	One or two pieces of fruit (with or without nuts)
BREAKFAST	Carbohydrate, like a bowl of cereal or 2 slices of enriched toast
MIDMORNING SNACK	Fruit or vegetable snack
LUNCH	Protein (tofu, beans), a green vegetable, and one other vegetable
MIDAFTERNOON SNACK	Vegetable or fruit snack
DINNER	Protein (tofu, beans), fruit, carbohydrate, enriched rice, vegetable
EVENING SNACK	Vegetable or fruit

NOTE ON NUTRITION:
FOLLOWING A HEALTHY VITAMIN REGIMEN

Will I be able to obtain enough vitamins for my baby and myself with my vegetarian diet?

You will be able to obtain more vitamins with a vegetarian diet than will most women on a non-vegetarian diet. That's because most vitamins are found predominantly in fruits and vegetables. You will get water-soluble vitamins (the B and C vitamins) in abundance whenever you eat anything that is grown in the ground—grains, beans, nuts, and all sorts of green vegetables. You will get your C vitamins in large quantities from fruits of all shapes and colors. The only exception to this is vitamin B_{12}, which will be more difficult for you to obtain as a vegetarian. You'll have to take a vitamin B_{12} supplement to maintain a healthy level during pregnancy.

You will obtain your fat-soluble vitamins (vitamins A, D, E, and K) from plant fats. You may be surprised to learn that plants have fats. They do indeed, but fortunately no plant fats are dangerous, like cholesterol. Your sources of these fat-soluble vitamins will be numerous and abundant. You will get your vitamin A from yellow and orange vegetables and your vitamin D from dairy products and from your own skin, which will be producing vitamin D when you venture out into the sunlight. You will get your vitamin E from grains, seeds, and nuts and your vitamin K from both alfalfa and within your own intestines, where your intestinal bacteria manufacture it.

As a vegetarian, you will surpass non-vegetarians in your ingestion of almost all vitamins. I say "almost" because you may need to supplement with vitamin pills if you fall into any of the following categories: if you are pure vegan, you must supplement with tablets of vitamin B_{12}; and if you are pure vegan and do not have access to daily sunlight, you may do well to supplement with vitamin tablets containing vitamin D. It is that simple. If you feel the need to supplement your diet with vitamin pills, you can do so without any worry—you'll be giving yourself the best of both worlds. If you haven't already, please read about the role vitamins play in the balanced vegetarian diet (chapter 2).

Should I start taking vitamins now?

Definitely. Though you may already obtain a sufficient quantity of vita-mins from your vegetarian diet, why take a chance? Call your doctor's of-fice and ask the nurse to recommend the prenatal vitamin that they prefer their patients to use. If they do not have a preference and suggest that you purchase your own over-the-counter vitamin until they check you, please follow the guidelines in chapter 2. You want to take vitamins with high levels of folic acid and low levels of vitamin A, as described in this text. Vitamins are not a substitute for a healthy diet; they are a com-plement to one. Vitamins do not take the place of your carbohydrates, protein, or fats; they are the spark that helps you metabolize your other nutrients more efficiently. No matter how good your diet, you can never be sure you're getting enough of *all* the vitamins you need. This is espe-cially true when you are newly pregnant and suddenly develop all sorts of food dislikes, aversions, and cravings that change your usual diet. This early phase of pregnancy is the critical time for your baby to receive folic acid to decrease its chance of developing spina bifida. You are making a wise decision by acting aggressively in this matter.

How do I choose the right prenatal vitamin?

When you go to your pharmacy or health food store, you will be able to find numerous varieties of vegetarian prenatal vitamins, many of which are free of unnecessary dyes and chemicals. There is no United States committee dictating which vitamins and minerals must be present in a vitamin supplement for it to be classified as a "pregnancy" vitamin.

Following is a general summary of nutrients you will commonly find in your prenatal vitamin:

Folic acid	800–1,000 mcg (1 mg)
Iron	30–90 mg
Iodine	0–150 mcg
Calcium compound	200–1,000 mg
Chromium	0–125 mcg
Copper	0–2 mg
Magnesium	0–450 mg
Selenium	0–100 mg

Zinc	15–25 mg
Vitamin A	3,000–4,000 IU
Vitamin D	400 IU
Vitamin E	30–150 IU
Vitamin C	60–300 mg
Vitamin B_1 (thiamine)	3–10 mg
Vitamin B_2 (riboflavin)	3–8 mg
Vitamin B_6 (pyridoxine)	6–20 mg
Vitamin B_{12}	12–32 mcg
Niacin	20–80 mg

A stool softener such as sodium docusate

Note:

- ◆ Your prenatal vitamin may contain a sufficient amount of folic acid so that you do not need another folic acid supplement.

- ◆ It is common for vegetarians to have lower blood levels of iron. Please make sure that your vitamin includes at least 90 milligrams of iron.

- ◆ It is important that your total intake of vitamin A from supplements does not exceed 25,000 IU from retinol. Please try to purchase prenatal vitamins that contain beta-carotene (a substance from plants that converts to vitamin A in the body), rather than traditional vitamin A (retinol) that is derived from animal sources.

- ◆ Some vitamins are measured in terms of international units and others in terms of milligrams or micrograms. This terminology must just be accepted.

Many vitamins contain healthy amounts of all needed nutrients; however, the amount of folic acid may be suboptimal. Some vitamins have only 400 micrograms of folic acid, while over twice that amount would be beneficial. Under certain circumstances, vitamins containing more than 1,000 micrograms (1 milligram) of folic acid require a prescription. To obtain an optimum amount of vegetarian prenatal vitamins, simply take your complete daily prenatal vitamin with 400 to 800 micrograms of folic acid and supplement this with an extra 500-microgram folic acid tablet, and voilà! You will have a vitamin regimen with approximately 1 milligram of folic acid.

The calcium in your prenatal vitamin may prevent you from fully absorbing your iron. If your blood count shows that you are anemic, your doctor may advise you to take extra iron pills later in the day rather than at the same time you are taking calcium.

If you are a vegan, your diet is totally plant based, which means you probably have a higher level of vitamins and minerals than most other people. You may, however, have lower levels of vitamin D and vitamin B_{12} because these are obtained predominately from meat or dairy foods. Try to supplement your diet with vitamins containing these.

You will need to take vitamins throughout your pregnancy and at least one time each day. Try to purchase vitamins you need to take only once or twice daily. If you purchase vitamins that require you to take four tablets four times daily, or thirty-two tablets each day, it may become both burdensome and nauseating to maintain this regimen throughout your pregnancy.

Prescription vs. Over-the-Counter Vitamins

When some vitamins contain 1 milligram of folic acid, they must be categorized as prescription drugs. That is why over-the-counter vitamins most often contain less than 1 milligram of folic acid. If your vitamin contains less than 1 milligram, supplement this with extra folic acid tablets. Prescription vitamins might actually be less expensive for you if you have an insurance prescription plan. Conversely, over-the-counter vitamins often offer more options, especially those vitamins that

- are vegetarian.
- are not coated with dyes.
- are free of artificial sugars.

In general, women can obtain the same quality and quantity of vitamins in over-the-counter vitamin supplements but will need to make wise choices.

Will I be able to obtain sufficient prenatal vitamins and minerals from a vegetarian diet without taking a vitamin supplement?

Almost all vegetarian women, on almost all days, will be able to. But how about those days you may be able to eat only salted tomatoes or pickled beets or chocolate?

> *There were some days during my first pregnancy that I was able to eat only salted peanuts. I could not stand the sight or smell of any other food. My knowledge of nutrition was overpowered by my desire for peanuts. I ate so many peanuts that I still dislike salted peanuts to this day.*

Food cravings and aversions abound during pregnancy, causing significant shifts in eating habits. Taking a vitamin supplement ensures that you are getting all the needed daily nutrients—which you may not be getting from a diet rich in salted tomatoes!

By taking your vitamins every day, you can feel sure that your baby is getting optimum nutrition every day of your pregnancy.

Protein Supplements

People have told me that I should start taking protein supplements or I will not obtain sufficient protein for my baby as a vegetarian. Is that true?

It absolutely is not true, for two reasons. The first is that as a healthy vegetarian, you should be getting more than enough protein. The second is that you should not take protein supplements because these will add an extra burden on your body's metabolism, while your healthy plant-based diet is totally nutritionally adequate for your baby and you during your pregnancy. This diet will be able to sustain both the growth and the development of your baby, as well as the changes in your reproductive tissues. It is important to note that vegetarian pregnant women on well-rounded plant-based diets are not protein deficient. Therefore, the purpose of taking a protein supplement would be just to add extra protein, not to fulfill any dietary deficiency.

One medical author reviewed and compiled the results of thirteen medical studies in which pregnant women used energy/protein supplements during their pregnancies. The supplements were considered "balanced," which means that less than 25 percent of their energy contents were derived from protein. The final results of the studies, evaluated together, showed that the women taking the protein supplements gained a minimal extra quantity of weight, 1.5 pounds, compared to the mothers who did not take the protein supplements. There was also a 1-ounce increased weight gain in the newborns of the mothers who took the protein supplements. The babies of these mothers were not healthier, and there was no difference in the rate of premature births, stillbirths, or fetal deaths between the protein supplement and nonprotein supplement groups of women. As there is no need for you to take these protein supplements, it is best that you not take them. You will fare better by eating natural grains, nuts, vegetables, and beans rather than these preprocessed concentrated foods.

I do strenuous athletic training. Will my vegetarian sources of protein be sufficient for me during my pregnancy?

As long as your diet is a healthy vegetarian one (and not a fast-food vegetarian diet of french fries and refined sugars), you should have plenty of protein to sustain your health and fitness during pregnancy. Many athletes are convinced that it is the protein in their diet that enhances their athletic performance, whereas it is really their carbohydrates that are sustaining them while they exercise. Your dietary protein needs will increase when you exercise, but not to that large a quantity. An individual performing strenuous endurance exercises should increase protein intake to approximately 1.3 grams of protein per kilogram of body mass. This amount of protein can be readily obtained from a diet that is deriving 12 to 15 percent of its energy from protein. Even a diet of pure vegetables—without nuts, eggs, beans, grains, or dairy products—supplies enough protein-derived energy to more than meet those needs.

An individual doing strength training should increase daily protein intake to 1.7 grams of protein per kilogram of body mass. This can be derived from a diet of 20 percent protein content, which is still within the reach of every educated vegetarian woman. For example, if you weigh 120 pounds, you weigh 55 kilograms. Therefore, you would need 95 grams of protein daily on the days that you are lifting weights, which would probably be every other day. You can obtain 42 grams of protein from 8 ounces of baked tofu and the rest from your cereal, beans, vegetables, and dairy.

AN OUNCE OF PREVENTION:
NUTRITION AND BIRTH DEFECTS

Can a vegetarian diet help prevent spina bifida in pregnancy?

A vegetarian diet most definitely will help you to prevent spina bifida. This disorder is caused by both genetic tendency and dietary deficiency—specifically deficiency of folic acid and other B vitamins.

Spina bifida is one manifestation of a group of serious defects called "neural tube defects." These defects affect the brain and spinal cord of a baby and include spina bifida, anencephaly, and encephalocele. This disorder and the other neural tube defects develop around the fourth week of fetal development, *even before a woman knows that she is pregnant!* A good vegetarian diet is generally high in folic acid (obtained from both food and vitamins). If you're taking adequate levels of folic acid, you can rule out the risk of your baby developing spina bifida from lack of this essential nutrient. Because these defects develop so early in pregnancy, women should start increasing their intake of folic acid as soon as they plan to conceive.

The term *spina bifida* refers to a disorder in which there is an opening between the spinal cord and the outer body coverings. An infant born with this defect may have loss of feeling or paralysis in the lower body and lack of urinary and bowel control.

The incidence of spina bifida varies depending upon a mother's age as well as her genetic history:

Within the general population	1.5	/ 1,000 live births
In children of women over age 35	2	/ 1,000 live births
In children who have a sibling with spina bifida	5–30	/ 1,000 live births
In children who have one parent with spina bifida	11	/ 1,000 live births
In children with a cousin with spina bifida	3–10	/ 1,000 live births

I know that spina bifida is present in my family. Can taking folic acid help me prevent this defect in my baby?

Numerous medical studies have shown that if you take folic acid while trying to conceive and during your first six weeks of pregnancy, you will decrease your chances of having a child with spina bifida, even if it runs in your family.

The chance of having a child with spina bifida is greatest in women of English and Irish descent. If these same women immigrate to the United States, the incidence of spina bifida in their newborns decreases. This indicates that both genetic and environmental factors can increase the prevalence of this disorder. If you had a previous child with spina bifida, you should take 4 milligrams (4,000 micrograms) of folic acid divided into four doses each day. It is best to take this dosage while trying to conceive and during the first two months of pregnancy, and divided in four doses. Folic acid is one of the B vitamins. As such, it is water-soluble and is flushed out of the body rapidly. By dividing the dose into four segments, you will maintain a uniformly high level of folic acid throughout the day.

Should I take folic acid even if I don't have any history of spina bifida in my family?

It is estimated that four thousand infants are born in the United States yearly with neural tube defects. It is possible to prevent over 70 percent of these disorders if women ingest higher levels of folic acid during the early phases of their pregnancies. The U.S. Public Health Service recommends that all women take at least 400 micrograms of folic acid daily when they are planning to conceive, trying to conceive, and throughout their entire pregnancy.

Folic acid is naturally present in all green vegetables. It is also added to many brands of cereal, bread, and orange juice. Vegan foods are the richest sources of folic acid, but as long as your diet includes a variety of foliage, beans, grains, and fortified foods and beverages, you'll be getting plenty of this crucial nutrient. Numerous plant foods contain folic acid, including artichokes, asparagus, avocados, beets, broccoli, cabbage, chickpeas, collard greens, cowpeas, cranberries, hummus, lentils, lettuce, lima beans, long beans, okra, parsnips, peas, pinto beans, soybeans, spinach, squash, tempeh, turnip greens, and yellow beans.

When you note how many plant-derived foods contain folic acid, you can appreciate the fact that you as a vegetarian do not have to eat liver to obtain this needed vitamin.

I have been told that too much vitamin A can lead to birth defects. I am vegetarian, so I eat many yellow and orange fruits and vegetables containing vitamin A. Should I decrease these foods during my pregnancy?

There is definitely an association between a pregnant woman's ingestion of high doses of vitamin A and the occurrence of birth defects in newborns (see chapter 2). This association, however, is related only to the *vitamin A present in vitamin tablets,* which is derived from animal sources. The birth defects that can result from taking high doses of vitamin A pills do not occur when your vitamin A comes from natural vegetarian sources. You can take vitamin A supplements and still eat vitamin A–rich vegetarian foods without causing harm to your baby—just make sure your vitamin supplement contains less than 25,000 international units of this vitamin if it is in the form of retinol (this is derived from fish oil and animal livers). Prenatal vitamin manufacturers are gradually converting the vitamin A content of their vitamin supplements from retinol to beta-carotene. Please read the label before you purchase yours.

If you eat large quantities of yellow and orange vegetables, the only problem you may experience is "carotenosis"—a yellowish discoloration of your skin. These vegetables contain pro–vitamin A in the form of beta-carotene, and that causes the yellowish discoloration. Carotenosis is often seen in people who drink large quantities of carrot juice, but fortunately, it is not dangerous to either a mother or her baby. If you decrease your intake of vitamin A–rich vegetarian foods, your skin color will return to normal.

Is it true that male children of vegetarians have an increased chance of developing congenital abnormalities?

There is only one study from England that has reported an occurrence of a particular abnormality in the male children of vegetarians. The study evaluated almost 7,000 male newborns. Approximately 1 out of every 150 male children were born with hypospadias. Hypospadias is a disorder in which the urethra, the urinary opening at the end of the penis, is located along the shaft of the penis rather than at the tip. A child affected with this problem will be able to urinate, but the direction of the urine stream will be at a different angle. Fortunately, when this male grows older, he will not encounter problems with sexual relations or reproduction.

The incidence of hypospadias in those males born to vegetarian mothers was five times the rate of that of males born to non-vegetarian women. But also note that the rate in the sons of meat-eating women who took iron was twice that in the sons of women not taking iron. The incidence of hypospadias in the sons of women who had the flu in early pregnancy was three times the rate of that in sons of nonaffected women.

Why should this congenital problem occur at a higher rate in sons of vegetarian mothers? One reason is that vegetarian diets often contain higher levels of natural plant estrogens, called "phytoestrogens." Phytoestrogens are compounds present within plants that are structurally similar to the estrogen hormones found in humans. They are present in large quantities in soy products, such as soy milk, tofu, miso, soybeans, and tempeh. Phytoestrogens are also present in sweet potatoes.

It is important to note that sons of women living in the Orient, where women consume large quantities of soy, do not have a higher incidence of hypospadias. The higher rate of hypospadias in the sons of carnivorous women who took iron supplements indicates that the causes of this problem may be multifactorial, possibly related to a combination of iron supplements, viral infections, and the ingestion of foods containing phytoestrogens.

What can you do? While you are trying to conceive, and for the first three months of your pregnancy, limit your intake of soy so that it is not your main source of protein. Also, unless you are anemic, limit your intake of extra iron supplements until after your first month of pregnancy. You will be taking vitamins with iron throughout pregnancy to prevent anemia, as will most pregnant women (see chapter 2), so limiting your iron supplements in the first month will not harm you.

CHAPTER 2

Vegetarian Nutrition During Pregnancy

In pregnancy
you will strive to optimize every nutrient in your diet
and to eliminate every toxin from your foods.

You want to consume only what is best for your baby,
yet the nutritional information you find
is conflicting in content
and narrow in scope.

Some books tell you it is safe to be vegetarian while you are pregnant,
yet others do not.
Some doctors say you must eat meat while you are pregnant,
others tell you that you need to consume fish,
and all sincerely believe
you need more protein.

Yet your heart and your instincts tell you it is safe to be vegetarian.
You know that it is natural to be pregnant,
that it is natural to be vegetarian.
And that the earth
can give you all you need to create this new life.

You are a dedicated vegetarian.
Your soul is deriving wisdom from a higher source.
A source that strives for peace and justice.

The life inside you will achieve overwhelming good health.
It will grow in strength.
It will develop in wisdom.
It will flourish in peace.

And as this tiny life within you grows,
Both you and your baby will be blessed.
Because you will have attained the knowledge and the insight
to create your new life,
without taking life.

DIETARY GUIDELINES

How can I plan for healthy nutrition during my pregnancy?

The American College of Obstetricians and Gynecologists (ACOG) is the governing body that sets the policies followed by all obstetricians in the United States. The ACOG determines which procedures obstetricians should perform and which guidelines they should follow to achieve optimum outcomes for all pregnant women and all newborns within our country.

In 1996, the American College of Obstetricians and Gynecologists published the *ACOG Educational Bulletin Number 229, Nutrition and Women.* This was designed to help obstetricians obtain a foundation and a reference point to promote optimum nutrition and health within their patients. In 2000, it published its third edition of *Planning Your Pregnancy and Birth* to help pregnant women make good choices.

ACOG models its nutritional guidelines on three respected sources:

1. Recommended Dietary Allowances for Women
   Compiled by the United States government, this is the recommended nutritional requirements for *nonpregnant, pregnant, and nursing women.*

2. *Dietary Guidelines for Americans*
   This is a joint publication from the U.S. Department of Agriculture and U.S. Department of Health and Human Services. It is a guide of

specific desirable foods. The *Dietary Guidelines for Americans* recommends for *all individuals* and is not specific for pregnancy.

3. USDA Food Pyramid
   Created by the U.S. Department of Agriculture, the pyramid outlines desirable quantities for every food group. The Food Pyramid recommends dietary guideline for *all individuals* and is not specific for pregnancy.

We will review the information contained within each of these sources to show how each is easily adaptable to and actually supports a vegetarian lifestyle.

What are the Recommended Dietary Allowances for pregnant women?

The government lists and quantifies the levels of protein, vitamins, and minerals for nonpregnant women, pregnant women, and nursing women. Not all of these nutrients need be consumed on a daily basis, but if you tally up all your nutrition for a week and then divide by seven, this is the average amount of nutrients you should obtain each day.

	Nonpregnant Women	Pregnant Women	Nursing Women
Protein, gm	50	60	65
Vitamin A, mcg	800	800	1,300
Vitamin D, mcg	5	5	5
Vitamin E, mg	8	10	12
Vitamin K, mcg	65	65	65
Vitamin C, mg	60	70	95
Thiamine (Vitamin B_1), mg	1.1	1.5	1.6
Riboflavin (Vitamin B_2), mg	1.3	1.6	1.8
Niacin (Vitamin B_3), mg	15	17	20
Vitamin B_6, mg	1.6	2.2	2.1
Folic acid, mcg	180	400	280
Vitamin B_{12}, mcg	2	2.2	2.6
Calcium, mg	1,000	1,000	1,000
Phosphorus, mg	700	700	700

Magnesium, mg	320	360	320
Iron, mg	15	30	15
Zinc, mg	12	15	19
Iodine, mcg	150	175	200
Selenium, mcg	55	65	75

The Committee on Dietary Allowance Guidelines sets the standards for the Recommended Dietary Allowances (RDA). These guidelines set a minimum level of the important vitamins and minerals we all need, but they do not delineate any maximum level. Some vitamins and minerals taken in excess can be harmful. No specific nutritional need stands alone; rather, all function together to create a strong nutritional foundation. Each individual on a team is only as strong and healthy as the whole team—so it is with your nutrients.

How a Vegetarian Diet Surpasses RDA Standards

The RDA list demonstrates that during your pregnancy you will need higher levels of folate, vitamin B_6, vitamin C, thiamine, riboflavin, niacin, iron, and protein. A balanced vegetarian diet meets—and more often than not surpasses—these requirements quite easily. Following is an example of how simply standard vegetarian foods can fulfill the RDA guidelines.

60 gm protein	1 cup cooked split peas (16 gm) + ½ cup firm tofu (20 gm) + 2 slices whole-grain bread (9 gm) + 1 cup pasta (8 gm) + 2 cups broccoli spears (12 gm) (Note: Some cereals contain 10 to 20 gm protein/cup.)
800 mcg vitamin A (5,000 IU)	1 raw carrot (20,250 IU) or 1 cup cooked spinach (14,740 IU)
5 mcg vitamin D (200 IU)	1 cup rice milk (100 IU) + 1 cup soy milk (100 IU) + 1 cup 2% milk (100 IU) + 15 minutes of sunlight daily (400 IU)
10 mg vitamin E (15 IU)	1 tbsp wheat germ oil (52 IU) + 1 avocado (6 IU)
65 mcg vitamin K	1 cup cooked kale (975 mcg) or 1 cup broccoli (310 mcg)

70 mg vitamin C	1 medium-size orange (70 mg) or 1 grapefruit (100 mg)
1.5 mg vitamin B_1 (thiamine)	1 cup enriched cereal (1.5 mg)
1.6 mg vitamin B_2 (riboflavin)	1 cup frozen broccoli (1.5 mg) + ½ cup enriched bran cereal (0.4 mg) + 1 cup mushrooms (0.44 mg)
17 mg vitamin B_3 (niacin)	1 bagel (3 mg) + 1 cup enriched cereal (20 mg) + 2 tbsp peanut butter (4 mg)
2.2 mg vitamin B_6	1 cup enriched cereal (2 mg) + 10 oz frozen broccoli (0.4 mg)
400 mcg vitamin B_9 (folic acid)	1 cup steamed spinach (448 mcg), or 1 cup boiled lentils (358 mcg) + 1 cup romaine lettuce (76 mcg)
2.2 mcg vitamin B_{12}	1 cup cottage cheese (1.3 mcg) + 2 eggs (1.2 mcg) or 1 cup enriched cereal (6 mcg)
1,000 mg calcium	2 cups cooked spinach (490 mg) + 1 cup cooked black beans (140 mg) + 2 oz Swiss cheese (260 mg) + 2 tsp blackstrap molasses (344 mg)
700 mg phosphorus	1 cup cooked lentils (356 mg) + ¼ cup wheat germ (325 mg) + 1 cup 2% milk (232 mg) + 2 tbsp almonds (184 mg) + 14 spears asparagus (112 mg)
360 mg magnesium	1 cup firm tofu (236 mg) + 2 tbsp cashews (89 mg) + 1 cup hummus (71 mg)
30 mg iron	1 cup prune juice (3 mg) + 2 tbsp blackstrap molasses (7 mg) + 1 cup black-eyed peas (4.3 mg) + 1 oz sesame seeds (4.2 mg) + 1 cup enriched cereal (8.5 mg)
15 mg zinc	1 cup baked beans (3.2 mg) + 4 tbsp pecans (3 mg) + 1 cup hummus (2.7 mg) + 1 cup Kellogg's Raisin Bran (3.75 mg) + 3 oz American cheese (2.5 mg)

| 175 mcg iodine | ⅛ tbsp iodized salt or a sprinkling of kelp or seaweed |
| 65 mcg selenium | 2 tbsp Brazil nuts (380 mcg) |

How can I use the *Dietary Guidelines for Americans* to help me as a vegetarian during pregnancy?

The U.S. Department of Agriculture and the U.S. Department of Health and Human Services joined forces to create the *Dietary Guidelines for Americans*. This publication gives advice concerning foods and healthy living, rather than advice concerning specific nutrients. It provides you with an overview of the basic rules for healthy eating during your pregnancy.

DIETARY GUIDELINES FOR AMERICANS

- ◆ Eat a variety of foods.
- ◆ Balance the food you eat with physical activity—maintain a healthy weight.
- ◆ Choose a diet with plenty of grain products, vegetables, and fruits.
- ◆ Choose a diet low in fat, saturated fat, and cholesterol.
- ◆ Choose a diet moderate in sugars.
- ◆ Choose a diet moderate in salt and sodium.
- ◆ If you drink alcoholic beverages, do so in moderation.

These guidelines are perfectly compatible with a healthy vegetarian diet. They are also clearly better suited to a vegetarian diet, particularly a vegan diet. As a vegetarian, you will obviously see that the guidelines do not mention the need for people to consume animal flesh or animal protein. The guidelines encourage a diet rich in grain products, vegetables, and fruits—a diet that is the mainstay of vegetarian nutrition. The guidelines also discourage a diet with fats, saturated fats, and cholesterol. Vegetarians are well aware that there is no cholesterol in any food that did not originate from an animal.

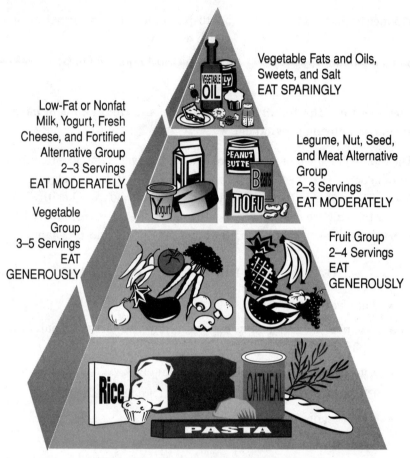

Vegetable Fats and Oils,
Sweets, and Salt
EAT SPARINGLY

Low-Fat or Nonfat
Milk, Yogurt, Fresh
Cheese, and Fortified
Alternative Group
2–3 Servings
EAT MODERATELY

Legume, Nut, Seed,
and Meat Alternative
Group
2–3 Servings
EAT MODERATELY

Vegetable
Group
3–5 Servings
EAT
GENEROUSLY

Fruit Group
2–4 Servings
EAT
GENEROUSLY

Whole-Grain Bread, Cereal, Pasta, and Rice Group
6–11 Servings   EAT LIBERALLY

Does a vegetarian diet meet the nutritional recommendations found in the USDA Food Pyramid?

As a vegetarian, you do not have to modify your diet at all. Actually, you are obtaining all of the nutrients you need, in some ways better than a non-vegetarian can. First, we should look at the pyramid:

The USDA Food Pyramid illustrates the desirable quantities of foods recommended daily from each of the five major food groups:

1. Breads and cereals.

2. Vegetables.

3. Fruits.

4. Dairy products.

5. Protein-rich foods such as dry beans, peas, nuts, eggs, meat, poultry, and fish.

It is important to note that the protein-rich food group is the only group containing foods derived from animal flesh. This group, however, *does not limit* the sources of protein to those of animal origin. It includes vegetarian sources such as beans, nuts, and eggs (for lacto-ovo-vegetarians). Although it does not mention the sources of protein vegetarians obtain from vegetables, these certainly qualify. The animal-derived sources of protein are included with vegetable-derived sources, and neither source is considered to be of higher nutritional value.

What are the basic nutrient categories I need to consume for my baby to be healthy during my vegetarian pregnancy?

The desire to maintain optimum nutrition throughout pregnancy is undeniably one of the most important goals each pregnant woman strives to fulfill. During your pregnancy, you will require an increased intake of several nutrients, but no reciprocal decrease in any other nutrient. For you to reach this improved nutritional level, you must either

- increase your total food intake; or
- increase your choices of foods with higher nutritive value.

As a pregnant woman, you need an adequate amount of *all* nutrients. There are two categories of necessary nutrients:

Macronutrients

These are required in large quantities as sources of energy and include

Carbohydrates: sugars, starches, fiber

Proteins: amino acids

Fats

Micronutrients

These are required in small quantities to help macronutrients function. They include

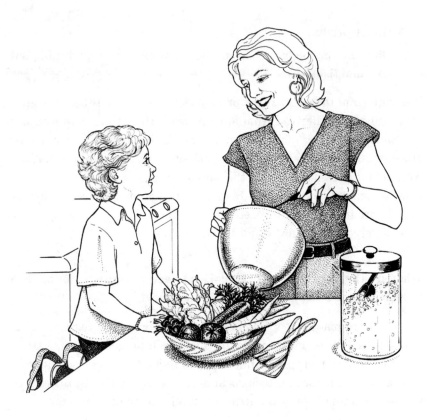

Vitamins: Water-soluble vitamins
Fat-soluble vitamins

Minerals: Macrominerals
Microminerals

CARBOHYDRATES

Will I be able to obtain the amount of carbohydrates I need during pregnancy with my vegetarian diet?

You definitely will be able to obtain sufficient quantities of carbohydrates as a vegetarian, but it will be up to you whether or not you obtain the healthiest quality of carbohydrates. Carbohydrates are abundant in our diets, as they are produced during photosynthesis within all plants and are the main source of energy for all individuals. They generally make up 50 to 60 percent of all of our diets, whether we are vegetarian or not. As a vegetarian, you will be able to obtain healthy carbohydrates from your fruits and vegetables. Vegetarian carbohydrate sources also come with the benefit of fiber, which helps us to eliminate and clean out toxins from our intestinal tracts. Nonhealthy sources of carbohydrates are simple sugars and refined starches, such as table sugar and white flour.

There are three types of carbohydrates—sugars, starches, and fiber. Simple sugars are the easiest carbohydrate for our body to digest, and as such, they cause our blood sugar levels to rise and fall rapidly. There are various types of sugars within our diets, and almost all are derived from plants. Glucose sugar is derived from starch, sugarcane, and milk sugar. Fructose sugar is derived from fruits and honey. Sucrose sugar is derived from sugarcane, molasses, beet sugar, maple syrup, and pineapple (because it is so sweet). Sucrose is used as table sugar. Lactose sugar is the only sugar derived from animal sources, and that source is milk.

Starches are digested at a slower rate than simple sugars and confer a more consistent "full" feeling when we eat them. Potatoes, corn, rice, root vegetables, and wheat are all starches. Present-day diets tend to be richer in simple sugars rather than healthy starches. This is not a healthy change, as starches generally contain a higher level of nutrients than do sugars.

Fiber is the indigestible cellulose component of fruits and vegetables. As a vegetarian, your high dietary intake of fiber brings great health advantages. Fiber contains a minimal amount of calories, yet it fosters good function of the intestinal tract and helps to better eliminate toxins from your body. There are several types of fiber, including cellulose, pectin (present in the rind of fruits), and carrageen. Fiber in the diet helps to decrease the cholesterol level in the blood. There is no fiber in meat, chicken, or fish, so vegetarians have a definite advantage over non-vegetarians in relation to their intake of fiber.

Sugars and Sweeteners

Should I decrease my intake of sugar while I am trying to become pregnant or during my pregnancy?

Sugars have no nutritive value other than being a source of energy and calories. Both sugars and starches are in the food category termed carbohydrates. Although it is recommended that 50 to 60 percent of your diet be composed of carbohydrates, no specific quantity is recommended by the authorities. That is because your body manufactures its own sugar—glucose—regardless of which foods you consume, be they carbohydrates, fats, or proteins. Therefore, you do not actually need to consume sugars to have them present in your body.

It is easy for your body to digest sugars, so they are an instant source of energy. They do not, however, contain protein, vitamins, or minerals. As a vegetarian, it is healthier to obtain much of the carbohydrate component of your diet from starch rather than from refined sugar. This is because the food sources of vegetarian starches also contain protein, vitamins, and minerals, whereas refined sugars do not.

I have heard that brown sugar and honey are healthier than white sugars. Is this so?

Although many people believe that brown sugar is a healthier form, it is actually just white sugar sprayed with molasses syrup. Similarly, many people believe honey is healthier, while in reality it is just a blend of fructose and glucose sugars.

There are actually many different types of sugars: sucrose, from sugarcane; fructose, from fruit; lactose, from milk; and maltose, from yeast acting on starch. All of these sugars are a source of rapid energy and calories, but they lack protein, vitamins, and minerals.

If I just eliminate desserts from my diet, will that help me decrease my sugar intake adequately?

I wish it were that easy. As a vegetarian, you have become very knowledgeable about foods and will be able to make all of your food choices count. Eating sugars, or refined carbohydrates, is not the way to do it. In our society, the elimination of sugars from our diets is a monumental task, accomplished only if we eat no processed foods and never eat out. Sugar is placed in, and camouflaged in, numerous food products. Sometimes the word *sugar* may be missing from a product label, but the words *sucrose, honey,* and *corn syrup* are there, and these sugars may be present in large quantities. Although you may not see the word *sugar,* many products may be filled with it. In this case, "a rose by any other name" tastes just as sweet. Varieties of sugars are abundant in many processed foods, including salad dressings, canned and packaged soups, sauces, cereals, ketchup, mayonnaise, chips, dips, artificial coffee creamers, and peanut butter. Canned vegetables also contain large quantities of sugars.

Now is the time to perfect your preparation of your grandmother's spaghetti sauce from scratch—without sugar!

Occasionally, I eat foods sweetened with saccharin. Can this be a danger for my baby?

The FDA tried to ban the use of saccharin in foods in 1977; however, this was not possible due to marked public resistance. Saccharin is a petroleum derivative that is three hundred to five hundred times sweeter than table sugar. In general, it is not considered safe, as it may be mildly to moderately cancer causing. Therefore, children and pregnant women should not consume foods or beverages that contain saccharin. If you are diabetic and must limit your intake of sugars, saccharin is definitely not your sweetener of choice.

If I were to drink beverages sweetened with aspartame, could that be dangerous to a baby?

Aspartame is a newer artificial sweetener and is actually somewhat more natural than cyclamate and saccharin. It also might be a little safer. Aspartame is a petroleum derivative and is a mixture of two amino acids, which are normally found in foods. It was accidentally discovered when a researcher tasted it and found out how sweet it was. It is two hundred times sweeter than sugar, and therefore only a tiny amount is needed as an additive to create a sweet taste.

Aspartame is not completely safe, as some people are sensitive to it. You should not worry if you consumed liquids containing aspartame before you knew you were pregnant, but once you know that you are pregnant, you should discontinue this chemical. One in fifteen thousand people lacks an enzyme to metabolize aspartame. In those women, the amino acid phenylalanine might build up in their system when they cannot metabolize it, and it can adversely affect their baby's intelligence. This disorder, known as "phenylketonuria" (PKU), is rare, but nevertheless it is advisable that you discontinue use of aspartame in your pregnancy, just in case you or your baby is a carrier.

Is the new artificial sweetener Splenda safe to use during pregnancy?

Splenda, also known as sucralose, is a derivative of the sugar sucrose and was approved for general usage by the FDA in 1998. McNeil Specialty Products studied the effects of sucralose on pregnant mice, rats, rabbits, and dogs and did not note any abnormalities in their newborns. Four of nine rabbits given high doses of sucralose, however, aborted their fetuses. Although the FDA report did not state the expected miscarriage rate for rats in laboratory conditions, I find this statistic of concern. Therefore, I believe it will be wise and prudent for you to avoid, or markedly limit, ingestion of sucralose during your pregnancy.

Which brand-name sweeteners contain which artificial sugars?

Aspartame is present in NutraSweet and Equal.

Saccharin is present in Sweet'N Low.

Sucralose is present in Splenda.

Sorbitol, mannitol, and xylitol are artificial sweeteners found in a variety of prepared foods. They contain no sugar but are very high in calories. They are not called sugars; they are called sugar alcohols and often contain more calories than traditional sugar.

PROTEINS

"If you're vegetarian, where do you get your protein?"

As a vegetarian, you have probably heard this question many times. But now that you are pregnant, you will be asked it so often that you may start to wonder yourself.

If you are a vegan, you obtain your protein from nutritious vegetables, beans, tofu, seeds, soy milk, grains, and nuts. If you are a lacto-ovo-vegetarian, your protein is in nutritious vegetables, beans, tofu, seeds, soy milk, grains, nuts, and dairy products. Vegetarians are usually quite knowledgeable about the nutritional content of a multitude of foods, so much so that most vegetarians know the following facts:

- ◆ Proteins are one of the major nutrients necessary for good health, along with carbohydrates, fats, vitamins, and minerals.

- Proteins make up 20 percent of our body weight.

- Proteins are the main component of our muscles, hair, nails, eyes, and skin. Protein is also the main component of the heart.

- Proteins are composed of building blocks called "amino acids." These are small nitrogen-containing compounds that join together to form larger proteins. Some amino acids must be obtained from our foods (essential amino acids), and others can be manufactured within our own bodies (nonessential amino acids).

- There are eight essential amino acids that we must obtain from foods in order to build protein. These are isoleucine, leucine, lysine, methionine, phenylalanine, threonine, tryptophan, and valine.

- The other, nonessential amino acids are produced within our own bodies, and we do not need to obtain them from foods.

- Amino acids are abundant in high-protein foods, yet almost all foods contain some amino acids.

- Animal-derived foods contain all eight essential amino acids within the same food.

- When combined, plant-derived foods contain all eight amino acids—and have none of the unhealthy cholesterol found in animal-derived foods.

How can I obtain the essential amino acids my baby and I need throughout my pregnancy?

All eight essential amino acids are found in vegetarian foods as well as in non-vegetarian foods. During pregnancy, you will just need to eat larger quantities of your protein-rich foods (including beans, nuts, grains, tofu, vegetables, eggs, and dairy products) than you might otherwise have preferred. On the positive side, these foods will be lower in fats, lower in pesticides, and lower in calories than the comparable protein-rich foods that a non-vegetarian needs to eat.

If you are a lacto-ovo-vegetarian, you will have no difficulty obtaining all of your eight essential amino acids, as eggs and dairy products contain these. If you are a vegan, however, you will need to eat a variety of protein-rich vegetables and grains in order to obtain all of your essential amino acids. That is because three of the essential amino acids—lysine, methionine, and tryptophan—are not present in every plant-derived food. That is not to say that if you are a vegan, you will have difficulty obtaining these amino acids. You certainly will not. You will simply need to obtain your full amount of amino acids from a variety of foods rather than from just one. That is fine, because as a vegetarian you have a variety of plant sources to rely on for good nutrition. As long as you give your baby and yourself all eight of the essential amino acids, you will both have the building blocks needed to create protein.

All eight essential amino acids are present in plant foods, but not necessarily all together in the same plant.

For example:

- Lysine is present in beans, wheat germ, eggs, fruits, and vegetables. It is not present in peanuts and grains.

- Methionine is present in beans, soybeans, peanuts, dairy foods, and eggs.

- Tryptophan is present in nuts, seeds, eggs, and dairy products. It is not present in corn, beans, and cereal grains.

There are more than enough choices within each of these popular vegetarian categories of foods for you to obtain all of your essential amino acids.

As a pregnant vegetarian, do I need to eat foods containing all eight essential amino acids in the same meal?

No, you do not need to eat them at the same time. For many years, a theory existed that vegetarians needed to study their diets and make sure that they consumed specific amino acid–rich foods with certain other amino acid–rich foods at the same time. This theory has since been disproved. The theory became popular when nutritionists observed that the meals predominantly vegetarian cultures chose often contained foods that, when combined, contained the full complement of all essential amino acids. Examples of such vegetarian meals would be corn and lima beans or rice and beans.

This theory was quite perceptive and helpful in showing how simply vegetarian individuals can obtain complete nutrition, but now we know that as long as people maintain a well-rounded diet containing each of the essential amino acids at some time, they need not eat them all within the same meal. As long as your diet contains all the essential amino acids on a long-term basis, your body will be able to build strong tissues.

Our bodies do not create protein right after we digest an amino acid–rich meal. Actually, if you do not exercise, your body might never create protein. It is not the amino acids that form muscles; it is exercise that transforms amino acids into protein and creates muscle mass. When you eat a protein-rich meal, the amino acids are broken down and stored within your body. When you exercise, your body draws on these stores to build muscle; yet if you are not active, the amino acids remain stored.

During the time that this "combining" theory was popular many people were dissuaded from becoming vegetarian. They felt they would have needed a Ph.D. in nutrition and a calculator in hand each time they went to the supermarket. Now we know that it's not necessary to combine proteins. Your vegetarian proteins are in no way inferior to non-vegetarian proteins, and your well-rounded vegetarian diet supplies you with all the amino acids you need for a healthy pregnancy.

Is the most important function of protein to form muscle tissue?

No, protein has many important functions that are necessary for your overall physical health. These include growth and maintenance of all body tissues, healing the body after illness and injury, production of blood cells, production of all energy after your carbohydrates and fats have been depleted, building of enzymes, formation of antibodies, production of hormones, and formation of hemoglobin. Individuals living in totally vegetarian cultures do not suffer from protein deficiency, which goes to show that the proteins derived from vegetation are more than adequate to successfully perform all of these bodily functions.

As a vegetarian, is it true that I can obtain my protein from typical vegetables and beans? Is the percentage of protein within these foods sufficient for my baby and myself?

Protein is present in almost all vegetables, but not in all fruits. As a vegetarian, you will need to eat a larger volume of food to obtain the recommended amounts of protein than will a non-vegetarian, but you will not need to increase your total number of calories. You will actually be consuming fewer calories and less fat from your protein than a non-vegetarian individual will. For non-vegetarians, many animal sources of protein come with "baggage"—namely, large quantities of cholesterol and many calories. Following is a list of several plant-based foods and the relative amount of protein contained within each of them.

Food	Serving Size	Protein (grams)	Calories from Protein (%)
Spinach, cooked	1 cup	5	48.0
Broccoli, cooked	1 cup	5	45.6
Tofu, firm	1 cup	40	43.6
Soybeans	1 cup	30	39.0
Lentils, cooked	1 cup	18	31.2
Soy milk	1 cup	10	26.0
Chickpeas, cooked	1 cup	15	22.0
Whole-wheat bread	2 slices	9	18.0
Peanut butter	2 tbsp	13	17.2
Potato	1 medium	4.5	8.0

My vegetarian diet contains less protein than the diet of my non-vegetarian friends. Does that mean my diet is inferior?

Although many non-vegetarians within our country consume high levels of protein, that does not mean your diet contains too little. From a health perspective, there is significant concern that people in industrialized countries who consume between 100 and 200 grams of protein daily are harming their bodies. People who consume these high intakes of non-vegetarian protein place a strain on their kidneys and their liver and store this excess protein as excess fat. Because this protein comes with high levels of animal fat, many non-vegetarians have an increased incidence of cardiovascular disease. In addition, high levels of animal proteins and fats are associated with an increased risk for various cancers.

The United States Recommended Dietary Allowance of protein for nonpregnant women is 50 grams daily, and many believe this standard may be too high. The World Health Organization sets the protein requirement at 25 grams daily.

What can happen if I do not get enough protein? How will I know if I am getting enough?

Too little dietary protein, termed "protein deficiency," can create a very serious condition. In indigent countries this condition is called "*kwashiorkor*" (Ghanian for "the evil spirit that infects the child"). Children with too little protein waste away. All of their bones become visible under their flesh, and their abdomens distend. This protein deficiency can lead to death if it is not treated. Marasmus, a combined deficiency of both protein and calories, is also prevalent in the third world. It develops when an individual is in a state of total starvation. Marasmus takes the lives of millions of individuals in the third world yearly.

These affected individuals are subsisting on only small quantities of rice and are deficient in both calories and protein. They are not consuming the abundance of beans, tofu, green vegetables, red and yellow vegetables, nuts, seeds, and grains that vegetarians and vegans in our country consume. Nor are they consuming the additional eggs and dairy products that lacto-ovo-vegetarians within our country consume. The current Recommended Dietary Allowance of protein in our country is 50 grams daily. This recommendation is increased to 60 grams of protein daily during pregnancy and to 65 grams of protein daily while women are nursing. Although these protein recommendations are high compared to the recommendations set by the World Health Organization, these levels are within the ranges commonly present in the diets of most healthy American vegetarians. You can easily achieve these levels of protein intake and have peace of mind knowing that you have obtained enough protein for your baby and yourself.

The vegetation on our planet is the predominant recipient of the energy from our sun. It is, therefore, the primary source from which all carbohydrates, vitamins, minerals, protein, fatty acids, and energy are derived for human nutrition. As humans, we have used three hundred different plant species for our survival for thousands of years. On a global scale, plants have provided 65 percent of all the protein used in this world for human nutrition. It is difficult to dispel the myth that we must receive our protein from animal sources rather than from vegetation, but with time, the population of our country will recognize that this is just a myth.

THE TRUTH ABOUT VEGETARIANS AND PROTEIN

- ◆ Vegetarians obtain enough protein from a standard, easy-to-prepare meal of wholesome vegetarian foods.
- ◆ Vegetarians do not have to spend complicated hours shopping for and preparing foods to obtain healthy levels of protein.
- ◆ Vegetarians do not need to gain excess weight to obtain enough protein.
- ◆ Vegetarians do not require animal protein to be strong and healthy.
- ◆ Vegetarians do not need animal proteins to develop muscles. It is strength training that develops muscles.

As a vegetarian pregnant woman, how does my protein intake compare to that of the average non-vegetarian pregnant woman?

The Recommended Dietary Allowance of protein during pregnancy is 60 milligrams daily. As mentioned previously, that value is quite high compared to the value recommended for pregnant women by dietary organizations in the rest of the world, yet it will not be difficult for you to obtain these levels, and it is best for you to try. You will in no way be deficient in protein compared to non-vegetarian women.

SUPERIOR TO MEAT-EATERS	
BETTER THAN MEAT-EATERS	
SAME AS MEAT-EATERS	X
CHALLENGE TO OBTAIN NUTRITION	
CAREFUL PLANNING RECOMMENDED	

The following list compares some vegetarian sources of protein with some non-vegetarian sources:

VEGETARIAN		**Non-Vegetarian**	
White beans, 1 cup	(17 gm)	Beef, 4 oz	(35–55 gm)
Tofu, firm, 1 cup	(40 gm)	Tuna, baked, 4 oz	(57 gm)
Black beans, 1 cup	(15 gm)	Pork, 4 oz	(55 gm)
Wheat germ, 2 oz	(30 gm)	Shrimp, 8 large	(10 gm)
Lima beans, 1 cup	(12 gm)	Chicken, roasted, 4 oz	(30–42 gm)
Vegetarian chili, 1 cup	(20–40 gm)		
Oat bran cereal, 1 cup	(10–26 gm)		
Granola cereal, 1 cup	(8–19 gm)		
Carob, 1 protein bar	(15–30 gm)		
Bagel, 1	(10 gm)		
Pasta, whole-wheat, 1 cup	(7 gm)		
Kidney beans, 1 cup	(15 gm)		
Tempeh, 4 oz	(18–30 gm)		
Veggie burgers, 4 oz	(5–24 gm)		
Milk, skim, 1 cup	(10 gm)		
Eggs, 2	(12 gm)		
Yogurt, low-fat, 1 cup	(15 gm)		

Milk contains 15 percent protein. Do I need to drink milk to give my baby sufficient protein?

For the first year of life, your baby will be sustained on a diet of human milk, which has only 5 percent protein. You may drink milk if you like it, but it is not essential for your baby's growth. I often wonder why we as Americans believe we need such high quantities of dietary protein to supply optimum nutrition to a fetus. I believe it is a matter of tradition. The high-protein myth is a very difficult one to dispel. If human mothers can sustain the lives of their newborns on a diet of only 5 percent protein, then it seems nature is telling us that a moderate amount of dietary protein is more than adequate. As vegetarians, our dietary choices have led us on new and unchartered courses, so we need to use our ability to reason, rather than tradition, to make our decisions.

FATS

As a vegetarian pregnant woman, how does my lipids (fat) intake compare to that of an average non-vegetarian pregnant woman?

As a vegetarian, your diet is low in unhealthy lipids and moderate in healthy lipids compared to the diet of a non-vegetarian. Several types of lipids are present within our diets—saturated fats, unsaturated fats, triglycerides, and essential fatty acids. Lipids can have both beneficial and detrimental effects within our bodies. The primary sources of lipids within our country are meats and dairy products. There are, however, some vegetarian sources of lipids, such as avocados, nuts, olives, peanuts, seeds, and soybeans. These contain the healthier types of fats. Although we think of lipids as being a negative element of our diets, they are necessary for us to achieve optimum health. The reason fat intake correlates so closely with weight gain is that unit for unit, fats contain more calories than either proteins or carbohydrates. Fats supply 9 calories per gram of food, while proteins and carbohydrates contain only 4 calories per gram of food. Whatever portions of these calories are not used for immediate energy are stored as body fat.

What is the difference between saturated and unsaturated fats, and how will my vegetarian diet affect my intake of these?

Saturated fats are derived from animal sources, such as meats, chicken, butter, and dairy products. They are usually solid at room temperature, which is a good way to distinguish them from unsaturated fats. Saturated fats are the lipids that contain cholesterol and are basically detrimental to our health. There are other fats that are also solid at room temperature, called "hydrogenated fats." Margarine is a hydrogenated fat. Hydrogenated fats, which are not always derived from animal protein, are just as unhealthy as saturated fats. Both saturated fats and hydrogenated fats tend to raise blood cholesterol values and cause cholesterol-related heart disease.

Unsaturated fats are derived from plants and are much healthier than saturated fats. There are two varieties: monounsaturated fats, such as olive oil; and polyunsaturated fats, such as peanut oil, corn oil, safflower oil, soybean oil, and most other vegetable oils. These fats do not adversely affect an individual's cholesterol level; in fact, olive oil, a monounsaturated fat, helps to prevent cholesterol-related cardiovascular disease.

Essential fatty acids are another component of our lipids. We cannot produce these within our own bodies, so we must obtain them from outside sources. They are all in the category of polyunsaturated lipids and are quite healthy for us. The most frequently discussed essential fatty acid is the omega-3. This fatty acid is commonly found in cold-water fish; however, it is also found in flaxseed oil, canola oil, and soybean oil. It helps to lower blood triglycerides and to raise healthy protective cholesterol. Omega-6 is another essential fatty acid. It is present in corn, safflower, sesame, soybean, and sunflower oils and is necessary for a healthy metabolism.

If I were to eat oily vegetarian foods, such as spaghetti with olive oil and garlic, or an oily Caesar salad, would this be bad for my baby?

Although high in calories, oils derived from plant sources do not carry the same serious side effects as do oils derived from animal sources. Specifically, they do not put you at risk for atherosclerosis (hardening of the arteries), as do butter and other non-vegetarian source of fats. All plant-derived oils are devoid of cholesterol. The common misconception is that the word *lipid* or *fat* is synonymous with the word *cholesterol.* Each has a very different meaning, both chemically and from a health perspective. Lipids constitute a large group of compounds, of which cholesterol is only one. Some plant-derived oils have actually been shown to decrease the cholesterol content of blood vessels. Olive oil, peanut oil, and canola oil are the common oils that have such abilities. The advantageous effect of olive oil was initially discovered when doctors noted the excellent cardiovascular health of individuals eating a typical Mediterranean diet, filled with olives and olive oil. Olive oil is definitely beneficial from a cardiovascular perspective, and to a lesser extent, so is sunflower oil, corn oil, and safflower oil.

The following lists the foods that contain each type of lipid. You will be able to observe that the only vegetarian lipid in the unhealthy group is coconut oil.

LIPIDS

FATS	ESSENTIAL FATTY ACIDS
Saturated Fats	**Linolenic Acid (Omega-3)**
Beef	Flaxseed
Pork	Soybean
Lamb	Rapeseed (canola)
Poultry	Pumpkin
Coconut Oil	Walnut
Milk	
Butter	**Linoleic Acid (Omega-6)**
Cheese	Soybean
Yogurt	Safflower
	Sunflower
Polyunsaturated Fats	Corn
Soybean Oil	Wheat Germ
Safflower Oil	
Sunflower Oil	
Cottonseed Oil	
Corn Oil	
Sesame Oil	
Peanut Oil	

Monounsaturated Fats

Olive Oil

Canola Oil

Almond Oil

Peanut Oil

Will it be beneficial for my baby if I consume some cholesterol in my diet?

Your baby does need some cholesterol, but your body will manufacture cholesterol itself, so you do not need to ingest any cholesterol from outside sources. Cholesterol is necessary for you and your baby to support the health of your cell membranes, your liver, your nervous system, and your skin. Natural cholesterol is manufactured within your liver; however, any organ in your body, with the exception of your brain, can manufacture it. All of your lipids together provide you with calories for energy, and stored lipids offer a protective blanket. Your dietary lipid intake need not exceed 25 to 30 percent of your total caloric intake for you to fulfill all these needs. Excess cholesterol will form a deposit on the inner lining of blood vessels and can cause atherosclerotic deposits in the vessels of your heart and brain. As a vegetarian, you can feel confident concerning the advantage you have achieved by eliminating these detrimental lipids from your diet.

CHOLESTEROL CONTENT OF COMMON FOODS

ANIMAL FOOD Cholesterol Content (in milligrams per 100-gram portion)		PLANT FOOD Cholesterol Content (in milligrams per 100-gram portion)	
Egg, whole	550	All grains	0
Kidney, beef	375	All vegetables	0
Liver, beef	300	All nuts	0
Butter	250	All seeds	0
Oysters	200	All fruits	0

(continued on next page)

	ANIMAL FOOD			PLANT FOOD	
Cream cheese		120	All legumes		0
Lard		950	All vegetable oils		0
Beefsteak		700			
Lamb		700			
Pork		70			
Chicken		60			
Ice cream		45			

SOURCE: *Pennington, J.,* **Food Values of Proportions Commonly Used**
(New York: Harper & Row, 14th ed., 1985)

Even though I am vegetarian, should I supplement my diet with fish oils to obtain healthy omega-3 fatty acids?

People usually take omega-3 supplements to prevent cardiovascular heart disease. Actually, it could be dangerous for you to supplement your diet with omega-3 fatty acids during your pregnancy. Some fish liver oil supplements contain high levels of vitamin A and D, but the vitamin A is derived from animal sources rather than vegetable sources and can cause abnormalities in an unborn fetus. In addition, fish livers tend to concentrate toxic materials, and this is not the time for you to include toxins in your diet. The fish that are used to create omega-3 supplements are also many of the same fish that the FDA has declared hazardous to pregnant women owing to their high content of methylmercury. For example, mackerel is often a source of omega-3 fatty acids for vitamin supplements, yet the FDA considers it hazardous to pregnant and nursing women.

There are readily available vegetarian sources of omega-3 fatty acids. If you wish to supplement with omega-3 fatty acids, please use cold-pressed flaxseed oil capsules. Flaxseed oil is one of the richest sources of omega-3 fatty acid, and it will be healthier for you than fish-derived omega-3 fatty acids in all respects.

VITAMINS

Could you please explain what a vitamin is and how vitamins contribute to a healthy diet?

Vitamins were first discovered in the early 1900s. They are tiny nutrients the body uses to metabolize carbohydrates, proteins, and fats; help chemical reactions to occur; aid with digestion; and build resistance to disease. There are two main categories of vitamins, *water-soluble* and *fat-soluble*.

Vitamins are *organic* substances. This means that they contain carbon and are derived from other living sources, such as plants and animals. Vitamins differ from minerals in that minerals are *inorganic* substances. This means that minerals do not contain carbon and are not necessarily obtained from a living source, although they can be. Minerals are found mainly in soil, sand, and rock. Most vitamins, with the exception of vitamin K and vitamin B_{12}, cannot be created within the human body. The bacteria that live naturally within the intestinal tract of humans form both vitamin K and vitamin B_{12}. Unlike carbohydrates, fats, and proteins, vitamins are required only in small amounts. Most of the other vitamins are found so ubiquitously in nature that deficiencies of them are rare regardless of a person's dietary habits. Vitamins may be obtained through numerous food sources as well as through vitamin supplements. A 1976 act of Congress, however, stripped the FDA of most of its control of the regulation and labeling of vitamin supplements concerning required composition and potency.

Vitamins assist in numerous chemical reactions that our bodies must perform to survive. Cooking, storage, exposure to air, and the processing of foods often cause the loss of many vitamins that were originally present. For centuries, vitamin deficiencies have caused a tremendous amount of suffering, numerous diseases, and tragic deaths. These vitamin-deficiency diseases included beriberi, a deficiency of vitamin B_1 (thiamine); pellagra, a deficiency of vitamin B_3 (niacin); pernicious anemia, a deficiency of vitamin B_{12}; scurvy, a deficiency of vitamin C; and rickets, a deficiency of vitamin D.

Water-Soluble Vitamins

◆ Vitamin B complex
Thiamine, riboflavin, niacin, pantothenic acid, pyridoxine, folic acid, vitamin B_{12}

◆ Vitamin C
Ascorbic acid

Water-soluble vitamins are most commonly found in plant foods and less commonly found in animal-derived foods. Water-soluble vitamins are found in raw foods. When these foods are cooked or processed, they lose much of their nutritional value because the vitamins disperse in cooking water and in air. To maintain healthy levels of water-soluble vitamins, you need to eat them every day, because the body excretes them on a daily basis.

Fat-Soluble Vitamins

Vitamins A, D, E, and K are the fat-soluble vitamins, so called because they remain stored in the fat cells of our bodies for long periods of time. This is especially true in the cases of vitamins A and D. Because of the long period of time over which the body stores them, it is possible that a toxic overdose of these fat-soluble vitamins might occur. Therefore, megadoses of these vitamins should not be taken. Deficiencies of fat-soluble vitamins occur with less frequency than do deficiencies of water-soluble vitamins, not only because the body stores them, but also because they maintain their nutritional value during the cooking and preparation of foods.

Water-Soluble Vitamins	Fat-Soluble Vitamins
Vitamins B and C	Vitamins A, D, E, and K
Lost during cooking	Stable during cooking
Mostly from plant sources	From both plant and animal sources
Excreted daily in urine	Stored in body fat
Not present in animals	Stored in fat and liver of ingested animals
New dose required daily	New dose not required daily
Deficiencies occur	Deficiencies very rare

Are vitamin deficiencies or vitamin excesses more significant to a woman while she is pregnant than they would be were she not pregnant?

It's important to watch your vitamin intake during pregnancy to ensure that you develop no deficiencies or excesses. Either extreme may adversely affect your baby's development. For example, folic acid, one of the water-soluble B vitamins, is excreted daily in the urine. Women with low levels of folic acid during conception and early pregnancy have experienced an increased incidence of spina bifida in their newborns.

Similarly, an excess of vitamin A, a fat-soluble vitamin, can cause birth defects in newborns. These include defects of the brain, heart, and face; cleft lip and cleft palate; and mental retardation. These tragedies due to excess vitamin A occur only through vitamin A derived from animal products, not that derived from vegetarian foods, because these are two different forms of the vitamin.

I know that B vitamins are important during pregnancy. What are the B vitamins, and why are they so important during pregnancy?

Following is a brief overview of the B vitamins, to give you a foundation of knowledge before we discuss each vitamin individually.

- All B vitamins are water-soluble and are not stored in the body fat.
- Because the B vitamins are all water-soluble, they can be lost when cooking in water and in steam.
- Vitamin B deficiencies occur easily—while fasting, dieting, eating refined processed foods, or eating large quantities of sugar.
- B-complex vitamins are commonly all found together in nature within the same plants.
- Bacteria living in our large intestine produce some vitamin B_{12}.
- Bacteria, fungus, and yeast are all capable of producing B vitamins.
- Overdoses of B vitamins do not usually occur.
- Excess B vitamins are excreted in the urine, giving it a yellow color.
- Many vitamin B deficiencies can occur, but no vitamin B toxicities occur.
- The richest natural source of B vitamins is brewer's yeast.
- Wheat germ and bran cereal are excellent sources of B vitamins.
- Green leafy vegetables and milk supply modest amounts of B vitamins.

- Animal products have scant amounts of B vitamins, except for vitamin B_{12}.
- Vitamin B_{12} is the only B vitamin found mainly in animal foods.
- Antibiotics deplete vitamin B_{12}–producing bacteria from the intestines.
- Ingestion of lactobacillus supplies the intestines with bacteria to produce its own B vitamins.
- Vitamin B is necessary for health of the skin, hair, eyes, and liver.
- Vitamin B functions are interrelated. It is beneficial to take them together.
- Deficiencies of B vitamins include fatigue, nervousness, depression, loss of appetite, cracks at the corners of the mouth, burning of the mouth or tongue, hair loss, constipation, and nerve sensitivity.

What can I do as a vegetarian to prevent the loss of all the water-soluble vitamins, B and C, from my foods?

You need to be aware that both cooking and storage of raw fruits and vegetables may cause them to lose water-soluble B vitamins and vitamin C. To help you retain the water-soluble vitamin content within your fruits and vegetables:

- Eat your fruits and vegetables raw when possible.
- If you are cooking vegetables, keep them crisp. This way they retain most of their vitamin content.
- Steam your vegetables, in preference to boiling them.
- Cut vegetables in large pieces rather than in small pieces, as small pieces have more surface area exposed to water and, therefore, greater loss of the vitamins.
- Leave the peel or skin on your vegetables.
- Use your leftover water as vegetable stock for gravy or soup, as all of your vitamins may be contained within this liquid.
- Serve your foods immediately after preparation.
- Cover and refrigerate the leftover fruits and vegetables immediately.
- Keep your pots tightly covered while cooking vegetables.

- Refrigerate foods high in vitamin C and store them in airtight containers, as this will help to maintain the vitamin content. Do not store them in water.

- When you prepare frozen foods, bring those foods directly from the freezer to the boiling water. Do not thaw them slowly.

- After you squeeze juice from an orange, drink it immediately. Juice will lose much of its vitamin C when exposed to air.

Vitamin B_1, Thiamine

You will have no difficulty in obtaining vitamin B_1–rich foods as a vegetarian, but the way you cook these foods may affect your true intake. In general, vegetarians consume more thiamine than do non-vegetarians. You will need to be cautious as to how you prepare your foods, because vitamin B_1 is easily destroyed by boiling foods or by the moist heat used to steam foods. It is also depleted from your body if you eat it along with a diet high in sugar, coffee, black tea, nicotine, or alcohol. The vegetarian food sources of thiamine are abundant and include wheat germ, whole wheat, enriched flour, brown rice, spinach, cauliflower, nuts, sunflower seeds, beans, peanuts, peas, avocado, many dried fruits, and blackstrap molasses.

Thiamine helps the body produce energy, convert ingested carbohydrates into fats, maintain the function of the nervous system, and conduct nerve impulses. There are no vitamin B_1 toxicity states, because it is a water-soluble vitamin and any excess intake is excreted in the urine daily. Deficiency states can occur, as may occur with many of the B vitamins. Deficiency of thiamine can lead to beriberi. Children with this deficiency suffer from confusion, fatigue, insufficient growth in their limbs, decreased heart function, and brain degeneration. The deficiency occurs in children growing up on an empty-calorie diet of white bread, soda, sweets, and fast foods. The Recommended Dietary Allowance of vitamin B_1 is 1.1 milligrams daily, but in pregnancy your recommendation is increased to 1.5 milligrams daily.

HOW DO YOU FARE AS A VEGETARIAN WITH VITAMIN B$_1$ INTAKE?

SUPERIOR TO MEAT-EATERS	X
BETTER THAN MEAT-EATERS	
SAME AS MEAT-EATERS	
CHALLENGE TO OBTAIN NUTRITION	
CAREFUL PLANNING RECOMMENDED	

FOOD SOURCES OF VITAMIN B$_1$

VEGETARIAN		Non-Vegetarian	
Toasted wheat germ, ¼ cup	(0.47 mg)	Broiled tuna, 4 oz	(0.32 mg)
Sunflower seeds, ½ cup	(0.65 mg)	Salmon, 4 oz	(0.31 mg)
Fortified instant breakfast, 1 pkg	(0.30 mg)	Pork, 3 oz	(0.78 mg)
Soy milk, 1 cup	(0.39 mg)	Cured ham, 4 oz	(0.80 mg)
Soybeans, dry-roasted, ½ cup	(0.37 mg)	Bacon, 4 oz	(0.38 mg)
Oatmeal, 1 cup	(0.75 mg)		
Sesame seeds, ½ cup	(0.72 mg)		
Seminola, 1 cup	(1.35 mg)		
Vegetarian breakfast links, 2	(1–7 mg)		
Walnuts, ½ cup	(0.23 mg)		
Müeslix, 1 cup	(0.50 mg)		
Pistachio nuts, ½ cup	(0.53 mg)		
Green peas, 1 cup	(0.42 mg)		

Spinach noodles,
1 cup   (0.39 mg)

Hummus, 1 cup   (0.23 mg)

Vegetarian egg roll, 1   (1–1.22 mg)

Wheat bran, ¾ cup   (0.38 mg)

Product 19 cereal,
1 cup   (1.50 mg)

Brazil nuts, ½ cup   (0.70 mg)

Food for Thought: Many vegetarian foods are rich in vitamin B_1. The main non-vegetarian foods rich in this vitamin are derived from pork. As a vegetarian, your intake will be excellent compared to the relative intake of vitamin B_1 by a non-vegetarian.

Vitamin B_2, Riboflavin

As a vegetarian, your ability to obtain foods rich in riboflavin will exceed that of a non-vegetarian. Fortunately, riboflavin is fairly resistant to the effects of heat and moisture, so this vitamin is not that easily destroyed during cooking. It is, however, sensitive to light—especially sunlight. That is why milk fortified with riboflavin should always be kept in the refrigerator, as the light will destroy its vitamin content. Some riboflavin-rich foods include brewer's yeast, seaweed, wild rice, dried peas, beans, peanuts, sunflower seeds, dark leafy green vegetables, asparagus, broccoli, spinach, collard greens, mushrooms, and avocado.

Your baby and you require riboflavin to help your cells produce energy and to use oxygen. Because riboflavin is a water-soluble vitamin, any excess is excreted in the urine, so there are no vitamin B_2 toxicity states. Severe deficiencies of riboflavin, however, may cause inflammation in the mouth, cracks at the corners of the lips, sore tongue, burning eyes, cataracts, weight loss, hair loss, and a general lack of energy. There are no life-threatening deficiency disorders of riboflavin, as normal intestinal bacteria produce some riboflavin even if the quantity in an individual's diet is small.

The Recommended Dietary Allowance of vitamin B_2 for women is 1.3 milligrams daily. In pregnancy the recommended allowance is 1.6 milligrams daily.

HOW DO YOU FARE AS A VEGETARIAN WITH VITAMIN B₂ INTAKE?

SUPERIOR TO MEAT-EATERS	
BETTER THAN MEAT-EATERS	X
SAME AS MEAT-EATERS	
CHALLENGE TO OBTAIN NUTRITION	
CAREFUL PLANNING RECOMMENDED	

FOOD SOURCES OF VITAMIN B₂

VEGETARIAN		Non-Vegetarian	
Brewer's yeast, 1 tsp	(1.25 mg)	Turkey giblets, 4 oz	(1.03 mg)
Spinach, 10 oz	(0.39 mg)	Cow tongue, 4 oz	(0.40 mg)
Miso soup, 1 cup	(0.70 mg)	Cow liver, 4 oz	(4.65 mg)
Product 19 cereal, 1 cup	(1.70 mg)	Mackerel, 4 oz	(0.61 mg)
Veggie burger, 2.5 oz	(0.60 mg)	Veal, 4 oz	(0.40 mg)
Kellogg's granola bar	(0.38 mg)		
Eggs, 2	(0.50 mg)		
Special K cereal, 1 cup	(0.70 mg)		
Steamed broccoli, 1 cup	(0.70 mg)		
Asparagus, 10 oz	(0.37 mg)		
Low-fat yogurt, 8 oz	(0.49 mg)		
Milk, 1 cup	(0.42 mg)		

Food for Thought: Vitamin B₂ is present in many different vegetarian foods but is not present in large quantities in any one food. Brewer's yeast is the richest source of vitamin B₂. The non-vegetarian sources of riboflavin are predominantly those of animal organs, such as heart, liver, and kidney. As a vegetarian, you fare relatively well in obtaining vitamin B_2, because non-vegetarian sources of vitamin B_2 are limited (unless you like liver).

Vitamin B_3, Niacin

You will have no trouble as a pregnant vegetarian finding excellent sources of niacin in your diet. Niacin is one of the most stable of the B vitamins and is not severely affected by heat, cooking, or light. You may also be producing niacin within your own body, by converting the amino acid tryptophan into niacin. In converting natural grain to white grain, however, up to 90 percent of the niacin is removed. To compensate, many manufacturers add niacin back and call the food "enriched." Always choose whole-grain breads and flour products enriched with niacin over grains that have been processed. Some vegetarian sources of niacin include peanuts, dry beans, peas, wheat germ, whole grains, enriched breads, avocados, dates, figs, prunes, milk, and eggs (your baby converts tryptophan in eggs to niacin).

Niacin has many functions. It helps your baby and you produce energy; maintain a healthy intestinal tract, skin, and tongue; and regulate blood sugar. As an adult, you are helped by niacin's producing hydrochloric acid in your intestinal tract; forming estrogen, testosterone, progesterone, and cortisone; stimulating your circulation; and preventing leg cramps, lowering blood pressure, and reducing cholesterol and triglyceride levels. There are no vitamin B_3 toxicity states. (If you consume high levels of niacin, usually by ingesting niacin vitamin supplements, you may experience a "flushing" sensation.) A niacin deficiency can cause pellagra. Symptoms of this disorder include diarrhea, skin irritations, skin pigmentations, light sensitivity, muscular weakness, and impaired brain function.

The Recommended Dietary Allowance of niacin is 15 milligrams daily. During your pregnancy, the recommended daily intake is 17 milligrams.

HOW DO YOU FARE AS A VEGETARIAN
WITH VITAMIN B$_3$ INTAKE?

SUPERIOR TO MEAT-EATERS	X
BETTER THAN MEAT-EATERS	
SAME AS MEAT-EATERS	
CHALLENGE TO OBTAIN NUTRITION	
CAREFUL PLANNING RECOMMENDED	

FOOD SOURCES OF VITAMIN B$_3$

VEGETARIAN		Non-Vegetarian	
Roasted peanuts, 1 cup	(20.56 mg)	Liver, 4 oz	(12.16 mg)
Oat cereal, 4 oz	(22.00 mg)	Leg of lamb, 4 oz	(7.14 mg)
Product 19 cereal, 1 cup	(20.00 mg)	Turkey, 4 oz	(5.77 mg)
Shiitake mushrooms, dried, 4 oz	(15.88 mg)	Beef, 3 oz	(8.40 mg)
Prunes, 4 oz	(2.22 mg)		
Avocado, 1	(3.32 mg)		
Bran flakes, 4 oz	(20.00 mg)		
Cornflakes, 4 oz	(20.00 mg)		

Vitamin B$_6$, Pyridoxine

Vitamin B$_6$ is abundant in vegetables, so it will not be difficult for you to obtain sufficient quantities for both your baby and yourself. Unfortunately, when foods containing vitamin B$_6$ are exposed to sunlight or are processed and cooked, much of the vitamin is destroyed. For example, raw sugarcane has a large amount of vitamin B_6, but refined sugar has none. Whole wheat has a large amount of vitamin B_6, yet refined wheat has almost none. Pyridoxine is a very important vitamin for women. It is involved in balancing hormones and regulating water shifts in women's bodies. It is a natural diuretic. Women require higher quantities of vitamin B_6 when their estrogen levels are elevated—such as during pregnancy, when they are on oral contraceptives, and when they take postmenopausal hormones. Examples of vitamin B_6–rich vegetarian foods are egg yolks, soybeans, dried beans, peanuts, walnuts, bananas, cabbage, cauliflower, potatoes, prunes, and avocados.

Vitamin B_6 assists in many metabolic changes within the body. It also functions within the brain to convert tryptophan into serotonin, which is a natural mood elevator. During pregnancy, women have an increased need for vitamin B_6. It assists in maintaining the correct hormone balance and the correct fluid balance. It may also help in relieving some of the nausea and vomiting of morning sickness. This vitamin also helps to form your baby's nervous system. Vitamin B_6 deficiency states can occur, manifesting as muscle weakness and as nerve system symptoms such as irritability, insomnia, nervousness, confusion, and tingling of the fingers and toes.

The Recommended Dietary Allowance of vitamin B_6 is 1.6 milligrams daily. During your pregnancy, for the reasons noted above, recommended intake is increased to 2.2 milligrams daily.

HOW DO YOU FARE AS A VEGETARIAN WITH VITAMIN B_6 INTAKE?

SUPERIOR TO MEAT-EATERS	
BETTER THAN MEAT-EATERS	X
SAME AS MEAT-EATERS	
CHALLENGE TO OBTAIN NUTRITION	
CAREFUL PLANNING RECOMMENDED	

YOUR VEGETARIAN FOOD SOURCES OF VITAMIN B₆

VEGETARIAN		Non-Vegetarian	
Cereal, enriched	(0.50–2.20 mg)	Beef liver, 3 oz	(0.71 mg)
Banana, 1	(0.90 mg)	Chicken, 3 oz	(0.45 mg)
Corn, 1 cup	(0.51 mg)	Pork, 3 oz	(0.41 mg)
Tomato juice, 1 cup	(0.46 mg)	Tuna, 3 oz	(0.36 mg)
Yard-long beans, raw, 1 cup	(0.40 mg)		
Yellow bell pepper, 1	(0.31 mg)		
Veggie burger, 3 oz	(0.50–1.10 mg)		

Food for Thought: When individuals take megadoses of vitamin B₆, over 2,000 milligrams daily, they may develop tingling in their fingers and toes. Fortunately, there are no permanent effects from this dose excess, and the symptoms are easily reversed when intake is reduced.

Folic Acid, Vitamin B₉

I know that folic acid deficiencies can contribute to the incidence of spina bifida in a developing embryo. Will I have difficulty as a vegetarian obtaining a sufficient amount of folic acid in my diet?

Fortunately, folic acid is abundant in vegetarian foods. The word *folic* is derived from the Latin word *foliage*. This vitamin is found throughout nature in green leafy foliage such as spinach, greens, and kale. Folic acid is an exceptionally important vitamin for pregnant women because women deficient in folic acid experience an increased incidence of birth defects. This vitamin is very sensitive and is easily destroyed by heating, cooking, sunlight, prolonged storage of vegetables at room temperature, and most types of food processing. Therefore it is very important for your baby and yourself that you eat some of your greens fresh and in their unprocessed state. The vegetarian foods from which you may obtain folic acid include green leafy vegetables such as asparagus, beet greens, broccoli, chard, kale, and spinach. Folic acid is also found in other nonleafy vegetables, such as green peas, artichokes, lima beans, and okra. Other vegetarian foods that contain folic acid include brewer's yeast; bean sprouts such as sprouts of soy, lentil, and mung; wheat germ; and fruits such as oranges, cantaloupe, berries, pineapple, and bananas. The bacteria present in your own intestinal tract also produce folic acid naturally.

Folic acid is required for our bodies to form RNA and DNA for cell division. Because your fetus has so many rapidly dividing cells, your need for folic acid doubles during pregnancy. You also need folic acid to produce red blood cells and to produce protein. There are no folic acid toxicity states. If you consume over 15 milligrams of folic acid daily, you may develop restlessness and intestinal cramping, but these symptoms will correct themselves when you decrease your intake to the recommended levels. Adults who become deficient in folic acid may develop anemia, fatigue, bruises, cracks at the corners of their lips, and irritation of the tongue.

When a mother is deficient in folic acid prior to and during her pregnancy, her embryo has an increased chance of developing a neural tube defect. These defects are very serious and include spina bifida and hydrocephalus. Factors causing spina bifida and hydrocephalus include both hereditary tendencies and nutritional deficiencies, specifically a low level of folic acid.

The Recommended Dietary Allowance of folic acid for a woman is 180 micrograms daily. Your Recommended Dietary Allowance preceding and during your pregnancy is 400 micrograms daily. If you take a dose with added security, such as 1 milligram (1,000 micrograms) of folic acid daily, this can only be beneficial.

If there is any chance that you might become pregnant, it is worth your taking 1 milligram of folic acid daily. This can be obtained from prenatal vitamins and from additional supplemental folic acid tablets. While you are taking extra folic acid, you must be sure to consume adequate amounts of vitamin B_{12}, as high quantities of folic acid can mask deficiencies of vitamin B_{12}. The Center for Disease Control recommends that women who have had a previous child with a neural tube defect, such as spina bifida or hydrocephalus, should consume 4 milligrams of folic acid daily prior to becoming pregnant and while they are pregnant. There is no harm to a baby or a mother in taking these large quantities of folic acid, because as a water-soluble vitamin, folic acid never causes toxicity.

It is critically important for you to take folic acid before you try to conceive and when you become pregnant, because spinal cord and brain abnormalities develop in an embryo during the time period from conception through the first six weeks of pregnancy. This is even before a woman may have missed her first period and before her pregnancy test may be positive.

Some women are not aware that they have a deficiency of folic acid. If you fit into any of the following categories, it is important that you talk to your physician and start taking 1 milligram of folic acid daily to ensure adequate levels of this vitamin for your baby:

- You recently used oral contraceptives.

- You've been taking sulfa or tetracycline (these antibiotics destroy folic acid–producing bacteria that normally grow within the intestines).

- You drink alcohol.

- Your diet consists exclusively of meat, white flour, white sugar, and fats.

- You have psoriasis (these skin lesions actually deplete folic acid).

- You take seizure medication for epilepsy.

- You take megadoses of vitamin C (this vitamin depletes folic acid from the body).

HOW DO YOU FARE AS A VEGETARIAN WITH FOLIC ACID INTAKE?

SUPERIOR TO MEAT-EATERS	X
BETTER THAN MEAT-EATERS	
SAME AS MEAT-EATERS	
CHALLENGE TO OBTAIN NUTRITION	
CAREFUL PLANNING RECOMMENDED	

FOOD SOURCES OF FOLIC ACID

VEGETARIAN		Non-Vegetarian	
Lima beans, dried, 1 cup	(272 mcg)	Beef liver, 3 oz	(123 mcg)
Lentils, boiled, 1 cup	(350 mcg)	Beef, 3 oz	(3–10 mcg)
Navy beans, boiled, 1 cup	(254 mcg)	Pork, 3 oz	(4 mcg)
Almonds, ½ cup	(78 mcg)	Chicken, 3 oz	(3 mcg)
Enriched cereal, 1 cup	(100–400 mcg)		
Banana, 1	(118 mcg)		
Chicory greens, fresh, 1 cup	(179 mcg)		
Spinach, 1 cup	(164 mcg)		
Yard-long beans, 1 cup	(250 mcg)		
Brussels sprouts, 10	(85 mcg)		
Romaine lettuce, 4 oz	(145 mcg)		
Egg, 1	(22 mcg)		
Milk, 1 glass	(12 mcg)		
Cheddar cheese, 1 oz	(5 mcg)		

Food for Thought: Your body stores extra folic acid in the liver for six to nine months. For this reason, pregnant woman should consume large quantities of folic acid, 400 micrograms to 1,000 micrograms, for months prior to becoming pregnant.

Vitamin B$_{12}$

Vitamin B$_{12}$ is rarely found in foods other than meats. Will I have difficulty obtaining a sufficient amount of vitamin B$_{12}$ as a vegetarian?

It's true that a vegan diet does not offer the same quantities of vitamin B$_{12}$ found in lacto-ovo-vegetarian or non-vegetarian diets. However, it is also true that vegans are rarely deficient in vitamin B_{12}. It is amazingly simple for a vegan to obtain sufficient quantities of this vitamin. Human beings have four main sources of vitamin B_{12}. The first source is animal-derived foods, such as meat, fish, eggs, yogurt, and organ meats. The second source is vitamin B_{12} produced by bacteria within an individual's own intestines. The third source is vitamin B_{12}–enriched food, such as cereal. The fourth source is vitamin B_{12} supplements.

Although vitamin B_{12} is currently the most likely vitamin in which vegans may become deficient, historically this was not the case. That is because bacteria are really the source of all vitamin B_{12}, not plants or animals. For centuries, these bacteria were present on the surfaces of unwashed plants, and prior to the institution of modern sanitation, vitamin B_{12} produced by bacteria was abundant on the surface of numerous plants. Nowadays, this vitamin is washed off the surface of our vegetation.

Those who eat animal-derived foods, including eggs and dairy products, are not deficient in vitamin B_{12} because the animal food sources have eaten soiled vegetation with vitamin B_{12} on the surface, and now these animals have absorbed it into their own bodies. In addition, the bacteria living within the intestines of these animals produce vitamin B_{12}. These animals then store the bacteria-derived vitamin B_{12} within their tissues, and the person eating this meat consumes the vitamin B_{12} indirectly.

Vitamin B_{12} is necessary for the health of the entire nervous system. People who are deficient in vitamin B_{12} may develop pernicious anemia, a fatal disorder. These individuals suffer from and develop irreversible nerve damage, sensitivity and redness of the tongue, and psychological dysfunction. In children, vitamin B_{12} is needed for growth and to stimulate appetite. There are no known diseases caused by an overdose of vitamin B_{12}. Thousands of times more than the Recommended Dietary Allowance of vitamin B_{12} has been given to people through injections, with no harmful side effects.

Vegans are not the only individuals who must be concerned about vitamin B_{12} deficiencies. Some individuals consume enough of the vitamin, but their stomach has stopped producing "intrinsic factor," needed for absorption of vitamin B_{12}. This decrease in production of intrinsic factor may be a genetic tendency. It can also occur as a result of laxative abuse or just old age. Taking antacids or antibiotics can also lead to a vitamin B_{12} deficiency. Antacids counteract the stomach's hydrochloric acid, which is needed for the absorption of vitamin B_{12}, and thereby decrease the body's ability to absorb vitamin B_{12}. Antibiotics may destroy vitamin B_{12}–producing bacteria within the intestinal tract. Some people are predisposed to vitamin B_{12} deficiencies; they might have insufficient production of enzymes or hydrochloric acid in their stomach to help them absorb vitamin B_{12}, or poor absorption capabilities for vitamin B_{12} within the small intestine. Such individuals with absorption problems are symptom-free and therefore have no idea that this is occurring.

What are some of the sources of vitamin B_{12} for a vegetarian?

♦ Lacto-ovo-vegetarians obtain vitamin B_{12} from dairy products.

♦ Tempeh, a fermented soy product, contains its own fermenting bacteria that produce vitamin B_{12}. The quantities of vitamin B_{12} within each brand of these products might vary considerably.

♦ Some sprouts may have vitamin B_{12}–producing bacteria on their surface.

♦ Vitamin supplements fortified with vitamin B_{12} may be purchased from any health food store or vitamin shop.

♦ Foods fortified with vitamin B_{12}, such as cereals and vegetarian fortified meat substitutes, are widely available.

♦ Vitamin B_{12} is produced by your own intestinal bacteria.

Why is it that most vegans are not deficient in vitamin B_{12}?

It is not surprising that lacto-ovo-vegetarians maintain adequate levels of vitamin B_{12}, as they obtain reasonable quantities by eating dairy products and eggs. Vegans may absorb sufficient amounts of vitamin B_{12} from the bacteria within their intestines. The bacteria within the intestines of vegetarians may produce more vitamin B_{12} than the bacteria within the intestines of non-vegetarians. It takes between five and twenty years to use up the vitamin B_{12} already present within the body, so deficiencies generally do not develop quickly.

♦ Vitamin B_{12} is sometimes found in water, particularly well water, so people who consume well water may have an abundant supply of vitamin B_{12}.

- Vitamin B_{12} can be found in bean sprouts, alfalfa, turnip greens, lettuce, peanuts, and peas, though the source is most likely soil, not the vegetables themselves.

- Vegans may consume more of their vegetables raw and thereby obtain vitamin B_{12} present on the surface of the foods.

- Most vegans are health-conscious and know that they need vitamin B_{12} and other vitamin supplements to maintain good nutrition.

The *Journal of Pediatrics* published an article in 1992 reviewing the outcome in six infants whose vegan mothers had developed vitamin B_{12} deficiencies. The mothers of these infants excluded all foods of animal origin from their diets throughout their pregnancies and while nursing. They did not give their nursing infants any supplemental nutrition or vitamin supplements. These infants developed anemia as well as neurological complications, including irritability, loss of appetite, failure to grow and thrive, poor brain development, and delayed development. Although the mothers did not have visible signs of vitamin B_{12} deficiency, their infants were severely affected. If you choose to remain vegan throughout your pregnancy and want to exclusively breast-feed your infant, you must supplement your diet with vitamin B_{12}. As long as you maintain a consistently healthy vitamin B_{12} level, there is no reason to think that your vegan nutrition will be harmful to you or your baby during pregnancy.

The Recommended Dietary Allowance for B_{12} is minute, only 2 micrograms daily. During pregnancy, this recommendation is increased to 2.2 micrograms daily. If you were to consume 10 to 20 micrograms daily, that would be fine. If you are deficient in vitamin B_{12}, 1,000 micrograms daily will not harm you. As with all the B vitamins, vitamin B_{12} can never reach a toxic level.

HOW DO YOU FARE AS A VEGETARIAN WITH VITAMIN B$_{12}$ INTAKE?

SUPERIOR TO MEAT-EATERS	
BETTER THAN MEAT-EATERS	
SAME AS MEAT-EATERS	
CHALLENGE TO OBTAIN NUTRITION	
CAREFUL PLANNING RECOMMENDED	X

FOOD SOURCES OF VITAMIN B$_{12}$

VEGETARIAN		Non-Vegetarian	
Cereal, enriched, 1 cup	(2.0–6.0 mcg)	Beef liver, 3 oz	(68.0 mcg)
Miso, ¼ cup	(0.13 mcg)	Clams, steamed, 9 large	(89.0 mcg)
Vegetarian burger, 3 oz 3 oz	(2–7 mcg)	Sardines, 3 oz	(8.5 mcg)
Cottage cheese, 1 cup	(1.2 mcg)	Tuna, 3 oz	(2.0 mcg)
Eggs, 2	(1.2 mcg)	Pork, 3 oz	(0.5 mcg)
Milk, 8 oz	(1.0 mcg)		
Cheddar cheese, 1 oz	(0.3 mcg)		

Food for Thought: Strict vegans who consume no food derived from animal sources may not be getting sufficient vitamin B$_{12}$ from their diet, but it takes many years for even a strict vegan to become deficient in vitamin B$_{12}$. That is because vitamin B$_{12}$ is stored within our body for years, and the bacteria living within our intestinal tract produce it naturally. Tempeh, which is a fermented soybean product, and some bean sprouts are vegan foods that contain varying quantities of vitamin B_{12}. Still, it is essential that you reinforce your body's store of vitamin B_{12} with foods and supplements.

Vitamin C, Ascorbic Acid

You will do wonderfully as a vegetarian in obtaining vitamin C, because this vitamin is found exclusively in fruits and vegetables. The highest quantities of vitamin C are obtained from fresh, uncooked fruits and vegetables. However, as this vitamin is very water-soluble, if you boil your vegetables, you will easily lose it. The "C" in vitamin C stands for citrus fruits. Vitamin C is abundant in oranges, grapefruit, strawberries, lemons, limes, cantaloupe, cherries, strawberries, and papaya. It is also abundant in broccoli, Brussels sprouts, tomatoes, asparagus, peppers, and cabbage.

Vitamin C is necessary for individuals to maintain the collagen connective tissue that holds their organs and body tissues together. Collagen is present in skin, joints, cartilage, and vertebral disks. It is vitamin C that gives the body support. Vitamin C also helps maintain healthy blood vessels, heal wounds, boost the immune system, fight virus, bacteria, and fungus, and raise the level of good HDL cholesterol. There are no vitamin C toxicity states, although megadoses of vitamin C, over 40,000 milligrams daily, may contribute to diarrhea and anemia. You should not eat chewable vitamin C tablets, as the ascorbic acid in them may erode the enamel of your teeth.

Scurvy is a disease caused by a deficiency of vitamin C. In 1500 B.C.E., it was first noted that people who did not eat citrus fruits lost energy, had difficulty breathing, had gum infections, developed tooth decay, and often died. In later years, scurvy often affected sailors. British sailors in particular were given limes to eat while at sea to prevent disease, which is why people started calling them "limeys."

The Recommended Dietary Allowance for vitamin C is 60 milligrams daily. During your pregnancy, your recommended dose will be increased to 70 milligrams daily. If you are fighting an infection, a dose of 500 milligrams four times daily is safe and beneficial.

HOW DO YOU FARE AS A VEGETARIAN WITH VITAMIN C INTAKE?

SUPERIOR TO MEAT-EATERS	X
BETTER THAN MEAT-EATERS	
SAME AS MEAT-EATERS	
CHALLENGE TO OBTAIN NUTRITION	
CAREFUL PLANNING RECOMMENDED	

FOOD SOURCES OF VITAMIN C

VEGETARIAN		Non-Vegetarian
Cantaloupe, ½ melon	(90 mg)	None
Kiwi fruit, 3	(75 mg)	
Red pepper, 1	(141 mg)	
Strawberries, ½ cup	(44 mg)	
Cauliflower, 1 cup	(90 mg)	
Broccoli, 1 cup	(140 mg)	
Green bell pepper, 1	(66 mg)	
Tomato, 1	(28 mg)	
Cabbage, 1 cup	(34 mg)	

Food for Thought: Vitamin C is easily absorbed from your intestines, but it passes through your body quickly—usually within three to four hours. It is best to take vitamin C supplements and eat vitamin C–rich foods several times during your day rather than taking all tablets at one time. Green bell peppers have twice as much vitamin C as does citrus fruit; red peppers have three times as much vitamin C as citrus fruit; and hot peppers contain even more vitamin C per unit weight than do oranges. In addition, hot peppers have been reported to increase the blood's ability to dissolve dangerous blood clots. Chilies help burn calories by boosting your postmeal metabolism.

Vitamin A

You will not have any difficulty whatsoever finding an abundance of vegetarian sources of vitamin A. This fat-soluble vitamin is present in all yellow and orange fruits and vegetables. As a pregnant woman, however, you must be aware that although vitamin A is essential for good health, excess quantities of some forms of this vitamin can cause fetal deformities. The forms of vitamin A that can cause birth defects are found only in animal sources and from vitamin supplements. The vitamin A you obtain from fruits and vegetables is different from the form derived from animal sources and cannot cause fetal abnormalities.

Vitamin A is necessary for optimal vision. Without sufficient vitamin A, the retina of the eye cannot function properly. An individual who is deficient in this vitamin will develop night blindness. This vitamin is also required for healing body tissues, skin repair, and good dental health. Because vitamin A is an antioxidant, it also functions to neutralize toxic cancer-causing oxygen radicals produced by the waste products of tissue metabolism. If you apply vitamin A to your skin, it will help to reduce wrinkles and to clear your acne. This vitamin is also needed in children, as it is essential for the formation of new bones. An individual deficient in vitamin A may experience loss of appetite and dry, itchy, bumpy skin, particularly on the backs of the arms. If you are deficient in vitamin A, your hair may become weak and dull, and your scalp may develop dandruff.

The two forms of vitamin A are beta-carotene and retinol. *Beta-carotene* is the form of vitamin A present in yellow and orange fruits and vegetables, as well as green leafy vegetables. *Retinol* is the form of vitamin A found in animal sources.

Beta-carotene	Retinol
Carrot	Liver
Squash	Fish liver oil

Sweet potato

Yam and pumpkin

Apricot, cherry

Mango, peach, papaya

Spinach, broccoli, seaweed

Egg yolk

Dairy products

Beta-carotene, or pro-vitamin A, is derived from yellow and orange fruits and vegetables and from leafy vegetables. It is converted to fully formed vitamin A within the intestines. Excess beta-carotene can cause yellowing of your skin but cannot cause any serious health problems. *Excess ingestion of fruits or vegetables containing vitamin A does* not *cause fetal abnormalities.*

Retinol, or fully formed vitamin A, is derived from animal sources, such as liver, fish oil, eggs, and dairy products. It is the only form of vitamin A in which *an excess can cause toxicity and fetal abnormalities.* This form of the vitamin is used to manufacture many vitamin A tablets. Excess ingestion of these vitamin tablets can also cause fetal abnormalities.

Vitamin A is a fat-soluble vitamin; therefore it can be stored in the liver, fat tissues, and kidneys for months. More than 25,000 international units of vitamin A is considered excessive. An excess of vitamin A, in the range of 25,000 to 50,000 international units daily, can result in significant birth defects affecting a baby's bones, urinary tract, and brain. The baby may also develop cardiovascular anomalies, small eyes, cleft lip and palate, mental retardation, and malformation of the features of its face.

The Recommended Dietary Allowance for vitamin A is 800 micrograms, or 5,000 international units daily. During your pregnancy, the recommendation is unchanged. If you plan to nurse, your recommended dose will be increased to 1,300 micrograms, or 8,125 international units daily.

HOW DO YOU FARE AS A VEGETARIAN WITH VITAMIN A INTAKE?

SUPERIOR TO MEAT-EATERS	X
BETTER THAN MEAT-EATERS	
SAME AS MEAT-EATERS	
CHALLENGE TO OBTAIN NUTRITION	
CAREFUL PLANNING RECOMMENDED	

FOOD SOURCES OF VITAMIN A

VEGETARIAN		Non-Vegetarian	
Cantaloupe, ½ melon	(9,230 IU)	Beef liver, 3 oz	(45,380 IU)
Sweet potato, 1	(9,240 IU)		
Carrot juice, 6 oz	(47,381 IU)		
Apricot, 1	(4,490 IU)		
Tomato, 1	(2,170 IU)		
Broccoli, 1 cup	(4,000 IU)		
Peach, 1	(1,330 IU)		
Milk, 8 oz	(500 IU)		
Butter, 1 tbsp	(430 IU)		
Cheddar cheese, 1 oz	(300 IU)		
Egg, 1	(260 IU)		

Food for Thought: The vitamin A present naturally in fruits and vegetables is not the type of vitamin A that causes abnormalities in a fetus. Because vitamin A derived from vegetarian food sources is so much safer than that derived from non-vegetarian sources, vegetarians fare better than non-vegetarians in their vitamin A intake.

Vitamin D

As a vegetarian or vegan, you will have no difficulty obtaining a sufficient amount of the fat-soluble vitamin D. There are three kinds of vitamin D. The first is found in animal-derived products like fish liver oil, egg yolks, liver, butter, or salmon. The second kind of vitamin D is manufactured within the skin when individuals come in contact with the ultraviolet rays of the sun. That is why vitamin D is often called the "sunshine vitamin." The third kind of vitamin D is the synthetic form and is used to fortify milk, some breakfast cereals, and other foods.

Your body needs vitamin D in order to use calcium. Regardless of how much calcium you ingest, you cannot use it if you do not have an adequate supply of magnesium and vitamin D. This vitamin is very important for children as well as for a developing fetus, because it helps form healthy bones and tissues. Since the body stores vitamin D, a daily dosage should not exceed 1,500 international units. People with vitamin D toxicity suffer from excessive thirst, diarrhea, nausea, headache, and weakness. Rickets is a disease that results from a deficiency of vitamin D. Children with rickets have weak bones that can eventually lead to skeletal deformities. They also develop tooth decay.

Individuals with limited exposure to sunlight may not be able to manufacture sufficient vitamin D in their skin. Such individuals might include those who work indoors, have darkly pigmented skin, live in a cloudy or polluted area, or live where there is a long winter season. Also affected might be those who wear many layers of clothing or who cover their bodies for religious reasons.

The Recommended Dietary Allowance for vitamin D is 200 international units (5 micrograms) daily. This is the same dose recommended during pregnancy.

HOW DO YOU FARE AS A VEGETARIAN WITH VITAMIN D INTAKE?

SUPERIOR TO MEAT-EATERS	
BETTER THAN MEAT-EATERS	
SAME AS MEAT-EATERS	
CHALLENGE TO OBTAIN NUTRITION	X
CAREFUL PLANNING RECOMMENDED	

FOOD SOURCES OF VITAMIN D

VEGETARIAN		Non-Vegetarian	
Soy milk, 8 oz	(100 IU)	Sardines, 3 oz	(1,000 IU)
Fortified cereals, 1 cup	(40 IU)	Cod liver oil, 1 tsp	(460 IU)
Milk, 8 oz	(100 IU)	Salmon, 3 oz	(350 IU)
Egg yolk, 1	(25 IU)		
Butter, 1 pat	(2 IU)		

Food for Thought: You can produce a healthy level of vitamin D within your own body by going out in the sunlight for twenty to thirty minutes a day, three days a week. There is no reason why vegan or vegetarian women within the United States should develop bone weakness or cause a vitamin D deficiency to develop within their infants. By taking vitamins, eating vitamin D–fortified foods, and obtaining twenty to thirty minutes of indirect sunlight every other day, you will avoid any risk of vitamin D deficiency for either you or your baby.

Vitamin E, Tocopherol

Vitamin E is found in both plants and animals, so it should not be a challenge for you to consume adequate amounts on a vegetarian diet. The vitamin was actually first isolated from wheat germ oil. The best plant sources of vitamin E are vegetable seeds or oils derived from nuts. When the vitamin is used as a topical lotion, it is absorbed through the skin. Although it is a fat-soluble vitamin, some vitamin E is lost when foods are fried, blanched, or cooked. This vitamin is found abundantly in vegetable oil, wheat germ oil, nut oil, butter, egg yolks, and milk fat.

The word *tocopherol* was derived from the Greek words *tokos* and *pherol,* meaning "offspring" and "to bear." Tocopherol literally means "to bear children." Animals that are deficient in vitamin E cannot reproduce; however, there does not appear to be a similar effect in humans. The main benefit of vitamin E is its role as an antioxidant to prevent free radicals produced by your tissue metabolism from contributing to the development of cancer. Vitamin E is not stored in your body as easily as are the other fat-soluble vitamins, so toxicity of this vitamin does not occur or is extremely rare. Deficiency of vitamin E is rare, and the symptoms are vague. Individuals who are deficient in vitamin E develop anemia, deposits of fat in their muscles, and loss of muscle strength.

The Recommended Dietary Allowance of vitamin E for nonpregnant women is 8 milligrams (12 international units) daily. During pregnancy, this requirement is increased slightly to 10 milligrams (15 international units) daily. The dose recommended during nursing is 12 milligrams daily.

HOW DO YOU FARE AS A VEGETARIAN WITH VITAMIN E INTAKE?

SUPERIOR TO MEAT-EATERS	X
BETTER THAN MEAT-EATERS	
SAME AS MEAT-EATERS	
CHALLENGE TO OBTAIN NUTRITION	
CAREFUL PLANNING RECOMMENDED	

FOOD SOURCES OF VITAMIN E

VEGETARIAN		Non-Vegetarian	
Wheat germ oil, 1 tbsp	(20 mg)	Ground beef, 3.5 oz	(0.18 mg)
Sunflower seeds, 1 oz	(14 mg)	Pork chops, 3.5 oz	(0.26 mg)
Almond oil, 1 tbsp	(5.0 mg)	Chicken, ½ breast	(0.26 mg)
Almonds, 1 oz	(7.0 mg)	Turkey, 3.5 oz	(0.60 mg)
Avocado, 1	(6.0 mg)	Beef liver, 3.5 oz	(0.64 mg)
Safflower oil, 1 tbsp	(5.0 mg)	Chicken liver, 3.5 oz	(1.44 mg)
Mango, 1	(2.5 mg)		
Peanut butter, 2 tbsp	(3.0 mg)		

Food for Thought: Vegetarians can obtain their vitamin E from sources that are totally healthy, as opposed to the non-vegetarian sources of vitamin E, which also contain cholesterol.

Vitamin K

Vegetarians fare better than do non-vegetarians in obtaining fat-soluble vitamin K from their foods, because most vitamin K is found in plants.

Like vitamin B_{12}, it is also manufactured in the body. There are two kinds of vitamin K. One comes from plant and animal sources. The other kind, and the best source of vitamin K, comes from good bacteria living within your own intestines. If your intestinal bacteria are functioning normally, there is no need for any vitamin K supplementation. Vegetarians can find vitamin K in alfalfa, greens, kelp, blackstrap molasses, and safflower oil.

Vitamin K toxicity rarely occurs, as natural vitamin K is easily eliminated from the body. When vitamin K is given medically in very high doses to help blood clot, toxic levels may be reached. Deficiencies of vitamin K are rare and are more likely to occur if an individual is taking antibiotics or has an intestinal problem such as poor intestinal absorption, excessive diarrhea, or colitis.

To keep your intestinal bacteria functioning well, it is helpful to eat yogurt with a natural bacteria curd, such as Dannon yogurt. Alternatively, you can take *Lactobacillus acidophilus* supplements. These will help your body maintain a good supply of vitamin K–producing bacteria. Your body needs vitamin K for blood clotting.

The Recommended Dietary Allowance for vitamin K is 65 micrograms daily, and this recommended dose remains unchanged during pregnancy.

HOW DO YOU FARE AS A VEGETARIAN WITH VITAMIN K INTAKE?

SUPERIOR TO MEAT-EATERS	X
BETTER THAN MEAT-EATERS	
SAME AS MEAT-EATERS	
CHALLENGE TO OBTAIN NUTRITION	
CAREFUL PLANNING RECOMMENDED	

FOOD SOURCES OF VITAMIN K

VEGETARIAN		Non-Vegetarian	
Asparagus, 12 spears	(180 mcg)	Beef liver, 3 oz	(89 mcg)
Turnip greens, 1 cup	(364 mcg)		
Chickpeas, 1 cup	(224 mcg)		
Cauliflower, raw, 1 cup	(192 mcg)		
Soybean oil, 1 tbsp	(76 mcg)		
Tomatoes, 1	(28 mcg)		
Strawberries, 1 cup	(21 mcg)		
Spinach, raw, 1 cup	(158 mcg)		
Egg, 1	(25 mcg)		

Food for Thought: Vitamin K is not transferred from a woman to her baby at birth. Yet her baby does not have any bacteria within its own intestines, so it cannot produce its own vitamin K. It is for this reason that all newborns are given injections of vitamin K to prevent them from developing any vitamin K deficiency–related bleeding problems. Babies begin to produce their own vitamin K naturally during their fourth day of life.

MINERALS

Minerals are inorganic or inert elements. They are found in living tissues as well as in the nonliving structures on our earth. They are all basic molecules that cannot be broken down into any smaller substance. Approximately 4 to 5 percent of the human body is made up of minerals. Of that percentage, most of the minerals are located in the skeletal system. Minerals, required for the healthy function of the entire body, are divided into two categories: macrominerals and microminerals. All are necessary for good health and are classified on page 109.

The trace elements, or microminerals, constitute less than 0.01 percent of your total body weight, but just the same as the macrominerals, they are essential for normal body function. All must work together to complete myriad essential functions the body requires. Minerals help to

TWELVE MACROMINERALS		FOURTEEN MICROMINERALS	
OXYGEN	O	IRON	Fe
CARBON	C	FLUORINE	F
HYDROGEN	H	ZINC	Zn
NITROGEN	N	STRONTIUM	Sr
CALCIUM	Ca	COPPER	Cu
PHOSPHORUS	P	COBALT	Co
POTASSIUM	K	VANADIUM	V
SULFUR	S	IODINE	I
CHLORINE	Cl	TIN	Sn
SODIUM	Na	SELENIUM	Se
MAGNESIUM	Mg	MANGANESE	Mn
SILICON	Si	NICKEL	Ni
		MOLYBDENUM	Mo
		CHROMIUM	Cr

metabolize carbohydrates, maintain proper immune response, maintain body temperature, prevent cancer, and keep the heart functioning. Minerals are present in the foods we eat, the soil in which the foods are grown, and the water we drink.

How many minerals we consume from water depends on the kind of water we drink. Soft water (typical water found in most cities) may contain only high levels of sodium. This high sodium content is the reason soft water is not always healthy for people with high blood pressure. Hard water, however, contains many minerals, including calcium and magnesium, and is generally healthy for everyone. Many minerals are also present in soil, though modern agricultural practices have begun to deplete this mineral source. When farmers recycle soil from crop to crop, or when they refine and process their harvests, much of the mineral value in foods is lost.

There are Recommended Dietary Allowances for only a few minerals: calcium, iodine, iron, magnesium, phosphorus, and zinc. Although the other minerals are necessary, the government has not specified the minimum requirements for each. To maintain a healthy diet for your baby and yourself, it is best to eat foods made from whole grains grown in nourishing soil (preferably organic), instead of grains that have been refined and processed. Refined sugars, caffeine, and alcohol flush healthy minerals out of your body, so it's important to limit your intake of these as you plan for a healthy diet.

Calcium

I don't eat dairy products. Does this mean I won't be able to obtain a sufficient amount of calcium during my pregnancy?

Calcium is the most abundant mineral in nature. You will find it in a great variety of vegetarian foods, like nuts, seeds, broccoli, greens, soybeans, dried figs, apricots, and molasses. You don't need to rely on dairy products for your calcium requirements. Calcium is one of the most important minerals for your body. It contributes to the growth and maintenance of your bones, the health of your teeth, normal circulation, and the health of your body tissues. Calcium is not the only mineral necessary for your bones, as you also require vitamin D, phosphorus, magnesium, silicon, and strontium to keep your bones strong.

If you feel you're not getting enough calcium from your diet and you want to take calcium supplements, you should know this:

FORM OF CALCIUM SUPPLEMENTS

- Calcium citrate is your most easily absorbed calcium supplement.
- Oyster shell or bone meal (ground-up cow's bones, certainly not very appetizing) may contain chemical impurities such as lead and other heavy metals. These are therefore not your best sources of calcium.
- Calcium lactate or calcium carbonate (such as Tums) create an alkaline environment in your intestinal tract and can actually slow down calcium absorption. These are *not* your best form of calcium supplement.

In most individuals, calcium excess is not a health problem, although those with parathyroid dysfunction may deposit excess calcium within their muscles, bones, and soft tissues. Most of these individuals know of their problem and do not consume a high-calcium diet. However, some people may not know they have a problem with their parathyroid gland, and that is why most people should not take calcium supplements without a specific reason.

Calcium deficiency can occur, not only if your diet is low in calcium, but also if your diet is high in phosphorus. The ratio of calcium to phosphorus in your bones is 2.5 to 1. If your diet includes higher levels of calcium than phosphorus, it is more likely that you will maintain this healthy ratio and healthy bones. To do this, it is best if you maintain a ratio of phosphorus to calcium within your diet of 1:1. The diet of many Americans contains a phosphorus-to-calcium ratio of 4:1. Calcium is a positive ion, which means it will bind with negative ions. Foods that contain phosphorus form negative ions. So if you have excess phosphorus in your diet, it will bind calcium to it and you will excrete both of these minerals. If such a situation develops, you may actually lose more calcium than you took in, and you will deplete the calcium stored in your bones. Phosphorus is present in carbonated drinks, meat, eggs, and cheese spreads.

You will absorb higher levels of calcium if your diet contains adequate amounts of vitamin D, magnesium, dairy products, and vitamin C. Regular exercise also helps the body to absorb calcium. However, if you follow a high-fat or high-protein diet that is rich in phosphorus, it will be more difficult for your body to absorb calcium.

If you have a calcium deficiency, you may develop twitching, nerve sensitivity, brittle nails, insomnia, depression, numbness, and heart palpitations. Painful muscle cramps in the calves may occur often during pregnancy, particularly in women who are deficient in calcium.

The Recommended Dietary Allowance of calcium is 1,000 milligrams daily, and you don't need to increase your calcium intake beyond this amount during pregnancy.

HOW DO YOU FARE AS A VEGETARIAN WITH CALCIUM INTAKE?

SUPERIOR TO MEAT-EATERS	
BETTER THAN MEAT-EATERS	X
SAME AS MEAT-EATERS	
CHALLENGE TO OBTAIN NUTRITION	
CAREFUL PLANNING RECOMMENDED	

FOOD SOURCES OF CALCIUM

VEGETARIAN		Non-Vegetarian	
Soybeans, boiled, 1 cup	(178 mg)	Sardines with bones, 3 oz	(199 mg)
Tofu, firm, ½ cup	(258 mg)	Salmon with bones, 3 oz	(203 mg)
Blackstrap molasses, 1 tsp	(172 mg)	Steak, 3 oz	(10 mg)
All-Bran cereal, 1 cup	(200 mg)	Pork loin, 3 oz	(10 mg)
Turnip greens, 1 cup	(198 mg)	Chicken breast, 3 oz	(18 mg)
Broccoli, 2 spears	(143 mg)		
Yogurt, skim, 1 cup	(452 mg)		
Milk, 1 cup	(290 mg)		
Cheese, cheddar, 1 oz	(200 mg)		

Food for Thought: Animal protein creates an acidic waste product that binds with calcium in your body and pulls it out with the other wastes. Vegetarian women have much lower rates of osteoporosis than do women on meat-based diets. Vegetarians fare better not just from the amount of calcium they achieve in their diet, but also from the amount of calcium that they are able to retain.

Magnesium

Magnesium is easier to obtain from your vegetarian diet than it is from a non-vegetarian diet. The largest proportion of all the magnesium you consume comes from vegetable sources. Magnesium is required for photosynthesis to occur within all plants, so it's no surprise that dark green vegetables are a great source of magnesium. Bones and teeth act as reservoirs for magnesium and supply it to the rest of your body when it is needed. The main food sources of magnesium are green vegetables, nuts and seeds, whole grains, soy products, and mineral water.

Magnesium is a very important mineral mainly because it assists in several hundred enzyme reactions that occur within our bodies. It is also a natural tranquilizer that helps to relax muscles and lower blood pressure. If a woman develops toxemia of pregnancy, or preeclampsia (see chapter 9), she is given large intravenous doses of magnesium sulfate to lower her blood pressure and relax her muscles in order to prevent seizures.

It is exceptionally rare for magnesium toxicity to develop. Magnesium deficiency, however, can develop if you eat too many processed foods and sugars, boil all of your foods, consume a lot of alcohol and caffeine, or use diuretics. Magnesium deficiency can cause fatigue, irritability, insomnia, loss of appetite, rapid heart rate, twitching, and muscle tremors.

The Recommended Dietary Allowance is 320 milligrams daily for nonpregnant women. During pregnancy, this requirement increases slightly to 360 milligrams daily. The dose recommended during nursing is 320 milligrams daily.

HOW DO YOU FARE AS A VEGETARIAN WITH MAGNESIUM INTAKE?

SUPERIOR TO MEAT-EATERS	X
BETTER THAN MEAT-EATERS	
SAME AS MEAT-EATERS	
CHALLENGE TO OBTAIN NUTRITION	
CAREFUL PLANNING RECOMMENDED	

FOOD SOURCES OF MAGNESIUM

VEGETARIAN		Non-Vegetarian	
Okra, fried, 1 cup	(92 mg)	Beef, 3 oz	(28 mg)
Brazil nuts, ¼ cup	(88 mg)	Salmon, 4 oz	(30 mg)
Almonds, ¼ cup	(96 mg)		
Wheat germ, ¼ cup	(84 mg)		
Dates, 10	(58 mg)		
Dried figs, 5	(71 mg)		
Prune juice, 1 cup	(26 mg)		
Corn, 1 ear	(58 mg)		
Milk, 8 oz	(28 mg)		

Food for Thought: Magnesium is absorbed more easily when ingested on an empty stomach between meals. The amount of magnesium within your foods will vary depending upon the amount of magnesium in the soil where that vegetable, fruit, or seed has been grown. Magnesium can be lost when you boil foods, so save your cooking broth and add it to a soup or sauce—it's a simple way to enrich your food naturally. Hard water and mineral water are also valuable sources of magnesium.

Phosphorus

After calcium, phosphorus is the most abundant mineral in the body. It is present in every cell and, like magnesium, it is stored primarily in the bones and teeth. High-protein foods such as meat, fish, and chicken are rich in phosphorus, yet vegetarians have no difficulty obtaining their phosphorus from seeds, nuts, grains, yeast, wheat germ, and bran. Most fruits and vegetables also contain some phosphorus.

Phosphorus is involved in almost all the chemical reactions within your body. It helps to convert carbohydrates and fats into energy, create proteins for growth and tissue repair, produce RNA and DNA, contract muscles, and maintain healthy teeth and bones.

There is no known phosphorus toxicity. However, if your diet contains a lot of phosphorus-rich foods like soda, meat, and convenience foods, you may decrease your stores of calcium (see "Calcium"). Since phosphorus is so abundant in the Western/American diet, deficiencies are quite uncommon. When they do occur, they cause a loss of appetite, poor growth of bones and teeth, weight loss, anxiety, and stiff joints.

The Recommended Dietary Allowance is 700 milligrams daily. This dose does not change during pregnancy.

HOW DO YOU FARE AS A VEGETARIAN WITH PHOSPHORUS INTAKE?

SUPERIOR TO MEAT-EATERS	
BETTER THAN MEAT-EATERS	
SAME AS MEAT-EATERS	X
CHALLENGE TO OBTAIN NUTRITION	
CAREFUL PLANNING RECOMMENDED	

FOOD SOURCES OF PHOSPHORUS

VEGETARIAN		Non-Vegetarian	
Hummus, 4 oz	(137 mg)	Liver, beef, 4 oz	(458 mg)
All-Bran cereal, ½ cup	(294 mg)	Beef, 3 oz	(298 mg)
Baked beans, ½ cup	(132 mg)	Chicken, 4 oz	(217 mg)
Tofu, firm, ½ cup	(239 mg)	Sardines, 4 oz	(456 mg)
Black walnuts, ½ cup	(290 mg)		
Peanuts, ½ cup	(280 mg)		
Cashew butter, 2 tbsp	(146 mg)		

Food for Thought: Although the recommended dose of phosphorus is 700 milligrams, one 8-ounce glass of soda contains 500 milligrams of phosphorus. So when you start to pour that second glass of soda, think about switching to water instead!

Iodine

Will I have difficulty as a vegetarian in obtaining a sufficient amount of iodine for my baby?

Iodine is present in all foods that come from salt water. Iodine is also present in the soil that is near coasts, bays, and other saltwater sources. Ocean depths extend so far beneath the earth's surface that they reach the salt layers in our earth's crust—that is why fish, seaweed and kelp, and sea salt are so rich in iodine. Iodine is a mineral, and a deficiency of it can have serious consequences to an unborn fetus, to a child, and to an adult. We can also get iodine from foods like iodized salt and iodine-enriched breads.

Iodine is necessary for proper functioning of the thyroid gland. Thyroid hormones work to maintain a healthy rate of metabolism; produce energy; form nerves and bones; enhance reproductive capabilities; promote healthy hair, skin, nails, and teeth; and keep the mind alert. If you consume iodine only from dietary sources, you will not develop iodine toxicity. However, if your intake of iodized salt is excessive, you could be putting yourself at risk. You may also develop toxicity if you use cough and cold medications frequently—iodine is an expectorant and is often a main ingredient of these medications. Iodine toxicity actually suppresses thyroid function instead of stimulating it. So while you need iodine to help the thyroid function normally, consuming too much can weaken its effectiveness.

If your iodine level is too low, your thyroid gland will lose its ability to function—this is called "hypothyroidism." In this case, the thyroid gland becomes enlarged and forms a goiter, which means that the gland is no longer working. Hypothyroidism causes fatigue, weight gain, dryness of the hair, slower metabolism so you always feel cold, and decreased mental function. If women are deficient in iodine during their pregnancy, or if they develop an iodine toxicity that suppresses their thyroid gland, their infants may be born with hypothyroidism or mental retardation.

The Recommended Dietary Allowance of iodine is 150 micrograms daily. The recommended amount in pregnancy increases to 175 micrograms daily, and for nursing women, it increases to 200 micrograms daily.

HOW DO YOU FARE AS A VEGETARIAN WITH IODINE INTAKE?

SUPERIOR TO MEAT-EATERS	
BETTER THAN MEAT-EATERS	
SAME AS MEAT-EATERS	X
CHALLENGE TO OBTAIN NUTRITION	
CAREFUL PLANNING RECOMMENDED	

FOOD SOURCES OF IODINE

VEGETARIAN		Non-Vegetarian	
Kelp, 3 oz	(100 mcg)	Saltwater fish, 3 oz	(250 mcg)
Seaweed (wakame), 3 oz	(500+ mcg)	Shrimp, 1 cup	(90 mcg)
All plants—varies with iodine content of soil			
Saltine crackers, 6	(200 mcg)		
Lima beans, 1 cup	(70 mcg)		
Eggs—varies with iodine content of chicken feed			
Milk—varies with iodine content of feed			
Iodized table and cooking salt			

Iron

I don't eat red meat. Will it be difficult for me to obtain sufficient iron during pregnancy?

If you maintain a well-balanced and well-planned vegetarian diet, you will consume more than enough iron. Some vegetarian foods that are rich in iron are kelp, wheat germ, pumpkin and sesame seeds, blackstrap molasses, dried prunes, and almonds. Aside from these nutritional sources, there are many dietary factors that can help you increase your absorption of iron. Try eating vitamin C and citrus fruits with iron-rich foods—the acid in vitamin C helps your body to absorb iron. Certain foods—like caffeine, soy protein, whole grains, chard or spinach, and milk—can inhibit the body's absorption of iron. With the exception of caffeine, these foods contribute to a healthy vegetarian diet; however, when consumed with iron-rich foods, they prevent your body from absorbing that iron. The simplest solution is to exclude these foods only when you are preparing a meal that is rich in iron.

The primary function of iron is to form hemoglobin. Hemoglobin is a component of red blood cells, and it enables your blood cells to carry oxygen. Hemoglobin contains almost 70 percent of all the iron within the body. Your liver, spleen, and bone marrow store the rest of the iron as a reservoir until your red blood cells require more. Some people are susceptible to iron toxicity. Thalassemia is a genetic blood condition in which the red blood cells cannot hold normal levels of iron. People with thalassemia may accumulate excess iron in their liver, leading to serious liver scarring. However, people with normal blood cells can also develop iron toxicity, usually from taking too many iron supplements and from natural food sources. Any excess iron accumulates in the liver and causes scarring and cirrhosis. In the case of iron deficiency, anemia usually develops and causes weakness, fatigue, shortness of breath, a rapid heart rate, and an increased susceptibility to infections.

An individual absorbs only a small percentage of the iron ingested. There are two types of iron in the diet, *heme iron,* which comes from animal sources, and *nonheme iron,* which is found in plants, eggs, and dairy. Although nonheme iron is not absorbed as easily as heme iron, vegetarians can absorb plenty of iron from their diets and still maintain optimum health during pregnancy.

Many people criticize the vegetarian diet because they don't believe it contains enough iron. You may think that by taking iron supplements during your vegetarian pregnancy, you will be proving those critics right. You are not.

Should I start taking iron supplements once I know I'm pregnant?

Supplemental iron is very beneficial for most women during pregnancy, whether they are vegetarian or not. Ask your health care provider if there are any reasons you should not be taking iron. At the beginning of your pregnancy, your blood will be checked for anemia and your physician will let you know if you need supplements. As your baby grows, you should expect your blood count to vary, because your body is transferring much of your iron to your baby and placenta. If you take care to keep your iron levels stable through diet and supplements (if needed), you'll prevent the onset of anemia and feel much healthier by the end of your pregnancy. Some iron supplements cause a considerable amount of undesirable side effects, including intestinal upset, constipation, and blackening of the stool.

Most often, iron in the form of iron sulfate (also called ferrous sulfate) causes these side effects. If you take supplements in the form of ferrous gluconate or ferrous fumarate during your pregnancy, you will experience these side effects very mildly. Overall, the easiest forms to take are ferrous succinate and ferrous fumarate. Some are more user-friendly to the intestinal tract than others. It is important that you not take calcium supplements with your iron, as calcium will decrease your absorption of iron. Remember that your prenatal vitamins usually contain calcium and iron within the same pill. If you are taking an iron supplement, please do *not* take it the same time you are taking your general prenatal vitamin; give yourself a four-hour interval, or the calcium in the vitamin will decrease your absorption of iron.

For an example of how much iron you will use during pregnancy, an individual normally uses 1 milligram of iron daily. During a full-term pregnancy, however, a mother transfers 500 to 1,000 milligrams of iron to her baby. Most of this transfer (500 to 700 milligrams) occurs during the last few months of pregnancy. In comparison, a menstruating woman loses only about 35 milligrams of iron during her entire menstrual period. Another comparison is that a unit of blood donated to the blood bank contains 200 milligrams of iron. Therefore, a pregnant woman is transferring two to five units of blood to her baby during the nine months of pregnancy.

The Recommended Dietary Allowance of iron is 15 milligrams daily. During your pregnancy, this recommendation is increased to 30 milligrams daily.

HOW DO YOU FARE AS A VEGETARIAN WITH IRON INTAKE?

SUPERIOR TO MEAT-EATERS	
BETTER THAN MEAT-EATERS	
SAME AS MEAT-EATERS	
CHALLENGE TO OBTAIN NUTRITION	X
CAREFUL PLANNING RECOMMENDED	

FOOD SOURCES OF IRON

VEGETARIAN		Non-Vegetarian	
Blackstrap molasses, 2 tbsp	(7.0 mg)	Chicken liver, 4 oz	(9.6 mg)
Lentils, 1 cup	(6.6 mg)	Beef liver, 4 oz	(7.5 mg)
Black turtle beans, 1 cup	(5.3 mg)	Beef, 4 oz	(3.5 mg)
Chickpeas, 1 cup	(4.8 mg)	Pork, 4 oz	(1.2 mg)
Product 19 cereal, 1 cup	(18.0 mg)	Chicken, 4 oz	(1.2 mg)
All-Bran cereal, 1 cup	(9.0 mg)		
Kellogg's Corn Flakes, 1 cup	(6.0 mg)		
Lima beans, 1 cup	(4.5 mg)		
Prunes, dried, ½ cup	(2.8 mg)		
Apricots, dried, ½ cup	(3.1 mg)		
Broccoli, 2 stalks	(2.6 mg)		
Avocado, 1 medium	(2.0 mg)		
Asparagus, 12 spears	(1.8 mg)		

Food for Thought: It is a challenge for most women to obtain enough iron in pregnancy. Vegetarian women are no exception. Although many plant-derived foods contain iron, the amount you actually absorb is considerably less. A good way for you to increase your iron intake is to cook with a cast-iron skillet. Not only are we what we eat, but we are also what we eat off of. Stomach acids play an important role in iron absorption, so it's a good idea to limit your use of antacids so you can get the optimum amount of iron from your foods.

Fluoride

Vegetarians and non-vegetarians obtain the same levels of fluoride from their diets. Although fluoride is not an essential mineral, it is helpful in strengthening the bones and teeth. Taking fluoride cannot replace the importance of eating the right foods, restricting our intake of refined sugars, or brushing and flossing our teeth properly. Natural fluoride is present in our oceans in the form of sodium fluoride. This is why individuals living in coastal areas, such as the Caribbean, who eat large quantities of fish have stronger teeth and a lower incidence of cavities than people in most other areas of the world. Black tea is also a significant source of fluoride. Children in England obtain 1 milligram of fluoride daily just from drinking three cups of black tea.

Fluoride is added to drinking water in many locations at a concentration of one part per million. More than two parts per million can cause health problems, so taking excess fluoride is not recommended. Although fluoride is often added as a component of toothpaste, this is not as effective a means of preventing tooth decay as taking fluoride orally. When fluoride has been added to drinking water, it can reduce dental cavities 30 to 50 percent. Sodium fluoride is not given routinely to pregnant women because an excess of fluoride can cause fluorosis, or dark staining, of the child's teeth. Very high levels of fluoride can cause metabolic changes within the liver, kidneys, and adrenal glands.

There are no fluoride deficiency states, and there is no specific Recommended Dietary Allowance for fluoride.

HOW DO YOU FARE AS A VEGETARIAN WITH FLUORIDE INTAKE?

SUPERIOR TO MEAT-EATERS	
BETTER THAN MEAT-EATERS	
SAME AS MEAT-EATERS	X
CHALLENGE TO OBTAIN NUTRITION	
CAREFUL PLANNING RECOMMENDED	

FOOD SOURCES OF FLUORIDE

VEGETARIAN		Non-Vegetarian
Black tea, 1 cup	(0.3 mg)	None

Food for Thought: Sixty percent of all municipalities in the United States add fluoride to the drinking water. If you live in an area with fluorinated water, you receive at least 1 milligram of fluoride daily. If you drink black tea, you will have a higher cumulative dose. The average adult who uses this tap water for hot and cold beverages obtains between 1.5 and 4 milligrams of fluoride daily just from drinking tap water. You can find out from your city or town government if fluoride has been added to your water. If fluoride has not been added to your water supply or you drink only well water or bottled water, you may want to supplement your diet with a prescription vitamin containing fluoride.

Selenium

Our bodies require only small amounts of selenium, but it is essential to good health. The amount of selenium in foods varies depending upon the selenium content in the soil in which crops are planted and animals graze. Selenium-rich vegetarian foods include wheat germ, brewer's yeast, Brazil nuts, whole-grain breads, and molasses. Selenium is an antioxidant, and as such, it helps prevent the development of cancerous cells. It also prevents loss of tissue elasticity with aging and can improve the body's immune response. There are no clearly defined selenium toxicity states; however, a deficiency may lead to an increased rate of cardiovascular disease, stroke, certain cancers, and hypertension. Psoriasis, eczema, cataracts, rheumatoid arthritis, and an increased incidence of infection may also result from a selenium deficiency.

The Recommended Dietary Allowance of selenium is 55 micrograms daily. In pregnancy, this dose increases to 65 micrograms daily; for nursing women, it is 75 micrograms.

HOW DO YOU FARE AS A VEGETARIAN WITH SELENIUM INTAKE?

SUPERIOR TO MEAT-EATERS	
BETTER THAN MEAT-EATERS	
SAME AS MEAT-EATERS	X
CHALLENGE TO OBTAIN NUTRITION	
CAREFUL PLANNING RECOMMENDED	

FOOD SOURCES OF SELENIUM

VEGETARIAN		Non-Vegetarian	
Brazil nuts, 2 tbsp	(380 mcg)	Salmon, 3 oz	(12–30 mcg)
Wheat germ, 2 tbsp	(11 mcg)	Shrimp, 3 oz	(34 mcg)
Brown rice, 1 cup	(19 mcg)	Tuna, 3 oz	(69 mcg)
Firm tofu, 4 oz	(20 mcg)		
Sunflower seeds, 1 oz	(17 mcg)		
Low-fat yogurt, 1 cup	(8 mcg)		
Egg, 1	(15 mcg)		
Mushrooms, 1 cup	(8.6 mcg)		

Zinc

Zinc is a very important mineral for the body, and with just a little extra effort, you can consume the same amount of zinc as non-vegetarians do. Although zinc is abundant on the earth's crust, much of it has been lost from the soil due to food processing and agricultural practices. For vegetarians, the best sources of zinc are whole grains such as wheat, rye, oats, pecans, Brazil nuts, pumpkin seeds, gingerroot, mustard, chili pepper, black pepper, and tofu.

Zinc helps our skin to form collagen and to heal. It also aids in the digestion of protein, immune response, and reproduction. Excess doses of zinc from supplements may cause dizziness, poor coordination, and an irregular heart rate. Zinc deficiency is more common than you might expect. Phylates, a fiber found in certain whole grains, can actually bind with zinc and limit its absorption if consumed in very large quantities. That is why it is important not to go to extremes when eating foods within one food group, but rather to eat a well-rounded diet. We also lose zinc through skin wounds and burns and through weight loss. Strict vegans on high-grain, high-fiber diets take special care to supplement their diets with zinc. In children, zinc deficiency manifests in slow physical development and a poor appetite. Signs of zinc deficiency in adults are hair loss, dermatitis, acne, fatigue, poor appetite, and poor digestion. Because zinc helps to heal wounds, a deficiency may also decrease the body's ability to heal itself.

The Recommended Dietary Allowance for zinc is 12 milligrams daily. In pregnancy your recommended allowance increases to 15 milligrams daily; for nursing women, it increases to 19 milligrams.

HOW DO YOU FARE AS A VEGETARIAN WITH ZINC INTAKE?

SUPERIOR TO MEAT-EATERS	
BETTER THAN MEAT-EATERS	
SAME AS MEAT-EATERS	
CHALLENGE TO OBTAIN NUTRITION	X
CAREFUL PLANNING RECOMMENDED	

FOOD SOURCES OF ZINC

VEGETARIAN		Non-Vegetarian	
Pumpkin seeds, 4 oz	(4.5 mg)	Oysters, steamed, 4 oz	(209 mg)
Tofu, 1 cup	(4.0 mg)	Beef, 4 oz	(6.0 mg)
Beans, 1 cup	(2.0 mg)	Pork, 4 oz	(5.0 mg)
Brazil nuts, 10	(2.0 mg)	Chicken, 4 oz	(2.3 mg)
Green peas, 1 cup	(2.0 mg)	Tuna, 4 oz	(1.0 mg)
Peanuts, ½ cup	(1.8 mg)		
Beets, boiled, 4	(1.3 mg)		

Part II
Your Pregnancy Month by Month

CHAPTER 3

Your Month of Conception and Your First Month

Could it be?

Is the test correct?

Your heart rises in elation; your stomach sinks in fear.

Your emotions are so overwhelming.

Yes.

You are pregnant.

You are now a creator,

a giver,

and a supporter

of a new life.

You have waited your entire life for this moment.

The moment you could shout and scream

and tell the whole world,

"I'm pregnant!"

The tiny person beginning to grow inside you

is the center of your universe.

You will plan for it,

eat for it

learn for it

and live for it.
Its life has become yours.

And as a pregnant vegetarian woman,
you are truly special.
because you have the peace of knowing
that you will bring your child into this world
without taking another life.

YOUR FIRST PREGNANCY TEST

I'm beginning to feel nauseated, but I think it might be too early to take a pregnancy test. When should I take one?

If you are feeling nauseated now, this means that your body has released pregnancy hormones into your bloodstream. If you take the test now, it will probably be positive already. In general, women can take their first pregnancy test three weeks after the first day of their last period. Your test may be positive even before you have missed your period.

If you have a regular menstrual cycle (every four weeks), normally you would have ovulated two weeks after the first day of your last period. Your egg and your partner's sperm will fertilize in your fallopian tube. This happily united pair then becomes a fertilized egg, which will proceed on its journey toward your uterus. As it is traveling down your fallopian tube, this fertilized egg is also growing into a many-celled embryo. The embryo will then enter your uterine cavity—like a champion marathon runner entering the Olympic stadium, proud and strong! Its journey will have taken a total of six to seven days. It is only after your fertilized egg has entered your uterine cavity and has implanted into your uterine muscle and blood vessels that placental hormones enter your bloodstream and can be detected with a blood or urine pregnancy test.

So you see, successful conception takes a month. Your pregnancy will be detected by a blood or urine test three weeks after your last period, representing one week after your fertilized egg has implanted.

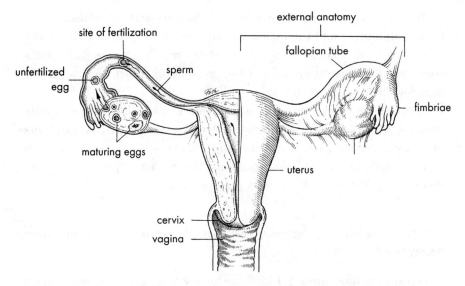

Your baby's six-day voyage as a fertilized egg down your fallopian tube.

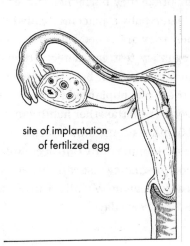

Which pregnancy test should I use?

Most over-the-counter pregnancy tests are quite similar and work using the same basic principle. It will be best for you to use a brand name pregnancy test and one that seems simple to use. If the manufacturer tells you to use your first morning urine sample, please follow their protocol. Your first morning urine sample contains the highest concentration of pregnancy hormones and will help you to detect your pregnancy earlier and more accurately.

If your test is initially negative within the time span recommended by the manufacturer, and you look at the kit again twenty minutes later and it is positive, it is best not to trust the later result. Some negative tests convert to false positive results just upon standing. It will be best for you to follow the initial directions.

If you are not sure that you are performing or reading the test results correctly, do not become discouraged. Remember that you never did this before, you are not a lab technician, and you are very excited. Please call your midwife or your doctor, and her office staff will probably recommend that you come in for a quick pregnancy test.

Is a blood or serum pregnancy test more accurate than a urine pregnancy test?

In certain circumstances, a blood pregnancy test may be more accurate and may detect your pregnancy hormones earlier than a urine test can. Because cells from your baby's placenta, called "chorionic cells," produce these hormones, they are called "human chorionic gonadotropins" (HCG). A blood pregnancy test can detect pregnancy when your HCG level is 50 international units. Your body achieves these levels just two or three days after your egg has implanted in your uterine lining.

A urine pregnancy test, on the other hand, can detect pregnancy when your HCG level is 100 international units. Normally it takes five days after implantation for these amounts of HCG to accumulate in your urine.

Sometimes a blood pregnancy test can also detect the hormones from a tubal (or misplaced) pregnancy, while a urine pregnancy test is not able to detect these for several days.

What signs of pregnancy might I expect to feel, and when?

During the first three weeks after the first day of your last period, you will feel fairly normal. That is because for the first two of these weeks, your egg has not yet even left your ovary. By the fourth week after the first day of your last period, even before you have missed your period, you may begin to feel surges of hormones rushing through you that may cause

- ◆ morning sickness or sickness throughout the day.
- ◆ an inability to eat certain foods, especially fried fatty foods, foods that have strong odors, and foods that are high in protein.

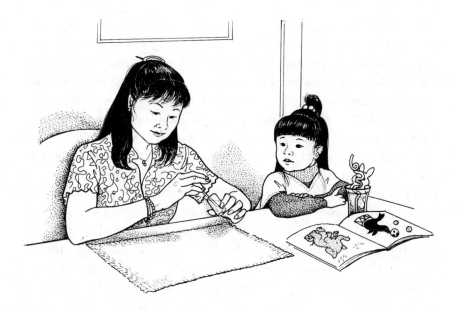

- ◆ extreme fatigue.
- ◆ breast pain and swelling.
- ◆ a bloated feeling and physical appearance.
- ◆ mood swings.
- ◆ all of the above-noted symptoms at the same time!

Every woman is different, so please do not worry if you are the one pregnant woman who feels great.

ONCE YOU ARE PREGNANT

My pregnancy test is positive! What should I do now?

First, feel joy and ecstasy. Feel on top of the world. You are special, and it is fine for you to cry tears of happiness. You are blessed. Your baby may be able to feel your spirit, so give that tiny person a sense of your inner peace and overwhelming love.

When you come down to earth again, please start taking care of yourself. If you have not begun taking folic acid vitamin tablets yet, it is best to start. Take at least 500 micrograms to 1 milligram of folic acid each day. This will help you decrease your chances of having a child with spina bifida (see chapter 1). Also, you had best start taking one standard vegetarian vitamin tablet with iron daily early in your pregnancy. This is because you may not be able to maintain your healthy diet now, until you reclaim your hormones. So at least you will be getting vitamins in tablet form. Then, make an attempt to change as many of your foods as possible to organic and natural products, as you do not want to consume any unnecessary pesticides at this time. Do not have any X rays taken, of any part of your body, without consulting your physician. It will be best for you to stop taking any medications you do not need, whether these are prescription or over the counter. If you believe that you need to take medications, call your physician to make sure the ones you are taking are safe for your baby. Often there are safer pharmaceutical alternatives. Also, if you have been taking any health food store herbs, teas, homeopathic remedies, or megavitamins, stop until you can consult your physician as to their safety. Please do not take vitamins containing more than 25,000 international units of vitamin A daily (refer to chapter 2). Your food sources may contain large amounts of vitamin A, but high doses of vitamin A from synthetic sources can be dangerous for your baby.

Try to stop smoking cigarettes, and do not use marijuana at all. You absolutely must not use any street drugs at this time, especially cocaine, heroin, crack, and psychotropic drugs. Do not drink any alcoholic beverages, including beer or wine. Last but not least, eliminate as many artificial chemicals from your diet as possible, including saccharin, cyclamate, and aspartame.

RECOGNIZING SERIOUS SIGNS

This is my first pregnancy. There are so many changes to my body, how will I know if I am having a serious problem?

If you ever experience any of these symptoms, you should call your doctor or midwife right away—weekday or weekend, day or night, rain or shine. The earlier your doctor knows about anything out of the ordinary, the better he will be able to take care of you.

- ◆ Vaginal bleeding of any type. Any bleeding, even spotting or bleeding after intercourse, might be important.
- ◆ Any lower abdominal pains, cramping, or spasms.

- Any sharp, sudden pains on either the right or left side of your abdomen.

- An inability to hold down foods or liquids for twenty-four hours.

- Any stream of fluid coming from your vagina, be it clear, blood tinged, greenish, or yellow in color.

- Faintness or dizziness.

- Shortness of breath.

- Pains when taking a deep breath.

- Developing fever over 100 degrees.

- Swelling and puffiness in your face, hands, or feet.

- Heart palpitations.

- Burning sensations when you urinate, or blood in your urine.

- Vision changes, including seeing double, spots, or flashing lights.

- Blood in your bowels or bleeding with a bowel movement.

DATES TO REMEMBER AND COUNT

Should I remember the exact day I think we conceived?

It may really be helpful if you can. It may not seem important at this time, but these dates often become very important when you approach, or pass, your due date. Please try to write down the first day of your last period. It is also a good idea to record the number of days your cycle usually extends, from the first day of one period to the first day of your next period. If you know the date or dates you believe you may have conceived and the date your pregnancy test became positive, this will make your final due date much more accurate. Of course, you may not deliver on this date, but you will probably deliver on a day quite close to it.

Knowledge of these dates may also be an invaluable source of information if at some point your doctor or midwife needs to take specific blood tests or ultrasound evaluations that correlate with a specific week of your pregnancy. Much later in your pregnancy, your doctor will use these dates as references to confirm that your baby is near, at, or past its due date. The date of conception may also help to determine if your doctor needs to induce your labor or perform a cesarean section.

Your Weeks of Pregnancy

How long am I really pregnant?

Pregnancy lasts an average of 280 days, when counting from the first day of your last menstrual period until the day you deliver. When you and your doctor count how far you have progressed in your pregnancy, this will be in terms of weeks or months—with each month being a 'four week month.' When you try to divide your 280 days using the traditional counting system of weeks and 'four-week' months, you'll end up with a pregnancy of 40 weeks, or ten months! Although months really last 30 to 31 days, pregnancy is not counted that way because it is difficult to keep track of 30-day increments. Because this concept of being pregnant ten months is inconsistent with our mind-set, other methods of counting the duration of pregnancy are often utilized.

One method, the one I have used in this book, starts counting your months of pregnancy from your fourth week after the first day of your last period. This is actually quite logical, because for the first two weeks after the first day of your last period, you will not even ovulate, and after you do, your egg will be in transit down your fallopian tube for an entire week. It is only after these three weeks that your fertilized egg will finally implant in your uterus.

For consistency, the following chapters will conform to this counting system, a system probably used by your doctor and many books you are reading, but not necessarily all.

Month of Conception: Zero to four weeks.

Month One: Four to eight weeks.

Month Two: Eight to twelve weeks.

Month Three: Twelve to sixteen weeks.

Month Four: Sixteen to twenty weeks.

Month Five: Twenty to twenty-four weeks.

Month Six: Twenty-four to twenty-eight weeks.

Month Seven: Twenty-eight to thirty-two weeks.

Month Eight: Thirty-two to thirty-six weeks.

Month Nine: Thirty-six to forty weeks.

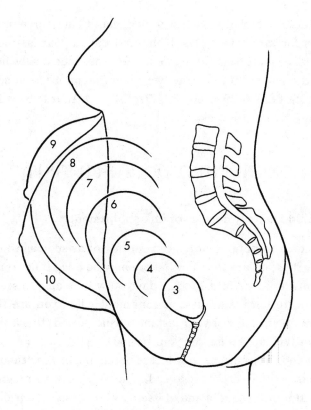

Monthly uterine expansion.

It's natural for you to think of pregnancy beginning at conception—this is when your body tells you a new life is growing inside you! Because your embryo will be fully implanted in your uterus by the fourth week, it will be easier for you to track your baby's development if you start counting months after the month of conception.

Calculating Your Due Date

Should I try to calculate my due date? How should I go about it?

You should definitely try. It will be exciting for you to calculate it, and you will probably be surprised at how accurate you are. Be prepared, however, because your physician may need to change your date if your ultrasound points to a markedly different date. Here is a simple way to find out your due date:

From the first day of your last period, count back three months and then count forward seven days. If the first day of your last period was September 27, count back three months to June, specifically June 27. To calculate the day within your delivery month, count ahead seven days from June 27: 6/28, 6/29, 6/30, 7/1, 7/2, 7/3, 7/4. Your baby will be born July 4, give or take two weeks.

YOUR FIRST DOCTOR'S VISIT

When should I call my doctor for an appointment?

Please make an appointment to see your doctor as soon as you find out, or believe, that you are pregnant. There may be a lag time from the day you call your doctor's office to the day you will be able to see her. It is best for you to have your first appointment when you are five to six weeks past the first day of your last menstrual period (this is one to two weeks after the day you missed your period).

Even if your home pregnancy test is barely positive, with just a minimal change in color—it is best to call. A weakly positive pregnancy test can be an important sign in and of itself, as it may signal a problem with your pregnancy. Seeing your doctor will be reassuring for you.

Nowadays, most physicians have their own ultrasound machines right in their office and will be able to view your pregnancy right away. They will be able to perform a vaginal or abdominal ultrasound to confirm that your pregnancy is in your uterus and not in your fallopian tube. They will also be able to determine how far along you are in your pregnancy and if your fetus, placenta, and gestational sac are developing normally.

YOUR MONTH OF CONCEPTION

During your month of conception, from the first day of your last period through the next four weeks, your chosen egg will develop within your ovary, leave your ovary, meet the sperm destiny chose for it, become fertilized, and implant into your uterine cavity. Quite a month!

During the third week, your egg is making its passage down your fallopian tube. At this three-week mark, your egg will meet with a group of friendly sperm, approximately two hundred million of them, only one of which will fertilize it. Together they fertilize and form the beginnings of a new life together. As a fertilized egg, your united egg and sperm will continue their passage down your fallopian tube and enter your uterine cavity to implant into your uterine wall.

The journey from your fallopian tube to your uterus takes about two weeks. It is when the fertilized egg implants into your uterine lining that the hormones it is producing will enter your bloodstream and you will be able to detect them on a pregnancy test.

YOUR BABY DURING THE MONTH OF CONCEPTION

- As your fertilized egg is traveling down your fallopian tube, it will start dividing and, from just one cell, it will transform into a cluster of rapidly dividing cells.

- As this cluster of cells grows, its central region becomes a hollow cavity.

- Cells on the outer surface of this cluster will burrow into the lining of your uterus and become your placenta.

- Cells near the hollow center of this cluster will become a specialized group of cells that will become your baby. This specialized group of cells is now called your "embyro."

- Your embryo can be seen as a tiny bulge within the central hollow cavity and contains all the tissue for your baby's body.

- Your tiny embryo's tissues will differentiate into three layers to form all its essential structures:

    Its outer layer, or *ectoderm,* will form its hair, skin, nails, brain, nerves, and teeth.
    Its middle layer, or *mesoderm,* will form its heart, kidneys, bones, and muscle.
    Its inner layer, or *endoderm,* will form its lungs, liver, and intestinal tract.

YOUR FIRST MONTH

Once your embryo has implanted into your uterine lining, many changes occur to both your embryo and yourself in rapid succession. As the placenta implants and develops, it infuses hormones into your bloodstream. These hormones may make you feel nauseous and may already be detectible on a pregnancy test. Your tiny embryo will start to develop a ridge of tissue down its back, becoming its brain at the top and its spinal cord at the bottom. So much is happening. Its eyes, ears, stomach, pancreas, intestines, and kidneys start to differentiate and form. Tiny limb buds pouch out to form arms and legs, and its tiny heart will start to beat.

YOUR BABY DURING THE FIRST MONTH

- Your baby, or "embryo" grows from $\frac{1}{10}$ of an inch in length to almost 1 inch. This is the length from the top of your baby's head to the bottom of its backside.

- Your baby's head is large. You can see the tip of its nose.

- Its early heart has divided into two chambers and has begun to beat.

- Its arms and legs have started to bud and grow.

- The major organs have begun to form.

- The beginnings of all essential structures have differentiated from each other.

- Its eyes are not yet opened, but black pigmentation can be seen under the skin covering the eyelids.

- Its intestinal tract is also forming.

- Its tiny jaw and mouth emerge, though the chin is not yet fully developed.

- Openings for the nostrils are visible.

- Its muscles have started to develop.

- Its lungs are tiny solid structures, with bronchi branching out from its throat.

CHANGES YOU MAY NOTICE IN YOURSELF THIS MONTH

- ◆ Morning sickness or sickness throughout the day. This may range from mild waves of nausea to a nearly constant feeling of sickness. You may experience the need to vomit and may even become dehydrated. You may also feel

    nausea with movement.

    nausea upon the sight or odor of foods.

    the need to nibble foods all day to stop nausea.

    the need to vomit after meals.

    the inability to eat certain foods, particularly fried or fatty foods, foods with strong odors, and foods high in protein.

- ◆ Breast soreness. This may range from mild soreness and swelling to pain when your clothes touch your breasts.
- ◆ Your skin may become oilier or drier.
- ◆ Your hair may become drier.
- ◆ You may have heartburn due to increased stomach acid, whether or not you have eaten.
- ◆ You may produce too much saliva and need to cough or spit more than usual.
- ◆ The pressure of your uterus on your bladder may cause you to urinate more often than usual.
- ◆ Fatigue and bloating may be common.
- ◆ Your moods will swing, and you may feel more emotional than usual.

Will I look different right away? Will everyone at work know that I am pregnant?

Even before your abdomen begins to enlarge, the people close to you might be able to tell that you are pregnant. Although your baby is so tiny and your uterus is just barely enlarged in the first month, the effect of your ovarian and placental hormones on the rest of your body may be overwhelmingly apparent. Your skin may become sallow, greenish, or pale, and you may appear tired, ill, swollen, and bloated. Generally, people at work won't know you are pregnant until you begin to show— usually in your third or fourth month.

KEEPING A JOURNAL AND TAKING PHOTOS

At no other time in your life will you experience the profound change that pregnancy brings. When you become pregnant, you anticipate not just the birth of a new life, but also the birth of a new woman—a mother! It's an exciting time for you, but it can also be overwhelming. That is why keeping a journal can be a rewarding exercise. Writing down your thoughts and recording your progress will help you prepare for the new life you're about to begin. Take pictures of yourself, too, to tuck inside

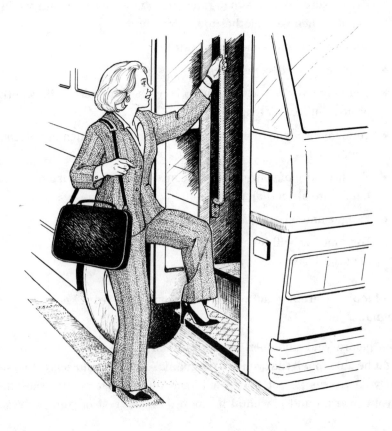

your journal. You may feel bloated and unattractive during much of your pregnancy, but later when you look back at these pictures, you'll see how beautiful and feminine you were, glowing with good health and joy.

Your journal will also be a wonderful thing to share with your child when he or she is older. Imagine reading about the day your mother first felt you move inside her!

MORNING SICKNESS

I have severe morning sickness. Sometimes it lasts all day! How can I sustain my baby and myself when it's so difficult to eat?

Morning sickness is completely natural—approximately two-thirds of women experience nausea and vomiting during pregnancy. Studies indicate that morning sickness is a sign of how a mother's body protects its embryo from foods that could possibly cause a miscarriage or create an abnormality. They observe that the symptoms of morning sickness are worse early in a woman's pregnancy, when the fetal organs are forming. Scientists deduce from this that a woman's body rejects certain foods because they may have harmful effects on fetal organ development. Studies that focus on specific food aversions during pregnancy show that pregnant women have the greatest food aversions to meat, fish, poultry, and eggs, as well as fried and fatty foods and coffee. Based on this, scientists have suggested that animal products could be dangerous to pregnant women and their embryos, possibly because they often contain parasites, pesticides, and other disease-causing organisms. What these studies conclude is that aversions during pregnancy to animal-derived foods have helped protect pregnant women and their unborn children for hundreds of generations. Is this not the wisdom of a woman's body?

Non-vegetarian pregnant women and their families are usually quite concerned about this aversion to animal protein and fats. They find it difficult to accept the concept that for thousands of years, if a pregnant woman felt sick eating meat, she would simply not eat meat. Our bodies have an innate wisdom that has helped us to perpetuate human life. Please have faith in the wisdom of your body. As a vegetarian, you will be able to nourish your baby very well because most of your intake will be from healthy food groups. Your body has an innate wisdom concerning which foods you should eat during pregnancy and which foods you should not. Women of all lands and of all generations have some type of food aversion during pregnancy, yet human life perpetuates itself. The instinctive wisdom of most women's bodies creates a craving for vegetarian-type foods during pregnancy, although non-vegetarians do not recognize that.

If you have been eating a well-balanced vegetarian diet in the months preceding your pregnancy, you will have the foundation to produce a strong, healthy baby. In every study evaluated, scientists have shown that women who have more morning sickness are less likely to miscarry, have a decreased chance of having a stillbirth, and give birth to children of normal weight. These same studies also show that you're likely to have morning sickness again in your next pregnancy. You might not think this is good news, but when you realize that this sickness is really your body's way of protecting and nurturing your pregnancy, you won't mind the nausea so much!

Do you know if wristbands for nausea during pregnancy are effective?

Many women have used wristbands successfully to relieve nausea. The most effective ones are those manufactured for the prevention of morning sickness. There are several manufacturers of these bands, and most are reasonably priced. Wristbands work on the acupressure principle. A plastic stud embedded in the band should be positioned on the inner surface of your wrist, as this is the acupressure site approximately 2 centimeters below the creases of your wrist. Pressure on this site will relay a message back to your brain to help relieve nausea. The bands may not totally alleviate your nausea, but they can reduce it significantly. Studies have shown that three times as many women obtain relief from nausea during pregnancy while wearing these kinds of bands as do those who do not wear them.

I have heard that vitamin B_6 is helpful in decreasing the symptoms of morning sickness. Is this so?

Medical studies have shown that if a woman takes 25 milligrams of pyridoxine (vitamin B_6) every eight hours for three days, she will experience significant relief of her morning sickness nausea. Vitamin B_6 does not make much difference if your nausea is mild, but if you have severe nausea and vomiting, you will have greater relief.

For years a drug called Bendectine, which contained vitamin B_6 and an antihistamine, was used throughout the country for nausea and vomiting associated with pregnancy. It helped women significantly, but in 1983, the pharmaceutical manufacturer of Bendectine withdrew the drug from the market because of an onslaught of lawsuits. The company won every lawsuit but decided to stop manufacturing the product to avoid any future legal action. Though no longer available in the United States, it is still widely used in Canada.

If you decide to take vitamin B_6 tablets, remember that B_6 is a water-soluble vitamin and therefore will be excreted rapidly in your urine. It is best to take it every eight hours so you can keep your levels consistent. Also, please give the vitamin a chance to work before you decide whether or not it is effective. It will take several days for you to start feeling the benefits. Eating foods rich in vitamin B_6 and taking supplements will definitely help you to cope with this difficult phase of your pregnancy.

Will I have a naturally low level of vitamin B_6 as a vegetarian?

Your natural levels will actually be higher than those of a non-vegetarian—a vegetarian diet helps you elevate vitamin B_6 levels. In vegetarians, who have a high-cellulose diet from eating fruits and vegetables, the natural bacteria within the intestines are able to manufacture their own vitamin B_6. In addition, the best dietary sources of vitamin B_6 are predominantly vegetarian foods, including wheat bran, wheat germ, soybeans, cantaloupe, cabbage, molasses, brown rice, eggs, oats, peanuts, and walnuts. People on high-protein diets excrete B_6 more rapidly, and their food sources are not as rich as these vegetarian foods are.

Will ginger really help to relieve my morning sickness?

Since ginger is a natural digestive aid, it may help you to obtain some relief. The ancient Greeks ate ginger after a large meal to aid digestion. They would eat an entire gingerroot wrapped in bread—this was the birth of gingerbread. Ancient Chinese sailors also used ginger, though in their case it was used to prevent motion sickness. In England and the American colonies, ginger was incorporated into a stomach-soothing drink, ginger beer, which then became known as ginger ale.

One gram of ginger is considered effective for relief of morning sickness. Try making a soothing cup of ginger tea. Grate 2 teaspoons of gingerroot and add 1 cup of boiling water. Let this steep for ten minutes before you drink it, and don't worry if you drink some of the unstrained fragments of ginger. One cup of this strong ginger tea contains 250 milligrams of ginger. Drinking a glass of ginger ale (1,000 milligrams of ginger) may also ease your nausea.

GOOD VEGETARIAN FOODS FOR MORNING SICKNESS

If you are like so many other pregnant women with morning sickness, you actually feel better when you eat these foods:

Dry crackers

Dry cereal such as cornflakes or Kellogg's Frosted Flakes

Baked apples and pears, fruit cobblers

Strawberries and rhubarb (sweet and sour)

Ginger tea

French toast

Pancakes

Baked potatoes with butter or sour cream

Carrots and peas with lemon or mayonnaise

Pickled tomatoes, carrots, hard-boiled eggs

Pasta

Spaghetti sautéed in olive oil and garlic

Hummus tahini with lemon and pita bread

Lemon tea with sugar and lemon/lime soda

Steamed vegetables with grated ginger

Steamed vegetables with lemon

Tofu and vegetable stews

Rice pilaf with lemon and garlic

Bland noodle soups

Salted tomatoes

Angel food cake

Avocado with lemon

Carrot juice

Cheese toast

Pickles

Guava juice

Warm apple cider

Olives

It's best to nibble on all of these foods very slowly. Eating quickly may push your body into waves of sickness. Try eating frequent small meals. Sip liquids slowly and let food ease down into your stomach. This is the perfect time to begin a vegetarian lifestyle.

What will happen to my baby if I cannot tolerate eating any foods that are high in protein?

If eating foods high in protein nauseates you, don't worry. Studies show that the protein a pregnant woman eats does not pass directly to her baby. Your body metabolizes the protein you eat and then stores it in your cells. It is subsequently broken down at a later date and passed on to your baby.

Proteins are quite difficult for your body to metabolize. In your first three months of pregnancy, your body expends less energy transferring your stored protein to your baby than it does breaking down new ingested protein. If you eat new protein, your body has to assimilate this protein and then break it down again to give to your baby. Once your morning sickness dissipates, you can start eating protein again and build up your body stores.

NOTE ON NUTRITION: PESTICIDES AND OTHER POLLUTANTS IN FOODS

Am I giving more pollutants to my baby because I eat so many fruits and vegetables?

Actually, the reverse is true: You are giving your baby a lower quantity of pollutants than a non-vegetarian mother would. Studies have shown that vegetarians have much lower levels of pollutants in their bodies than meat-eaters. You are doing the far better thing for your baby by maintaining a meat-free diet during your pregnancy.

Foods derived from animal sources, particularly meat, fish, and dairy products, are the most likely foods to bring cancer-causing pollutants into our bodies. These pollutants contain dangerous organochlorines, compounds containing carbon and chlorine that are dangerous to people as well as insects, including DDT, PCB, and dioxins.

Why do people who ingest meat-based foods have such high levels of pesticides?

Pesticides are deposited on soil and plants to prevent insects from ruining crops. Once these pesticides are deposited, they remain in our soil for over forty years. When we eat plants we wash off the pesticides, but when cows, pigs, lambs, and chickens eat plants, they obviously do not wash off the pesticides. These grazing animals consume large quantities of pesticides in their diets and then store them in their fat tissue. People eat meat and fat from animals, and there is no way they can remove the pesticides. That is why meat-eaters have much higher levels of pesticides in their bodies than vegetarians do.

What can I do as a vegetarian to decrease my levels of pesticides and pollutants?

If you are not a total vegetarian, please buy meat or fish that comes from farms that raise animals on organic produce. If you are a total vegetarian, wash the surfaces of all your fruits and vegetables. Do not eat imported fruits and vegetables, as pesticide regulations in some countries may be less stringent than those in the United States. It is best that you eat in-season locally grown fruits and vegetables and that you choose organically grown and pesticide-free produce. You should try to use coffee, tea, and sugar that have been grown and packaged in the United States.

Remember that pollutants remain in the fat tissue of animals for years, and humans are no exception; as animals, we also retain pollutants in our bodies for years. If you've maintained a healthy vegetarian lifestyle up to this point, you and your baby are off to a great start.

PESTICIDES AND POLLUTANTS: IMPORTANT FACTS FOR A VEGETARIAN

- ◆ Meats contain fourteen times more pesticides than plant foods.
- ◆ Dairy products contain five and a half times more pesticides than plant foods.
- ◆ Meat and dairy products are the source of 60 to 85 percent of all the pesticides present in humans.
- ◆ Meat, fish, and dairy are the main sources of toxic chemicals in our food supply. These chemicals include pollutants such as PCB, DDT, and dioxin.
- ◆ A study of Eskimo women, whose diets include large quantities of fatty fish, showed that their pesticide levels were ten times higher than the levels of Canadian women whose diets were lower in animal fats.

◆ Meat and dairy products account for 95 percent of the pesticide DDT found in our bodies.

◆ Livestock need sixteen pounds of feed to produce one pound of their own flesh, which means that each pound of beef has been produced from sixteen pounds of pesticide-covered vegetation.

◆ Significant quantities of the pesticide DDT pass from a cow's body fat into its milk.

◆ High levels of the pollutants DDE and PCB have been found in the breast milk of mothers who consume high levels of fatty meat or fish.

◆ Newborn hypotonia (poor muscle tone) and hyporeflexia (poor reflexes) have been related to PCB exposure.

◆ Studies show that pesticides accumulate and remain in the body fat of humans for decades.

◆ Several medical studies show that vegetarian women maintain lower levels of pesticide in their bodies and their breast milk than do non-vegetarians.

AN OUNCE OF PREVENTION: KNOWING ABOUT INFECTIONS

TORCH Infections

What are TORCH infections?

TORCH refers to a group of infections that harm an unborn child if a woman contracts them during her pregnancy. If you have contact with or come down with any of these infections, it is not a given that your baby will be affected, but you should know what these infections are. They include toxoplasmosis, rubella (German measles), cytomegalovirus, and herpes virus (genital herpes). Other serious infections that can pass through the placenta to your baby include varicella (chicken pox and shingles), Fifth's disease (parvovirus), syphilis, Coxsackie virus B3 and B4, tuberculosis, hepatitis B, and HIV.

Not all infections can pass through your placenta to affect your baby. Most of the common bacterial infections, like strep throat or urinary tract infections, will not harm your baby. However, viruses are tiny organisms that can pass through the placenta and affect your baby. Fortunately, the flu—a group of common viral infections—is not usually caused by a virus that passes through to affect a baby. Also, in some cases, you may have an infection that causes a fever. Though you may not pass that infection to your baby, a high fever can put a strain on your baby's health.

If you have come in contact with or develop any kind of infection, inform your health care provider. She will know immediately if you have need for concern. Some serious infections can be prevented if you receive treatment immediately following contact with an infected individual, and some can be treated effectively even after you are infected.

Toxoplasmosis

Approximately one in every one thousand infants born in the United States is infected with toxoplasmosis. Toxoplasmosis is an infection caused by *Toxoplasma gondii,* a tiny parasite that lives in the body and intestines of certain animals. Humans can catch it in three ways: by eating raw or undercooked fish or the meat of an infected animal; by contact with the feces of an animal that has excreted it (changing a cat's litter is one of the most well-known ways of catching this infection); and by contact with soil on which an animal has deposited the toxoplasmosis organism or its eggs. Studies have shown that eating undercooked meat is the primary way most people contract toxoplasmosis. Contact with infected soil and travel outside of Europe and North America is the second greatest risk factor.

At your initial pregnancy visit, your doctor will test you for toxoplasmosis. If you believe at any time later that one of the above risk factors may have compromised you, please let your doctor know so you can be retested. The symptoms of toxoplasmosis are vague, so if you contract it, there is only a 10 to 20 percent chance that you will know you have become infected. Symptoms generally include a flulike syndrome, with fever, aches, sweating, and swollen lymph nodes around the neck occurring one to three weeks after you have contracted the infection.

If you have ever worked in an animal shelter, there is a chance you have developed immunity to toxoplasmosis. Nevertheless, it is still important that you take precautions to avoid reinfection, because immunity levels vary. Women who work in veterinarian facilities, animal shelters, meat processing and packaging warehouses, and nurseries or landscaping centers have a greater likelihood of acquiring immunity to this disease, but also a greater chance of contracting it if they are not immune.

Toxoplasmosis is an infection that will pass through the placenta to your baby any time during pregnancy and actually does so more easily later in pregnancy. Studies show that if you contract this infection early in your pregnancy, there is a 14 percent chance your baby will become infected, but if you contract it during your last three months, the chances increase to 60 percent. However, in babies who become infected earlier, the infection is likely to be more severe and may be fatal. Most babies infected with toxoplasmosis do not show any signs of infection at birth. Later, however, 55 to 85 percent will gradually develop symptoms. These include impaired hearing and vision, mental retardation, rashes, seizures, and scarring of the brain. That is why it is so important to make sure you do not contract this disease, get tested if you think you have had contact, and take antibiotics and other treatments if you contract it during your pregnancy.

My son was given a pet rabbit. I was told that rabbits carry toxoplasmosis. Is that true?

Yes, rabbits can carry toxoplasmosis, but you do not have to worry that you will catch it—unless you eat this family pet! Rabbits, mice, rats, and other rodents can carry this parasite in their body tissues, but you can catch it only by eating their flesh. Toxoplasmosis does not live in the intestinal tracts of these rodents, as it does in cats, so they do not pass it in their feces.

As for other common household pets, birds can carry illnesses, but none are specifically harmful to a fetus. Dogs do not carry any illnesses that are harmful during pregnancy, but the ticks that live on dogs can. Ticks on dogs or deer can carry Lyme disease; fortunately, it is not common for a fetus to contract this infection. Nevertheless, check your dogs constantly for ticks if you live in an area where Lyme disease is prevalent and ticks are present.

Rubella (German Measles)

Rubella, or German measles, is a virus that passes through the placenta and infects virtually every organ in a baby's body. It causes growth retardation, small head size (microcephaly), encephalitis, hearing loss, blindness, and a multitude of other symptoms. Although an affected child may appear normal at birth, other symptoms may develop gradually, affecting its vision, hearing, growth, and intellect.

Rubella is not nearly as frequent a problem as it was in the early 1900s when it was first discovered in Germany. This viral infection is most commonly spread during the late winter and early spring. Symptoms develop over one to three days and include a rash, swollen lymph nodes, and fever. Since mass immunizations began, instances of rubella in our country have decreased 96 percent. However, some women may lose their immunity if they have not received a booster. It is best to have your immunity status checked before you become pregnant. You cannot receive a booster while you are pregnant.

Cytomegalovirus

Cytomegalovirus is currently the most common congenitally acquired infection in our country. It affects an average of 1 percent of all newborns in our country and is the leading cause of hearing loss in newborns. During pregnancy, this viral infection can pass through the placenta and affect a baby at any time during pregnancy. The virus is spread from one infected person to another through saliva, urine, blood, and sexual contact. Within one to two months of contracting the virus, the individual will have a silent infection, meaning there will be no symptoms. A large percentage of the population already has had contact with cytomegalovirus and has become immune. Although many women may show immunity to this disease, 0.1 to 1 percent of women may still pass on this congenital infection to their newborn. If you were not immune prior to your pregnancy and you contract the disease, there is a 10 percent chance that your baby will be affected. Newborns affected with this virus demonstrate a variety of symptoms, ranging from congenital deafness, jaundice, blindness, microcephaly (a small head), rash, and retardation.

Two percent of all pregnant women in the United States acquire cytomegalovirus during their pregnancies, but not all of the infants become infected. If you work at a school or day care center, or have other young children at home, your risk is higher because of your contact with the urine, saliva, and other body fluids of the children for whom you care. Eleven percent of women who start working at a school or child care center develop this infection within their first year of employment, although most women are not aware this has occurred. Many children have had contact with this virus and spread it unwittingly at a much greater frequency than infected adults because they are still in diapers or are being toilet trained.

Herpes Virus

I have recurrences of genital herpes. What are the chances I might pass this on to my baby?

Although 5 percent of all women in our country have genital herpes, only one baby out of every two thousand is infected with this virus at birth. In most instances, women pass this viral infection to their newborn during their first attack of genital herpes. Seventy to 80 percent of all babies who become infected with this virus do so at the time of delivery, but some may become infected while still in their mother's uterus.

What is the significance of having Type I or Type II herpes virus?

Eighty to 85 percent of all women with genital herpes have Type II herpes virus. This strain of the virus affects only the genital area of a man or a woman and is spread almost entirely through sexual contact. Type II herpes viral infections present with more blisters, more discomfort, and more frequent recurrences. In general, they are more difficult than Type I herpes in all respects.

Fifteen to 20 percent of all women with genital herpes have Type I herpes virus, which they have contracted either through sexual intercourse, from oral sex, or from their own oral herpes by touching a lesion on their own mouth and then touching their genital region. Type I herpes viral infections present with fewer blisters, less discomfort, and fewer recurrences. Although the physical effects are generally milder, outbreaks from this strain of the virus at delivery can affect a newborn as seriously as a Type II virus. The main difference is that if you have Type I herpes, your outbreaks will occur with less frequency and this will decrease your chances of infecting your baby.

I am not sure if my partner has herpes. Is this significant?

This is a very significant issue, because it is important that you not catch herpes for the first time during your pregnancy. If you have your first attack of genital herpes early in your pregnancy, you will triple your chances of having a miscarriage. If you have your first attack during the latter two-thirds of pregnancy, you will increase your risk of delivering prematurely. If you have a first attack when you deliver, your newborn will have a 50 percent chance of becoming infected at birth.

Both you and your partner need to be tested. Any suspicious lesions he has need to be evaluated, and he should have his blood tested for herpes antibodies. If he has, or has ever had, herpes, his body will have antibodies and the test will detect these. In this situation, please use condoms during genital contact for the remainder of your pregnancy and avoid having any sexual relations when he has an active outbreak. You will also need to be checked for antibodies, as you may already have the disease and may be a silent carrier. It is important for you to watch for any possible outbreaks yourself, so you can be careful not to infect your newborn at delivery.

How would I know if I carry herpes?

If you have herpes, you might develop either one or several blisters in your genital region, usually at the same site each time you have an outbreak. In some women, there is an early silent phase during which they experience itching or burning of their labia before blisters appear. When these blisters do appear, they are often surrounded by a reddened region and are quite painful and tender. During an outbreak, you may feel weaker and feverish and have swollen lymph nodes in your groin. During a first attack of herpes, the labial tissues may become so swollen and blistered that a woman cannot even urinate. Some women, however, do not have any symptoms with their outbreaks—these are called "subclinical outbreaks" or "silent outbreaks." Although these outbreaks are certainly easier for such women, the absence of symptoms means they won't know if they are having an attack near the time of delivery. That is why all women with a history of herpes need to be acutely observant for even minor symptoms to protect their baby.

I have frequent herpes outbreaks. Can I prevent an outbreak at the time of my delivery?

You can try to prevent outbreaks naturally by keeping yourself relaxed, mentally and physically. It is common for women to experience outbreaks more often if they are overtired, overworked, or overstressed. In particular, try not to worry about having an outbreak, because you do not want to add an extra level of stress to what should be an exciting and happy time of your life.

Four weeks before your due date, you should also ask your doctor to place you on an antiviral medication like Acyclovir, Valtrex, or Famvir. These medications decrease the frequency and intensity of herpetic outbreaks, which means you'll be less likely to experience an outbreak at the time of delivery. Studies have shown that all of these medications are safe for both you and your baby during pregnancy and have no negative effects on newborns.

If you have an outbreak of herpes at the time of delivery, you must have a cesarean section. A baby can contract the virus very easily during vaginal delivery, either from the blisters on your vagina or through contact with amniotic fluid that has touched a blister. Your newborn is quite vulnerable to infections—herpes is no exception. Once the virus has spread to its tiny organs, it can be fatal. This doesn't mean you cannot have a vaginal delivery if you are a carrier of herpes; as long as you don't have an active outbreak when you're ready to deliver, the chances are your baby will be fine.

As a vegetarian with herpes, are there any dietary measures I can take to decrease my chances of having a herpes outbreak?

Taking a daily supplement of L-lysine, an essential amino acid, during the last four to five months of your pregnancy can help to prevent recurrent outbreaks of herpes. Your chances of having a herpetic outbreak will decrease if you have a higher level of the amino acid lysine than the level of arginine in your diet. Unfortunately, as vegetarians, our ratio of lysine to arginine is not as high as it is in non-vegetarians. The average ratio of lysine to arginine in non-vegetarians is three to one. In vegetarians, the average ratio is only one to one. Once you start supplementing with lysine, please take it consistently, or you will increase your chances of having recurrent outbreaks. Along with a daily lysine dose of 500 milligrams, increase your dietary intake of lysine-rich foods. These include milk, cheese, yeast, beans, and eggs.

Other Infections
Chicken Pox

Chicken pox, or varicella, can be dangerous not only for your baby, but also for you during pregnancy. This infection does not occur often during pregnancy because most adult women had this virus in childhood and are now immune. (Even among those who do not recall having this infection as a child, 80 percent of women have immunity.) If you do not know your immunity status, have a blood test right away to determine if you are immune. If you are not immune, you will need to receive a varicella immune globulin injection, even though you are pregnant, once you have been exposed to this virus. This immune globulin will either prevent you from developing chicken pox or will lessen the severity of your infection if you do come down with it.

No one can predict how the chicken pox virus will affect you during pregnancy. Some women who catch chicken pox during their pregnancy develop severe cases that progress to chicken pox pneumonia or chicken pox encephalitis, both of which require hospitalization. Although non-pregnant women may have just the standard case of chicken pox with skin lesions and fever, your case may be much more severe while you are pregnant. Similarly, no one can predict whether your baby will be one of the 2 percent who are affected by chicken pox during pregnancy. The chicken pox virus can cross the placenta up until the twentieth week of pregnancy. After that point, you need to worry more for your own health than for your baby's. Even though it is unlikely that your baby will become infected at this late date, you may develop an overwhelming chicken pox infection that affects not just your skin, but, as I mentioned earlier, your lungs and your brain as well. If you develop chicken pox just at the time of delivery, your newborn may become sick because its immune system will not be sufficiently mature to fight the virus. Your entire medical team, including your obstetrician and your pediatrician, will be watching you both closely.

The small percentage of babies who develop serious side effects may have neurological impairment, blindness, and structural abnormalities of their arms, legs, or torso. After you recover from your infection, your gynecologist will recommend that you visit a high-risk obstetrician or radiologist for high-resolution ultrasounds. These may reveal some physical signs that your chicken pox has affected your baby. Think positively—most infants whose mothers contracted this infection during their pregnancy are born without any abnormalities.

Fifth's Disease

What are the symptoms of Fifth's disease, and how is it spread?

For many years, Fifth's disease was never diagnosed as a specific disease, as it is now. As a child, if you developed viral-type symptoms and a pinkish hue on your face, you may have had Fifth's disease. Your mother probably thought that you had the average flu. Sixty percent of all adults are immune; if you have yourself tested for parvovirus antibodies and they are present, then you had this infection previously in your life and you are not in danger of contracting it again. Children are the most frequent carriers, so if you are a teacher or child care worker and not already immune, there is a higher chance you will catch it if there are infected children in your classroom. Fifth's disease is transmitted through droplets of saliva. If you can, take time off from work until the virus runs its course through your school or day care center. You'll be much better off if you do not catch Fifth's disease during your pregnancy.

One-third of all people who contract this virus have no symptoms at all. The other two-thirds of infected people usually have fever, aches, and a pinkish "slapped cheek" coloration on their cheeks. Once you catch this virus, you are contagious, though these symptoms take about ten days after infection to develop.

Fifth's disease does pass through your placenta and can cause your baby's red blood cells to break down. When this happens, a baby becomes so anemic that it cannot carry enough oxygen from its umbilical cord to its vital body organs. Two to 9 percent of affected infants may lose their lives as a result. If you contract Fifth's disease, your physician will watch you closely throughout the entire remaining course of your pregnancy. You will be given repetitive ultrasound examinations to make sure your baby does not become swollen due to anemia. If it does, your doctor may perform a vaginal delivery or a cesarean section earlier than your due date so she can transfuse your baby with healthy blood cells. Once you are pregnant, ask your doctor to test your immunity so you can be prepared, if necessary, to protect your baby and yourself from exposure.

HIV

Why do I need to be tested for HIV?

It is very important for a woman to find out if she carries HIV because treatment with antiretroviral therapy can greatly reduce the chances that her baby will ever become HIV-positive. All people who are diagnosed with HIV never knew they had the virus until they were tested. No one ever thinks the test will be positive. If an HIV-positive woman is treated with zidovudine (a form of antiretroviral therapy) during her pregnancy and delivery, and her baby receives treatment during its first six weeks of life, the chances that the baby will become HIV-positive decrease from 25 percent to 5 percent.

I am HIV-positive and on antiretroviral medication. Will I need a cesarean?

Your antiretroviral medications and a cesarean section will greatly decrease the chances of your baby's becoming infected with the virus at delivery. Newborns can contract the HIV virus from their mother's body fluids at delivery. If the level of viral particles in your blood is high and if your baby comes in contact with a high volume of viral particles during a vaginal delivery, there is a greater chance it will become infected. Your medication is decreasing your viral load drastically, and by having a cesarean section two weeks before your due date, you can deliver before your membranes rupture and your body fluids have contact with your baby. Studies have shown that by taking antiretroviral medication throughout your pregnancy and having a cesarean section before labor starts, you will decrease the risk of HIV transmission to your baby to 2 or 3 percent.

Scarlet Fever

Scarlet fever develops after contact with a particular strain of the strep virus. If you come down with this strain, your skin will break out in tiny red pinpoint dots that have joined together and blanch white if you press them. Children develop this pink or scarlet manifestation with strep infection more often than adults do. Your baby cannot catch this variant of strep infection from you, so the strep infection is not any more dangerous for you during your pregnancy. If you develop a gnawing painful sore throat, most of the antibiotics needed to treat strep throat are considered safe to use during pregnancy.

Hand, Foot, and Mouth Disease

Hand, foot, and mouth disease is a viral infection that usually affects young children and occurs most often during the summer. An infected child will have a dozen or so blisters on the palms of the hands and soles of the feet. Blisters will also develop and ulcerate on the back of the throat. It is unlikely that you will come down with this infection, but if you were to, it would not harm you or your baby. There is no treatment for this virus, and it will resolve by itself.

CHAPTER 4

Your Second Month

As you progress in your pregnancy
you will experience a range of fears and joys.

You may recognize
objectively
that all is well, healthy, and normal.

But being pregnant is so different
from any experience you have encountered in your life
that you cannot help but question
the changes you are experiencing,
your body, your moods, and your energy levels.

Eventually,
you will begin to feel secure in your new life—
a life of constant changes.
You will begin to look forward to each new change,
and realize that changes are good.
You will accept that you are no longer able to direct
and control your life
in the ways you used to, before your pregnancy.

You will feel peace
that the path you are now on
will lead you where it knows you should go.

This new path has drawn you in and will lead you,
now and for the rest of your life.
It will control your love, emotions, compassion, and spirit,
for now they will be a bridge
from you to your child.
You will never again be only yourself.

Now that you have found this wisdom,
your mind, body, and soul
will begin to relax.
And you will enjoy this new mysterious journey
and accept and cherish all of its changes
as that which is meant to be.

YOUR BABY DURING THE SECOND MONTH

- Your baby's body will grow from 1 inch to 2 inches long from its head to the bottom of its backside.
- Your baby's head is quite large, and its forehead is prominent.
- Its face has started to develop a profile.
- The outer portions of its ears are beginning to grow.
- Its eyes and eye lenses are forming.
- It can open and close its mouth.
- Its fingers and toes have separated.
- Almost all of its internal organs are starting to form.
- Its intestines have begun to function.

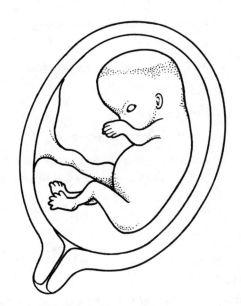

Your eighth week through your twelfth week is your second month of pregnancy. This is your baby at eight weeks.

◆ Its glands have started to produce hormones.

◆ Its liver is producing blood cells.

◆ Its nervous system has started to develop—your baby will make its first movement this month.

◆ Toward the end of this month, your baby's heartbeat may be audible with your doctor's handheld Doppler device.

CHANGES YOU MAY NOTICE IN YOURSELF THIS MONTH

You will experience all the changes you noticed during your prior months of pregnancy, plus a few new ones! Just when you feel that one symptom is ending, another will intensify. Remember that most of your symptoms usually represent signs of a strong and healthy pregnancy.

◆ Morning sickness throughout the day.

◆ Increased mood swings.

◆ A general bloated feeling.

- Pressure from your uterus on your bladder and just above your pubic bone.

- Acne, particularly on your chin.

- Thinner hair.

- Constipation.

- A wider, less-defined waist.

- A shift in your other organs as your uterus grows. Your uterus is not yet visible over the top of your pubic bone, but you may sense that you are larger.

WEIGHT WATCH

How much weight is healthy to gain? I do not want to gain too much.

The American College of Obstetricians and Gynecologists has set guidelines for weight gain during pregnancy.

- If your weight is normal at the beginning of your pregnancy, a weight gain of twenty-five to thirty-five pounds is optimum. That is three to four new pounds each month. If you eat exactly the same quantity of foods during pregnancy that you ate prior to becoming pregnant, you will probably gain twenty-five pounds.

- If you are twenty to thirty pounds overweight at the beginning of your pregnancy, a weight gain of fifteen to twenty-five pounds is optimum. That is two and a half new pounds each month.

- If you are more than thirty pounds overweight at the beginning of your pregnancy, a weight gain of zero to fifteen pounds is optimum. That is just about one pound each month. In this case, it is not necessary for you to gain any weight at all, as long as you do not actively try to lose weight. It is the quality, not the quantity, of your foods that is important for your baby's development.

I usually recommend that if you are overweight and do not wish to gain weight during pregnancy, you follow a "weight-maintenance, 2,000-calorie diet." Within the framework of this diet, you should be able to eat healthy foods, get enough vitamins, minerals, fiber, and protein, and still maintain a stable weight throughout your pregnancy.

Your 2,000-calorie vegetarian diet should include an abundant variety of fruits and vegetables, grains, seeds, beans, and nuts. If you are lacto-ovo-vegetarian, your diet should also contain dairy products and eggs.

I'm afraid I'm gaining weight too rapidly. I do not want to gain more than twenty-five pounds during my entire pregnancy.

Your body knows what is right for your baby. There are so many variations in each woman's rate of weight gain during pregnancy that there is no single definitive pattern. From my experience, the most typical pattern of weight gain is the following:

- ◆ Two to six pounds during the first twelve weeks.
- ◆ Five to eight pounds between the twentieth and twenty-fourth weeks.
- ◆ Five to eight pounds between the twenty-fourth and twenty-eighth weeks.

After the twenty-eighth week of pregnancy, most weight gain is due to fluid retention and growth of your baby, your placenta, and your uterus. Not much new body fat is formed in your body after the twenty-eighth week.

Where the Weight Is Going

Each of us gains weight differently. The chart on the following page will give you a sense of how much weight you may gain in each of your phases of pregnancy and where you'll see your weight increase.

Some women, such as myself, gain much of their weight during their first twelve weeks of pregnancy. This may happen if you are feeling nauseated all the time and feel better only when you are nibbling small amounts of food. You'll find that you are nibbling food all the time. Listen to your body and eat these frequent small meals. The wisest compromise is to nibble healthy low-fat foods, then keep your meals similarly healthy and low in fat. Good foods to snack on are crackers, canned unsweetened fruit, fruit cobblers, steamed vegetables with grated ginger, rice with lemon, and sliced and salted tomatoes.

WEIGHT GAIN IN POUNDS				
	10 WEEKS	20 WEEKS	30 WEEKS	40 WEEKS
SITE				
Fetus	0.01	0.7	3.3	7.5
Placenta	0.04	0.4	0.9	1.4
Amniotic Fluid	0.07	0.8	1.7	1.8
Uterus	0.3	0.7	1.3	2.1
Breasts	0.1	0.4	0.8	0.9
Blood Volume	0.2	1.3	2.9	2.8
Fluid Retention	0	0.1	0.2	3.7
Maternal Gain	0.7	4.5	7.7	7.4
TOTAL	1.4	8.9	18.8	27.6

Will I be able to gain enough weight with my vegetarian diet to sustain my baby and myself?

Absolutely. As long as you include healthy amounts of fats and carbohydrates in your diet, you'll have no difficulty. Both vegetarian and nonvegetarian diets have more than enough calories to support a pregnancy. It is simply a matter of making wise choices.

If you are twenty pounds less than your desired weight at the start of your pregnancy, you are considered underweight. Your recommended weight gain during pregnancy, according to the American College of Obstetricians and Gynecologists, is twenty-eight to forty pounds. That is an average weight gain of four to five pounds each month, almost one-sixth pound each day. To achieve this weight goal, you need to consume approximately 583 more calories daily than a woman who is not under-weight (3,500 calories of food creates one pound of body tissue). If you increase your volume of foods at each meal and eat healthy snacks, it won't be difficult to gain the extra weight you need to support your pregnancy.

HEALTHY WAYS TO INCREASE YOUR CALORIES

As a vegetarian, you can eat a wide array of healthy, calorie-rich foods:

◆ Nut spreads and butters

◆ Bean and lentil dishes

◆ Vegetables sautéed in olive oils and nut oils

◆ Oily salad dressings

◆ Chopped nuts in vegetarian stews

◆ Vegetarian meat substitutes

◆ Nuts and coconut desserts

◆ Whole-grain rice and beans

◆ Tempeh

◆ Fruits in the form of pies and cobblers

◆ Avocado, potato, rice, and bread

In addition, if you are a lacto-ovo-vegetarian, you can eat these foods:

◆ Cream sauces on vegetables

◆ Cheese fondues

◆ Milk shakes or full-fat milk

◆ Full-fat yogurt dishes

◆ Melted cheese over vegetables

◆ Cheese toast and cheese omelet

Oils may also help to increase your weight gain. Give the following a try:

◆ Deep-fried cauliflower and broccoli

◆ Indian vegetable fritters

◆ Broccoli rabe with garlic roasted in olive oil

◆ Oriental-style vegetables stir-fried in sesame oil

- Lo mein–style sautéed noodles
- Hash-brown potatoes and onions

There are an unlimited number and variety of vegetarian dinners that you can prepare with more oil and more fats to increase your total number of calories. Here are some good choices:

- Spaghetti in olive oil and garlic
- Tacos made from tofu or beans
- Grape leaves stuffed with rice
- Cabbage leaves filled with rice and nuts
- Vegetarian country stews
- Vegetable casseroles
- Fried rice and vegetables

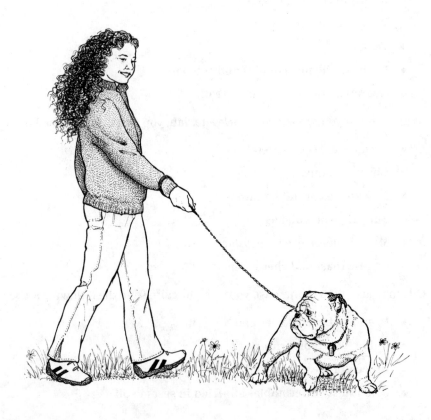

I gained seven pounds already and I'm embarrassed to get on the scale in the doctor's office. Will I have to be weighed through my pregnancy?

We all have different body types and weights. Your propensity toward weight gain, both before and during pregnancy, is never totally within your control. The measurement of your weight should be a guideline for *you* to help you achieve your own goals; it is not a reflection of your character or a reason for anyone to pass judgment on you. Remember, every woman must gain some weight during her pregnancy; in pregnancy, you are the life support to your baby, your placenta, your amniotic sac, and your uterus.

In the latter part of your pregnancy, checking weight gain is especially important. Excess weight at that time may actually be due to fluid retention; your doctor will look at your weight to make sure you have not developed toxemia of pregnancy. During my first pregnancy, I gained fifteen pounds within my first two months. I needed to nibble food every second so I would not feel nauseated. I was ashamed for the doctor to see this. During my third pregnancy, I lost fifteen pounds in these same two months because I was too nauseated to eat at all. Anyone who speaks harshly to you about your pregnancy weight gain does not understand what your pregnancy feels like to you.

Use your weight variations as a guideline for yourself. If you are gaining too much or too little compared with your own goals, modify your food choices. As a vegetarian, you will be well informed about the nutritional and caloric content of your own foods. Now is the time for you to follow a meal plan that suits your needs to help you achieve your nutritional goals. Remember: Nutritional goals come first, weight goals come second.

FATIGUE

I am so tired. Is this because my vegetarian diet isn't supporting me, or is it due just to the pregnancy?

A healthy vegetarian diet with sufficient vitamins, minerals, and calories will in no way contribute to your feelings of exhaustion. When your doctor evaluates your initial CBC (complete blood count), she will make sure that you are not anemic, which is often the cause of fatigue. Several components of the CBC, including the hemoglobin and hematocrit, will also show if your levels of iron or vitamin B_{12} are low.

Pregnancy is exhausting, whether you are vegetarian or not. Nature really wants you to rest now, but we all know that this is not always possible. To help you combat fatigue, try stretching in the morning to stimulate your circulation; at noon, make sure you take a break to eat and rest. See if there is a cubicle or rest area at work where you can just lie down for half an hour. Three P.M. is a usual pregnancy crash time, so try to drink juice or other liquids then to keep up your energy. When you get home from work, rest for an hour.

After you eat dinner, try to get some exercise. This may sound contrary to how you are feeling, but often when you feel so tired, exercise can increase your energy. You can go to a gym, go for a brisk walk, put on an easy exercise tape, or crank up the tape player and dance at home. Your body is caring for two people. I know that one is very tiny, but it is mighty and it takes all the energy it needs first. The profound fatigue during pregnancy is something every woman experiences no matter what her dietary choices are. The best thing you can do is accept that you are not superwoman. Trying to prove otherwise will make you just that more tired and stressed. I tried to do that, and no one will ever remember all the work I did, or that you will do. When I was pregnant with my third child, I acted chipper at work and chipper when I bathed the children, but by eight P.M. I would crash. My husband said he never saw a human being sleep so much. It is universal that pregnant women need more rest—it is the will of nature. Please give yourself as much time for rest and sleep as you can.

BODY CHANGES

I'm only two months pregnant and I feel as though I have lost my waist already. If my baby is so small now, how did this happen?

Even if you have not gained a single ounce of weight, fat tissue will start to collect on your abdomen almost as soon as you become pregnant. During your pregnancy, you will have an increase in your total body fat stores, not just a redistribution of it. This new fat that you store definitely will not be distributed uniformly throughout your body. Studies measuring total skin thickness as an indication of body fat content have shown that, in pregnancy, a woman's body fat increases 20 to 40 percent in some regions of her body, the waist being one of them. While these fat stores will not shed as quickly and easily as they appeared, they are normal in pregnancy; with a little effort, you should be able to drop them once your baby is born.

Is my vegetarian diet contributing to my breast soreness?

Actually, it might be, especially if you are a vegetarian who eats large amounts of mushrooms. Mushrooms can stimulate cystic changes in the breasts and can cause painful swelling and soreness in breast tissue. In pregnancy, your breast ducts and glands are growing in size and number from hormonal stimulation, and mushrooms can add to this stimulation, causing more soreness than usual in pregnancy.

Some mushrooms have a stronger effect on breast tissue than others. Tiny button mushrooms will not make them as sore as the large portobello, shiitake, or dried Oriental mushrooms. Non-vegetarians cannot imagine the varieties and quantities of mushrooms that vegetarians include in their diet. For many vegetarians, a portobello mushroom/ tomato sandwich is a dietary staple. There are times I have been awakened at night by breast soreness, only to recall the large plate of sautéed black mushrooms I had for dinner.

There is nothing unhealthy about a diet rich in mushrooms. Shiitake is a Japanese mushroom that contains a virus-producing interferon, a medication used to treat cancer. Reishi mushrooms have been eaten in the Orient for over two thousand years, and the Chinese believe they will bless you with eternal youth and longevity. Reishi mushrooms stimulate the body to produce blood cells that help fight infection and improve immunity. Dried Oriental mushrooms can supply the same amount of protein you would find in a portion of lean meat. If you're experiencing intense soreness in your breasts, limiting the amount of mushrooms you eat will most likely ease the pain, but you need not give up this delicious vegetable—just be aware of how it affects your overall health and well-being right now.

I find that I have much more saliva than usual, and I need to spit often. Why is this happening?

In some women, the salivary glands located on either side of the jaw and neck produce too much saliva during pregnancy. In most women this decreases by itself by the fourth month, but I have seen it last the entire nine months of pregnancy. There is no health risk involved, though I understand how annoying this is for you. The best thing that you can do is just accept it, I'm afraid. Please keep your cup with you and make sure that you are drinking enough liquid and eating enough salt to make up for all the liquids and sodium that you are losing.

FOOD CRAVINGS

Would I have fewer cravings if I were following a meat-based diet?

I do not believe you would. Normally in pregnancy, there is a pattern within which women crave the tastes of certain foods. For example, pregnant women are known to crave ice cream, sweets, candy (particularly chocolate), and fruits. They prefer strong tastes, such as sweets and vinegar. Though you could argue that most of these fall into the junk food category, you can see that the craving here is for a strong taste more than it is for particular nutrients. On the opposite end of the spectrum, pregnant women usually have their greatest aversions to meat, poultry, and certain seasonings, such as oregano.

Studies vary, however, as to the exact foods within each category that are the worst offenders. Approximately 38 percent of all pregnant women experience food cravings, and 68 percent experience food aversions. Much of the weight gain a woman experiences during pregnancy is due to a desire for strong taste, hence the well-known "pickles and ice cream" craving. Instead of wasting your "strong taste" binges on sweets, try less fattening strong-tasting foods that contain lemon, vinegar, herbs, or spices. Try preparing broccoli with lemon and garlic. Lightly sauté garlic in olive oil and dribble over steamed broccoli. Then generously squeeze lemon juice over the entire dish. Another simple dish is pickled vegetables, a marinade of vegetables pickled in vinegar and water that can be prepared in large quantities and kept for weeks. Then you can reach for these vegetables whenever you crave a strong taste. Prepare 3 cups water and 1 cup vinegar and add any variety of vegetables you wish—tiny tomatoes, carrot slices, green pepper slices, and baby cucumber—then let this marinade sit in your refrigerator for three days so the flavors can marry. You can also add shelled hard-boiled eggs. If you're craving something sweet, try fragrant beverages such as decaffeinated cinnamon tea, orange spice tea, or green tea with a generous twist of lemon.

Now is a good time to broaden your culinary horizons to include various herbs, spices, fruits, and vegetables that are popular in other cultures. Seek out low-calorie and healthy vegetarian recipes in Indian, Asian, and Middle Eastern cookbooks. The various spices used to create these ethnic dishes might help you satisfy your need for strong tastes, and the vegetables in these recipes will increase your vitamin B and fiber intake. Traditional Middle Eastern baba ghannouj or hummus tahini with parsley and lemon juice are two of my favorites—they taste delicious and have wonderful nutritional value.

NOTE ON NUTRITION:
HEARTBURN AND SAFETY OF ANTACIDS

I experience heartburn regularly—whether I eat or I do not eat. Could the heartburn be related to my vegetarian diet?

It is unlikely that your vegetarian diet causes or exacerbates your heartburn. Heartburn is common during pregnancy; your body produces more stomach acids and intestinal enzymes. It also takes longer for food to travel through the intestines during pregnancy. All of these bodily changes help women keep foods within their system longer to reap the most nutritional benefits possible.

But what if the body overdoes this protective mechanism? This is exactly what is happening when a pregnant woman develops heartburn. The heartburn is caused by a number of specific factors. First, the progesterone your body produces during pregnancy causes the muscular valve between your stomach and esophagus to relax. This progesterone also slows down your stomach's peristaltic contractions, so the gastric acid your stomach has created just lies there. Because it is not moving, this acid irritates the stomach lining. The result is accumulated gastric acid "reflux" upward into your esophagus. Added to these changes is the presence of your enlarging uterus, which may be putting pressure on your stomach. As a result, even more gastric acid gets pushed upward into your esophagus.

Although some foods may worsen your heartburn in pregnancy, all foods or even the absence of food may cause heartburn at any time in any person, regardless of diet. Fried, fatty, or spicy foods are typical offenders, as are citrus fruits and juices. Eating a large meal may also trigger heartburn. You can relieve your symptoms of heartburn if you

- eat frequent small snacks instead of large meals.

- walk around after eating, with your shoulders back and chest out.

- avoid lying down right after meals. When you do lie down later on, keep your head and shoulders elevated on pillows.

- drink frequent sips of seltzer.

- snack slowly on Italian ices to dilute and neutralize gastric acid and prevent the burning sensation.

My favorite treatment for heartburn is Italian ices. Most women eat ices at a slow enough rate to absorb their newly produced stomach acids.

Antacids

I am trying so hard to have a healthy pregnancy; is it really safe for me to take antacids?

Yes, it is considered safe to take them, but I believe it is even safer to avoid them. Antacids have never been shown to cause abnormalities in a fetus, but they can affect your body in other ways. Antacids can actually decrease your level of calcium; they can also decrease your absorption of iron. This is more significant for you as a vegetarian, since you may have a lower level of iron already. Antacids may also cause you to swell and retain fluids, because they are basically compounds of salts. All antacids are not the same, as they may contain a variety of salts, including calcium carbonate, calcium saccharin, aluminum hydroxide, or magnesium hydroxide. Your body may react differently to these various combinations.

It is best that you not take antacids containing aluminum, because these can pull calcium from your bloodstream into your intestinal tract, thereby decreasing the amount of calcium left for you and your baby. Just because medications are sold over-the-counter does not mean they are without risk. If your heartburn persists, the next line of medical treatment usually recommended will be Carafate. After that, doctors often suggest Tagamet and Zantac. These are considered safe in pregnancy, but your doctor will tell you which preparation is best for you.

AN OUNCE OF PREVENTION: VAGINAL AND BLADDER HEALTH

I have so much discharge now that I am pregnant. Is this normal? Is it safe to use a tampon?

It is common for pregnant women to produce a very heavy discharge. This does not mean that you have an infection; it just means that your hormones are healthy. Your hormones stimulate your cervical glands to produce a greater volume of secretions. To be on the safe side, have your doctor take a vaginal culture to check that the discharge has not been caused by a vaginal infection. One specific infection, *Hemophilus vaginalis,* may increase the chances of premature labor, so if you develop that infection, it needs to be treated. If you have an excessive amount of vaginal discharge, you may be leaking amniotic fluid, so do inform your doctor.

Once you are sure that your vaginal fluid is normal, the best thing to do is change your underwear often and use a light panty liner or minipad. If you decide to use tampons, use those with a low absorption level—they are less likely to cause toxic shock syndrome. You should change your tampons often and use them infrequently. It is best not to sleep with a tampon inserted, and please remember when you put one in!

I have a yeast infection, and I am so irritated; is it safe to use creams to treat it?

Yeast infections occur more commonly during pregnancy than at other times. Check with your doctor to make sure that your infection is in fact yeast, and then consider why you developed this infection. Yeast grows more easily when sugar is present in vaginal secretions, as yeast thrives on sugar. When you eat sweet foods, you are feeding any yeast present, so you would do well to eliminate cake, candy, soda, ice cream, and cookies to avoid an infection and to help clear one up. Don't eat anything that tastes sweet, even artificial sweeteners, as some yeast infections can live and thrive on diet sugars. The diet sugars may not be nutrition to you, but they can be to yeast.

Also, consider that yeast grows in a warm, moist, dark environment like a bacteriology chamber; your vagina is a similarly warm, moist, dark site, so it supports the growth of yeast. One helpful solution is to wear clothing that won't trap humidity or block circulation. Do not wear panty hose, Lycra-spandex pants, or tight jeans, and try to wear 100 percent cotton underwear, loose-fitting pants, and skirts until your infection heals. Yeast creams are safe to use, but it will be best if you first try natural means to rid yourself of the infection.

Yeast from your intestines can move from your rectal area into your vaginal area, causing infections. To avoid this, change your diet to decrease your production of internal yeast by eating unsweetened natural-curd yogurt. This yogurt is effective because it contains *Lactobacillus acidophilus,* which replaces yeast in your intestines. Please read the labels on the yogurt package, as not all yogurts have a natural curd. Dannon yogurt does, as do many organic yogurts found in health food stores. You can also buy tablets or granules of *Lactobacillus acidophilus* at health food stores and add them to cereals, yogurt, and a variety of other foods.

If these natural techniques are not effective, you can use over-the-counter yeast preparations, such as Monistat, in either vaginal suppositories or cream form. To administer the cream with an applicator, lie on your back and insert a tiny bit of the applicator tip into your vagina, with your finger alongside the applicator. By using this technique, you will not push the applicator in too far. Press out the cream and let it slide back and down into your vagina. Then apply the external creams to your outside tissues. If you are still not better after this, see your gynecologist for a prescription yeast preparation. There are many safe preparations, and there is no need for you to suffer.

I have had a yeast infection three times during my pregnancy. Why is it recurring?

Thirty percent of all women harbor yeast, *Candida albicans,* in their vagina, and many don't even know it. When women become pregnant, yeast can thrive and be recognized by its white curdlike discharge and its itch. Yeast grows easily in pregnant women because they excrete more sugar into their vaginal secretions, fostering its growth. A yeast infection occurs spontaneously, meaning you didn't have to catch it from anyone, but you may end up transmitting it to your husband, who may then transmit it back to you. Please follow the guidelines above to treat it.

Am I more prone to develop yeast because of my high-carbohydrate vegetarian diet?

As a vegetarian, you have a diet that may well be higher in carbohydrates and lower in fats and proteins than a non-vegetarian's. Make an effort to increase your intake of protein-rich foods such as tofu, cheese, beans, and eggs and avoid foods rich in simple carbohydrates such as cake, candy, ice cream, soda, honey, molasses, fruit, and fruit juice. You will have a better chance of preventing a yeast infection if you switch from simple to complex carbohydrates, foods such as potatoes, rice, breads, and other whole-grain nonsweetened cereals. Please read the labels on your cereals to make sure they are not high in corn syrup, dextrose, malt, or any other words meaning sugar.

Can I pass my yeast infection on to my baby at birth?

Yes, your baby may catch your yeast infection at birth and develop thrush, a yeast infection in the mouth and throat. This infection is easily treated with liquid antifungal drops that can be placed in your baby's mouth. However, it would certainly be advantageous for your baby if you are free of this infection prior to your delivery.

I have several venereal warts on my vulva. Can they be dangerous for my baby?

A sexually transmitted virus, human papillomavirus (or HPV), causes venereal warts. This virus, in fact, can be passed on to a newborn at delivery. You are not alone in having this virus: it's estimated that 2 to 5 percent of all pregnant women have it. When a woman contracts the virus, she may develop several small cauliflower-shaped wartlike growths on her vulva and vagina. Even if she has the visible lesions removed, other tiny nonvisible lesions might be present. The virus can also be the cause of Pap test changes and can also cause cancer of the cervix.

Some women who have had their warts removed years prior notice that they recur during pregnancy. That's because the virus can live in a dormant state for years. During pregnancy, a woman's immune response is suppressed and the warts start to grow again. During your pregnancy, you may not be able to receive the standard topical treatment for these warts—podophyllin, 5-fluorouracil, or interferon—so your gynecologist may decide to numb your skin and either freeze them, remove them surgically, or treat them with an acid solution. If your warts are tiny, she may just leave them alone, knowing that they will resolve after you deliver and your immune response is once again strong.

A newborn can become infected during delivery and can develop polyps on its larynx from the virus. Sixty percent of all babies who have laryngeal polyps were infected with HPV at birth. The chances that you will pass this infection on to your baby are remote, a .04 percent risk. Because the risk is so small, an elective cesarean section is not usually recommended. Your doctor will discuss with you what she feels is appropriate in your situation.

If I just developed venereal warts, does that mean my husband has been unfaithful?

Not necessarily, because although HPV is a sexually transmitted disease, you may have had contact with the virus years ago from a prior sexual contact and had no visible lesions all this time. The virus may have remained dormant and then reactivated itself during your pregnancy. Many women have had venereal warts ten years prior to their pregnancy, have had a ten-year wart-free interval, and then, during their pregnancy, have an outbreak of the warts, the virus having remained silent in their body tissues for many years.

I have *Trichomonas vaginalis*, and the doctor prefers to wait until next month to treat it. Is this serious?

Trichomonas vaginalis, a common vaginal infection, causes a yellow irritating discharge. It is considered a sexually transmitted disease; however, trichomonads live in water droplets, so you may have gotten this infection from contact with contaminated water. If you sat in a puddle on the edge of a swimming pool while you were wearing a skimpy bathing suit, and another woman with trichomoniasis just sat in the same puddle, you may have caught it from her. The trichomonas organism is a small protozoan with two active tails that enable it to wiggle around in vaginal fluid. Once you contracted this infection, your husband probably contracted it, too, although he may have no symptoms.

Several medications, metronidazole or Flagyl, used to treat the infection are considered safe after the first three months of pregnancy. Your doctor may want you to wait until you are even further along in your pregnancy to use them. Both your husband and you should be treated simultaneously and should avoid sexual relations during this time. Trichomonas infection will not harm your baby. Some concern always exists that any severe vaginal infection might irritate amniotic membranes and cause premature rupture of these membranes, so it is best that you receive treatment after your first three months of pregnancy.

I had one outbreak of genital herpes before I met my husband. I never told him about it, and I would like to keep this confidential. Must I tell my obstetrician?

It is critical that you tell your obstetrician. If genital herpes is undetected, it can have devastating effects on your newborn. Herpes virus can remain in remission for years and suddenly exacerbate. Pregnancy is one time this often happens. If you and your doctor do not recognize an outbreak and your membranes rupture, your baby can develop a life-threatening infection. During pregnancy, your body is stressed and immunologically weakened, and your doctor might want to place you on an antiviral medication during your last month of pregnancy to prevent an outbreak (see page 153).

I had vaginal irritation and my doctor detected *Hemophilus vaginalis*. Is this serious?

Bacterial vaginosis is caused by a group of bacteria that, if permitted to remain in a woman's vagina, may cause premature labor and premature rupture of her membranes. These bacteria are often termed *Hemophilus vaginalis, Gardnerella vaginalis,* and *Corynebacterium vaginalis.* They are very common infections, and 10 to 25 percent of all women have had one of them, presenting as a thin, gray, irritating vaginal discharge with a fishy or ammonia-type odor. After you have completed your first three months of pregnancy, your doctor may treat you with oral or vaginal antibiotics, metronidazole, or Flagyl, and may treat your husband, too.

I was treated for chlamydia. Could this affect my baby?

Chlamydia is not dangerous to a fetus during early pregnancy but may cause a problem if present during delivery. As it does not pass the placenta, it does not affect a baby in the uterus. Once a woman's membranes rupture, however, and a baby contacts chlamydia-containing vaginal fluid, it may develop conjunctivitis and scarring of its corneas. Chlamydia infections are common throughout the world, and in third world countries, where eyedrops are not routinely available for newborns after birth, affected newborns may develop severe scarring of their eyes, leading to blindness.

I may have had contact with gonorrhea. Is treatment dangerous during my pregnancy?

During your pregnancy, the treatment is not dangerous, nor is the disease. At delivery, however, it can cause conjunctivitis and serious scarring of the baby's corneas. If you test positive for this infection, the laboratory obtaining the positive test must report these results to the state. Health care workers will contact you to determine from whom you contracted this infection so that treatment can be given to all potentially infected individuals.

Can I use a douche? I am using a douche regularly, and I feel unclean without it.

You should *never* douche while you're pregnant. Years back, when women used to douche more often, some women lost their pregnancies and, in some cases, their lives as a result. The long probe used to douche is dangerous because it can reach as far as the cervix and cause a miscarriage. Also, when douche water is pushed into the vagina with pressure, it can go through the cervix and flow between the placenta and the inner uterine wall, which causes the placenta to separate. This separation, called "placental abruption," cuts off the baby's blood and oxygen supply. When oxygen supply is disrupted, a fetus cannot survive. In other cases, air can be pushed into the uterus with the douche water. The air forms a bubble that travels through the large veins in the uterus and the bloodstream, where it lands in the pulmonary blood vessels. This causes a pulmonary embolism, which can be, and has been, lethal.

If you wish to feel clean internally, the safest thing to do is just relax in a medium-temperature warm bath and let the water gradually rinse your vaginal region and cleanse the area naturally.

I am prone to bladder infections. People have advised me to drink cranberry juice to prevent these infections. Will this work?

If you are prone to develop bladder infections, you may be even more susceptible to them during your pregnancy. There are several things you can do to help prevent these infections. Drinking cranberry juice may help you rid yourself of the infection and may eliminate the need for you to take antibiotics. There is a component within cranberries that prevents bacteria, particularly *E. coli,* from adhering to your bladder wall. When these bacteria cannot attach to your bladder, they cannot grow, and you flush them out in your urine. Mixed-cranberry drinks, such as cranberry-apple juice, are not as effective, so please drink 100 percent cranberry juice or take cranberry tablets. You should also try to drink at least eight glasses of liquid daily to flush yourself out.

> *I eat little dried cranberries for just this purpose. I mix them with walnuts to combat their tart taste. Do not look for dried cranberries around Thanksgiving season—they are nowhere to be found!*

CHAPTER 5

Your Third Month

You have less energy now
and will want to rest more often.
You will wonder how this tiny fetus can have such
a strong effect on you.

This is all part of nature's plan.
Your body is exhausted,
and you must give it the relaxation it needs.
But you will realize that this quiet time is a gift.
It is a time for you to be excited, contemplative, and creative.
You are craving information and answers
about your life and the life of the baby within you.

During your peaceful moments,
nature is giving you the time you need to think about your pregnancy.
You will reflect so often about this tiny child
and your role as its mother.

And you will question,
Am I really giving my baby the health it needs?
Will all of my tests be normal?
Can I safely exercise, move, and even dance for joy?
Can I eat what I wish to eat?
Will my body change forever?

Will my husband still love me later?
Will I be a good mother?

There are so many questions,
and your biggest question is:

How will I know what is right for my baby?

You will just know.
You have been given the common sense
and the instinct
to best care for this new life.

What is right for other children or other mothers
is not necessarily right for your baby or for you.

Simple love will tell you what is best.
And with this love,
all of your choices
will be the right ones.

YOUR BABY DURING THE THIRD MONTH

- ◆ Your baby will grow from 2 inches to 4 inches from its crown to the bottom of its torso.
- ◆ Its weight will increase from 1 to 3 ounces.
- ◆ Its muscles are strengthening, so it will move around more.
- ◆ Its skin is almost transparent.
- ◆ A tiny nose and lips are developing.
- ◆ All of its internal organs are growing and maturing.
- ◆ Eyelids have started to form.
- ◆ Its little ribs and backbone are developing, but they are very soft.

Your twelfth week through your sixteenth week is your third month of pregnancy. This is your baby at twelve weeks.

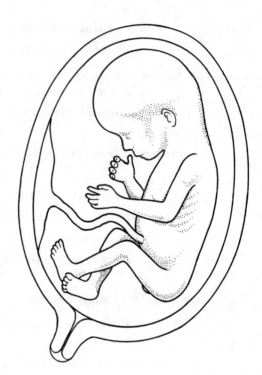

- Its neck will grow longer so the head no longer sits on the chest.
- Its ears move forward from the side of the head toward its face.
- The inner ears begin forming.
- Its fingers and toes start to develop tiny nails.
- Hair starts to grow.
- Calcium will begin to deposit in its bones.
- Its head is still quite large.

CHANGES YOU MAY NOTICE IN YOURSELF THIS MONTH

You will still be experiencing many of the changes of your prior months, plus the following:

- Your uterus will expand halfway between your pubic bone and your navel.

- You may need to start wearing maternity clothes.

- You may notice red, spidery-type skin lesions, called "telangiectasia," on your face, arms, and legs. These may appear as red branching spider lesions under the skin.

- You may develop dark pigment blotches on your forehead, upper lip, and the sides of your cheeks. These are "chloasma," often called the "pregnancy mask."

- Your palms may appear red.

- The skin on your abdomen, breasts, hips, and buttocks may begin to show stretch marks.

- You may develop skin tags on your neck and under your breasts.

- Your skin moles may become darker and larger—your doctor should examine these.

- Your breasts have become heavier, so you may need new bras.

- Your nipples and the surrounding areolae may become darker in pigment.

- Your breasts will continue to feel tingling and soreness.

- A pigmented line may become apparent down the middle of your abdomen. This is called the "linea nigra."

- The refraction of your eye lenses may change, making it difficult for you to see as clearly as you did before.

- You may start to feel the fluttering of fetal movement by the end of this month.

- It will become easier for your doctor to hear your baby's heart with a Doppler.

EXERCISE DURING PREGNANCY

I feel so much better when I exercise, but I do not want to do anything that will hurt my baby. My doctor says I am very healthy. Is it really safe for me to exercise?

The American College of Obstetricians and Gynecologists states that there has been no demonstrated increase in birth defects among pregnancies of women who continue to perform even vigorous exercise during early pregnancy. If you are the average pregnant woman, exercise is not only safe for you, it is healthier. According to the ACOG, there is no data in humans to indicate that a healthy pregnant woman should limit her exercise intensity or should need to worry about the rapidity of her heart rate. If your doctor believes you and your baby are healthy, you can continue exercising at your own pace, you do *not* have to be concerned about your heart rate, and you don't have to worry that you're hurting your baby.

The American College of Obstetricians and Gynecologists provides these recommendations about exercise during pregnancy:

1. Regular exercise (three times a week) is better than sporadic exercise.

2. After your first three months of pregnancy, don't lie on your back while exercising. Your uterus may press on the blood vessels bringing blood back from your legs to your heart and could decrease blood flow to your baby.

3. When doing aerobic exercise, don't push to the point of exhaustion.

4. When doing weight lifting, don't hold your breath. Use slow, controlled movements with small sets.

5. When using the treadmill, remember that your balance may be off, especially during your last three months of pregnancy, so be careful not to fall.

6. When using exercise machines, avoid direct trauma to your abdomen.

7. Make sure you increase your food intake while exercising, because you're burning more calories.

8. Make sure your environment is healthy, drink enough liquids, wear clothing that lets you perspire, and make sure the room in which you are exercising is not too warm.

9. After you deliver, you can phase back into your exercise program gradually over four to six weeks.

Although random individuals often tell pregnant women not to permit their heart rates to elevate above 140 beats per minute, the ACOG does not feel the rate of a woman's heartbeat will affect her baby's health whatsoever.

> *In my years of practice, I often noticed that those individuals who tell pregnant women not to exercise during pregnancy have never exercised themselves.*

What is happening to my baby when I exercise?

Various physiological changes occur in pregnant women during exercise. Certain positions will affect the blood flow to your uterus, your breathing pattern will change, your balance might be off, your joints and ligaments become looser, your body will regulate its temperature differently, and your metabolism will function differently.

The blood flow to your uterus changes while you exercise. During your first three months and your last three months of pregnancy, blood flow to your uterus may decrease when you lie on your back. This flow will increase again if you lie on either your right side or your left side. Try to avoid exercises that require you to lie flat on your back. When you stand still, you may actually cause the greatest decrease in blood flow back to your baby. If you need to stand still for long periods of time, keep moving your legs as though you are marching in place.

Your breathing patterns during exercise also change. Now that you are pregnant, you have a greater need for oxygen, *even at rest.* So unless you are very fit, there is less oxygen available for you to do aerobic exercise. Please do not start a rigorous exercise program now. You can continue the exercises you are used to doing, and if you wish to increase the intensity, please do so gradually.

As your uterus expands, your balance and your center of gravity may be off, which may cause you to fall forward. Be careful while you are exercising that you do not fall, especially on your stomach.

Your joints and ligaments may be looser and more prone to injury during your pregnancy. However, the only joints that have been proven to be more susceptible to injury during pregnancy are those in the hands. In any case, it is best to practice caution when performing exercises (like jogging or weight lifting) that may strain your joints.

Before you were pregnant, exercise would raise your body temperature. Now, however, your inner body temperature will not change when

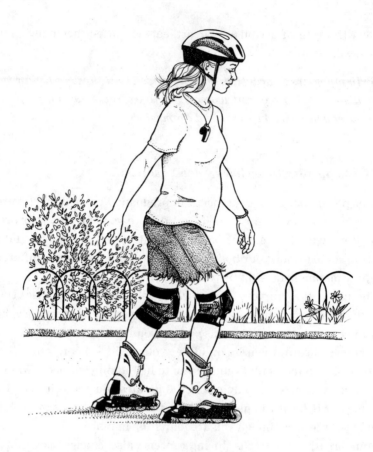

you exercise. Many studies have shown that your body experiences maternal adaptation to pregnancy. This means that although you may feel warm while you are exercising, the inner parts of your body remain cool, to protect your baby from heat. This is important, because body temperatures over 102.2 degrees due to fevers early in pregnancy have been shown to cause neurological problems in newborns.

When you are pregnant, you use more carbohydrates during exercise. Make sure your diet includes extra carbohydrates so you will have enough energy while you are exercising. If you feel weak or faint while you are exercising, it is a sign that your baby needs more fuel.

Will my baby's body be affected by my exercising?

Your baby's heart rate may increase five to fifteen beats per minute during vigorous aerobic exercise, but this has not been shown to cause any health problems for unborn babies. If you exercise strenuously, your baby may be born with less fat tissue. Otherwise, studies show that regular, healthy exercise does not put your baby at any risk.

SAFETY TIPS BEFORE YOU BEGIN

- When you exercise, always use caution. You do not want to overextend yourself or take unnecessary risks.
- If you start to feel uncomfortable, slow your pace or take a break. "No pain, no gain" is not your motto now.
- Taking your hands off your exercise machine to check your heart rate may cause you to lose your balance and fall. If you are concerned about its rapid rate, stop moving before you check it.
- Do not let yourself get out of breath. If you cannot talk while exercising, you need to slow down.
- Drink liquids if you feel dehydrated.
- Enjoy your exercise.
- Feel positive that your exercise is helping your baby and you.

In what instances should I avoid exercise?

It will be necessary to avoid exercise if you have signs of premature labor or contractions, premature rupture of your membranes, an incompetent cervix, vaginal bleeding, signs of poor growth in your baby, or medical problems such as hypertension, thyroid disease, heart disease, or lung disease. Please discuss with your doctor the kind of exercise you want to do, and based on your medical status, he will know what is safest for you.

> *A patient of mine ran in a marathon. She did not tell anyone she was pregnant and started bleeding and cramping after the race. She miscarried. We will never know if she was destined to miscarry or if the race was too strenuous for her.*

Rigorous exercise tests your physical strength, so be careful not to undertake any exercise that will put your baby's survival to the test. If you experience shortness of breath, dizziness or faintness, chest pain, an irregular heart rate or palpitations, pelvic pain, uterine contractions, or any bleeding or gush of fluid from your vagina, stop exercising and consult your doctor.

Safe Exercise for Baby and You

What type of exercise should I do now that I am pregnant?

That depends upon what you did before you were pregnant and what you would like to do now. Walking is wonderful exercise, so if you were not terribly active before, walking is a good way to begin. Try going for a brisk half-hour walk every other day. Yoga is very effective in building strength and balance. Do not let the slowness of the motions mislead you; yoga is a very healthy workout. Golf is a great sport, mostly because it involves a lot of walking. When you are standing at each hole, however, make sure you march in place to keep your blood flowing. Swimming is a good, safe exercise, but diving is out. You can swim throughout your pregnancy, but as you come close to your due date, discuss with your doctor whether it will be safe for you to be in the pool when your water breaks.

Bicycle riding is fine until you are three months pregnant. After that, consider using a stationary bicycle. If you fall on a moving bicycle, the handlebars will hit your uterus. Aerobics will be good exercise, too, if you follow a tape or class that is low impact. Higher-intensity workouts may push you too hard. Jogging is more strenuous on your body, but it is fine to continue during pregnancy if you keep to a lower-level pace. You'll be able to pick up your regular pace again once your pregnancy is over. If you play tennis, try playing doubles; with a partner you won't need to work as hard, but you will still get a good workout. When you train with weights, use slow, steady movements, do fewer repetitions, and make sure you breathe.

If you ski, be careful not to fall, and consider cross-country skiing instead of downhill. You may feel short of breath in the mountains because the air is thinner the higher you go, so try to avoid skiing at very high altitudes. I have had pregnant patients sustain leg injuries while skiing at remote mountain resorts, and obtaining proper medical care, especially in a foreign country, can be difficult. Please use good judgment when you undertake any potentially dangerous sport, as you will have many other years to advance your skills.

Exercises to Avoid

Are there any sports that I should not do?

Yes. You will be much safer if you stay away from scuba diving, water skiing, surfing, and any other sport that might qualify as "extreme." The appeal of these sports is often the risk factor. Now is not the time to start adventurous exercise, so try to stick to your regular routine.

Exercise will bring you much enjoyment, good health, and relaxation during your pregnancy. You may need to be more careful now, but I encourage you to keep exercise as part of your healthy lifestyle—it can be very rewarding for you as your pregnancy progresses.

DENTAL HEALTH

Will my teeth develop more cavities because I do not eat dairy products or because so much of my calcium will be going to my baby?

Your vegan diet will not make you more likely to develop cavities. Contrary to what most of us have been taught, cavities are not caused by a diet low in dairy products, they are caused by bacteria called *Streptococcus mutans* and *Streptococcus sobrinus*. A diet high in sweets supports the growth of these bacteria and thereby contributes to the bacteria-causing decay. In no other respect is the incidence of cavities related to diet. Whether your diet is vegetarian or carnivorous or whether or not you eat dairy has nothing to do with having healthy teeth.

If you have many cavities, there are some measures you can take to prevent your children from experiencing the same fate. First, feed them a healthy vegan diet, do not feed them with your utensils to avoid spread of bacteria, and encourage them to brush their teeth with fluoride toothpaste. Then limit their consumption of refined sugars and sugar-containing beverages.

My gums have become swollen, and my teeth feel looser. Am I going to lose my teeth? What is happening?

Please discuss this with your dentist. You may have an inflammation that requires treatment with antibiotics. If that is not the case, then you probably just have gingivitis of pregnancy. This will not cause your teeth to fall out. There is an old wives' tale that a woman loses a tooth for every pregnancy, but there is little truth to that. The dentist will ask you to floss more often to stimulate your gums and recommend that you gargle several times a day with slightly salted water to toughen your gums. Gingivitis during pregnancy may be very uncomfortable for you, but it will not make you lose your teeth and will resolve shortly after you deliver.

When I brush my teeth, my gums are bleeding. Is this happening because I am pregnant?

It may be: bleeding gums are common during pregnancy. The surface lining of your gums, the epithelium, becomes thinner during pregnancy, and the underlying tissues become swollen and filled with blood vessels. Together, these two changes will cause bleeding even when your gums are touched lightly. The swelling also leads to increased sensitivity. The bleeding may be an indication of a bleeding disorder, related or not related to your pregnancy. If you have an inflammation of your gums, this may also be a cause of bleeding. To narrow down the specific cause in your situation, it will be necessary for you to discuss the problem with your obstetrician. She will perform blood tests to evaluate your blood-clotting factors and your blood-clotting cells, called "platelets." She will also test your blood and urine for toxemia of pregnancy. If all of these tests show that you are normal, she will refer you to your dentist for an exam. You may need to use a softer brush until you deliver and your gums regain their usual strength.

I have a soft, swollen lump on my gum. The doctor said it is just a "pregnancy tumor" that will go away after my pregnancy. What causes this to develop?

No one knows why this kind of growth, called an "epulis," develops during pregnancy, and no one knows why it resolves after pregnancy. These tumors are soft, tender, swollen growths that sometimes grow to an inch in size. They may begin growing anytime during a pregnancy and generally shrink and disappear within the month after delivery. They usually appear pink or red, because they contain a large number of blood vessels, and can bleed profusely. It will bother you during your pregnancy because it will get in the way when you try to eat, may be painful, and may bleed. You may need to eat softer foods so as not to irritate it.

I need to have dental work done. What kinds of anesthesia will be safe for me?

You should try to avoid chemicals that will affect your entire body, such as nitrous oxide, unless you have no other options. When you receive nitrous oxide, or laughing gas, every cell in your body will be affected by it. Nitrous oxide has a systemic effect, meaning that the effect penetrates your entire body and every cell in your baby's body. If you receive Novocain, it will affect only your tooth region. If you are not allergic to Novocain, this is the medication you should choose.

When I had Novocain before, I developed a rapid heartbeat. Do you think I should have Novocain again, or should I try to have the work done without any medication?

That depends on your pain threshold and the extent of work you need. Less medication is always best. If you believe you will need medication, ask your dentist for Novocain without epinephrine. It is possible that when you felt that rapid heartbeat, it was from the epinephrine and not from the Novocain. If epinephrine entered small blood vessels in your gum, it would have gone to your heart and caused the rapid heart rate. Most pain medications for local injection are manufactured with or without epinephrine. Epinephrine may be beneficial if you are having a tooth pulled because it will help to decrease bleeding at the site. Unless your dentist thinks that you will have a large amount of bleeding, it is best that you take Novocain without epinephrine.

I was just at the dentist for treatment of a tooth abscess, and the dentist gave me an antibiotic. Is this safe to take?

That depends upon what the dentist gave you. If your dentist recommended an antibiotic, please ask him to confirm that it is safe for your pregnancy. You may need to check with your obstetrician as well about the specific antibiotic your dentist prescribed. Most antibiotics dentists prescribe are safe. These include antibiotics in the penicillin, Keflex, and erythromycin families. After the first three months of your pregnancy, tetracycline antibiotics should not be used because they can cause discoloration of your baby's teeth and problems with the growth of your baby's bones. If you do not use an antibiotic, your tooth abscess may not resolve on its own and you may end up with a more serious abscess requiring stronger antibiotics and hospitalization. It is best to take the antibiotic now when only a small dose is needed.

HYPOGLYCEMIA

I am hypoglycemic. Will my vegetarian diet make my condition more difficult to control during pregnancy?

A well-balanced vegetarian diet should not worsen your condition. The key to preventing hypoglycemia is for you to maintain a high level of fat and protein in your diet. Here is an example of how your cycle of hypoglycemia might perpetuate itself:

- You awaken in the morning and eat refined sugars, such as a doughnut.

- Your pancreas produces a surge of insulin to digest the carbohydrates from your doughnut.

- Your pancreas then oversurges and produces too much insulin.

- An hour or two later, you are hypoglycemic. You feel weak, you tremble, and you crave more sugar desperately. Your body produced too much insulin, and now your blood sugar is too low. You will instinctively eat more sugar because you will feel better immediately. Your oversurge of insulin is now balanced with the new sugar.

- Two hours later, however, you'll be hypoglycemic again owing to a repeat oversurge of insulin.

As a vegetarian, you can use several techniques to prevent yourself from getting into a hypoglycemic cycle. You can add foods that are high in fat or protein to your high-carbohydrate meal. Once a hypoglycemic cycle has occurred, you can break your cycle with foods that are high in fat or protein. It is best that you not eat high-carbohydrate meals. For example, when you eat apples, also eat cheese or tofu cheese; when you eat bananas, also eat natural peanut butter; when you eat pastry, also eat walnuts. It will be best for you to choose breakfasts that do not contain refined sugars, but instead eat toast with nut butter, an egg-white omelet with tomatoes, whole-grain pancakes with macadamia nuts, a tofu-and-egg omelet, or a bagel with tofu cheese.

There is no need for you to convert to a meat-based diet to prevent hypoglycemia. Many vegetarian foods have high levels of fats and protein and can help you avoid such a cycle. Basically, foods containing nuts, eggs, beans, tofu, and cheese are the best choices to eliminate hypoglycemia during your vegetarian pregnancy.

IF YOU HAVE FOOD INTOLERANCES

Lactose Intolerance

What is lactose, and what does it mean to be lactose intolerant?

Lactose is a sugar present in milk and other dairy products. Some people are born without the enzyme to digest the milk sugar known as lactose. Many people have this enzyme when they are younger but lose the capacity to produce it when they are adults.

If you are lactose intolerant, you will experience gas pains, diarrhea, vomiting, or severe abdominal pains when you eat dairy. Not every person is meant to drink milk, but you may be able to tolerate other dairy products. Lactose intolerance will not make you nutritionally deficient during your pregnancy as long as you are eating enough protein and calcium.

I am lactose intolerant and vegetarian, so I have no animal protein or dairy products in my diet. Will I be able to give my baby enough protein?

Yes, without a doubt. By being both lactose intolerant and vegetarian, you have almost become a vegan (although you may still eat eggs). Dairy products are not necessary for a healthy pregnancy. As a vegetarian who is lactose intolerant, you can obtain healthy and adequate amounts of protein from egg whites, tofu, soy products, beans, nuts, grains, and vegetables. The amount of proteins in these foods is more than enough for both you and your baby.

I am mildly lactose intolerant, but I like dairy products. What can I do to help my body digest dairy products now that I am pregnant?

As you are only mildly intolerant, you have many options to modify your body's absorption of lactose. You can take Lactaid during your pregnancy; it is considered safe. Lactaid helps your body digest lactose sugar in the absence of the lactose enzyme. You can also drink chocolate milk. Many people who are mildly lactose intolerant are surprised that they can tolerate chocolate milk. This is because chocolate helps the body to metabolize lactose more easily. If you drink small but frequent quantities of regular milk, rather than a large portion at one time, you may be better able to digest it. Try ¼ cup of milk per meal. To keep dairy in your diet, give different dairy products a try. Many people experience lactose intolerance with one dairy product but not with another. Trial and error is the only way you will know which products your body can tolerate.

Citrus Intolerance as a Vegetarian

My body cannot tolerate citrus fruit. As a vegetarian, will I still be able to obtain sufficient vitamin C for my baby?

Yes, you will just need to obtain it from a variety of sources. Vitamin C is found in citrus fruit, but it is also present in a variety of fruits and vegetables. There is no vitamin C in any foods that are derived directly or indirectly from animal sources. Vitamin C will be very important for you during your pregnancy because it is essential in the formation of collagen, the tissue your baby needs to create its skin, ligaments, cartilage, vertebral disks, and capillaries. It will also help fortify your immune response and protect you against bacterial, viral, and fungal infections (see page 98).

Fortunately, there are many noncitrus sources of vitamin C, including cherries, papaya, cantaloupe, and strawberries. The vegetable sources of vitamin C are red and green peppers (your best source), asparagus, broccoli, Brussels sprouts, cabbage, garlic, potatoes, parsley, sauerkraut, sprouts, tomatoes, and leafy green vegetables. You must remember that vitamin C is water-soluble, so much of it will be lost if you cook your vegetables in water. Therefore steam your vegetables in a double boiler, rather than boiling them directly in water. Also, if copper is present in your water or in your cookware, this will diminish the vitamin C in your food, so definitely do not boil vitamin-containing vegetables in copper-lined cookware. (Please read chapter 2 to learn more about vitamin C and its role in your healthy vegetarian diet.)

Gluten Intolerance as a Vegetarian

I have celiac disease, and I suffer from diarrhea whenever I eat wheat products. Will I be able to obtain adequate nutrition for both my baby and myself on a vegetarian diet?

Maintaining a gluten-free diet will always be a challenge for you, particularly because the American diet relies so heavily on wheat. In many ways, however, a vegetarian diet favors a gluten-free diet. Though you are not able to eat any grains that contain gluten (such as wheat, oats, barley, and rye), there are many nongluten grains—including corn, rice, buckwheat, and millet—that you can eat. These are easy to incorporate in a vegetarian diet, and you can pair them with so many other healthy vegetarian foods: all fruits, vegetables, nuts and seeds, and dairy and egg products. The possibilities are endless.

You will undoubtedly find it difficult to eat out in restaurants, since wheat-based fillers are added to many other foods and sauces. To avoid triggering your gluten intolerance, try eating at restaurants that serve Asian, Indian, Middle Eastern, or Latino cuisine. These types of foods are often healthier and offer a wider array of both vegetarian options and grains.

As a pregnant vegetarian with gluten intolerance, you should follow medical guidelines and eliminate wheat, oats, barley, and rye from your diet. This is critical, because almost 50 percent of women with celiac disease who did not watch their diets during pregnancy experienced complications. These include anemia, a higher miscarriage rate, a higher incidence of low-birth-weight infants, and a higher risk of having a newborn with intrauterine growth retardation.

NOTE ON NUTRITION: PEANUTS AND TOXINS

As a vegetarian, I obtain much of my protein from peanut butter, but I recently found out that peanuts contain a toxin. Should I stop eating peanuts?

It is true that peanuts contain a toxin, so it will be better for you to vary the nuts you eat and limit your intake of peanuts. You do not need to give them up entirely. Aflatoxin is a mold that grows on the surface of peanuts and has been shown to be toxic and lead to liver cancer. Aflatoxin contaminates peanuts and, to a lesser degree, corn and several other plant foods. This contaminant is present on both domestic and imported peanut products and cannot be eliminated entirely from these food sources. If you buy a bag of peanuts in their shells, you can actually see this mold on the peanut shells—but you cannot see it in the peanut butter. Although this toxin is known only to cause cancer, and not to cause birth defects, it is best to decrease the quantities of any toxin in your diet.

Medical studies have shown that vegetarians ingest a higher quantity of this cancer-causing mold. One study showed blood levels of 62 percent in vegetarians compared to 22 percent in non-vegetarians. It is common practice for many vegetarians to eat larger quantities of peanut butter and peanuts than non-vegetarians. You should rotate your intake of nut spreads; try replacing peanut butter with other nut butters made from pecans, almonds, and pistachios.

Why are peanuts the only nuts with high levels of this toxin?

Peanuts are the only nuts that are not true nuts. Other nuts are really a one-seeded fruit. They grow on trees and contain the seeds for a new plant. Most true nuts have a woody shell and are protected from the environment. Peanuts are beans containing seeds in a pod. The peanut plant grows close to the soil and burrows stalks into the soil, so the peanuts themselves grow under the ground. At that location, they are subject to attack by fungus and mold.

AN OUNCE OF PREVENTION: GENETIC DISEASE SCREENING

I have heard there are hereditary diseases that parents can unknowingly pass on to their children. How do I know if I have any of these?

Each of us has thousands of ancestral genetic traits. Both you and your husband give one set of these traits to your children. If both you and your husband carry a genetic trait for a disease, this will create a one in four chance that your children may actually develop the disease. Various ethnic and racial groups carry genes for specific diseases.

Sickle-Cell Anemia

If you are of African American descent, there is a one in ten chance that you carry the sickle-cell trait. If both you and your husband carry this trait, there is a one in four chance that your child may have the disease. The actual disease causes red blood cells to elongate into a "sickle" shape. These sickled red blood cells obstruct blood vessels, which causes anemia and great pain. A simple blood test can detect if you carry the trait for sickle-cell disease.

If you are of African, South Indian, or Middle Eastern descent, you should be tested to see if you are a carrier for the sickle-cell trait. The sickle-cell trait is often present in people whose ancestors came from countries where malaria was present. Individuals with the sickle-cell trait have resistance to malaria and over the centuries have had better survival rates in tropical countries.

Cystic Fibrosis

One in twenty-five people of northern European and Ashkenazic Jewish ancestry carry the trait for cystic fibrosis. Your child must receive the trait from both your husband and you to develop the disease, which causes a buildup of thick mucus in the lungs and other organs.

Spina Bifida

Spina bifida is a multifactorial disease. This means that some people are more prone to inherit and develop this disease, but other factors can modify that risk. Spina bifida is most common among individuals of Irish and English descent (see page 51). A diet rich in folic acid can help prevent its occurrence (see page 90). Your doctor will check your blood between your sixteenth and twentieth weeks of pregnancy to see if your baby has spina bifida.

Mediterranean Anemia

This disease is also known as thalassemia or Cooley's anemia. It is most common among individuals of Italian, Greek, Chinese, or Filipino descent. If you carry the gene for this disease, your red blood cells will be small and will not be able to hold as much iron as the average person's red blood cell. You will always be anemic. If your child inherits the trait from both you and your husband, the illness may be very severe.

I am vegetarian, and I carry the trait for thalassemia. I have been told not to take iron because my tiny red blood cells cannot retain iron. Now that I am pregnant, my doctor is advising me to take iron. Will this help to raise my iron levels?

Usually, an individual with thalassemia should not take extra iron. Because of your condition, it is normal for you to have a lower blood count than a person without thalassemia. Your hemoglobin level of 10 grams is as healthy for you as a level of 12 to 14 grams is for most other people.

Since your tiny red blood cells cannot accommodate much iron, excess is diverted to your liver, where it can cause scarring and cirrhosis. When you're pregnant, however, your situation changes and it will be best for you to supplement your diet with iron tablets. You may not need the iron, but your baby and its placenta definitely do. Also, you need to prepare for blood loss at delivery when your placenta separates. The typical dose for supplements is one or two tablets of 32 milligrams of elemental iron daily.

Your physician will prescribe the correct dose for you. She will also have your husband's blood evaluated to see if he is a carrier of thalassemia. If both of you were to pass the thalassemia trait to a child, a more serious form of the disease could develop. Vegetarians frequently have lower hemoglobin counts to begin with because their diets contain less iron. This is one time it will be good for you to increase your hemoglobin level by taking iron supplements and eating iron-rich vegetarian foods before you or your baby develop a serious case of anemia (see page 119).

Jewish Genetic Diseases

Even if only one of your ancestors was Jewish, you should be tested for this group of diseases. Regardless of what your religious beliefs are, you still carry the genetic traits of your ancestors.

Gaucher's Disease: Children receiving this trait from both parents collect a fatty material in their liver, spleen, bone marrow, and brain.

Cystic Fibrosis: People of Ashkenazic Jewish ancestry have a higher chance of carrying the trait for this disease, in which dangerously thick mucus builds up in the lungs.

Tay-Sachs Disease: Children receiving this trait from both parents build up chemicals within their nervous system that lead to blindness, paralysis, and eventually death at a very young age.

Canavan Disease: Children who receive this trait from both parents usually die in infancy due to spongy degeneration of the brain.

Niemann-Pick Disease: Children receiving this trait from both parents usually die by two years of age due to the buildup of a chemical called "sphingomyelin" in their brain.

More than 95 percent of Jewish people who subsequently have a child with one of these diseases had no prior family history. When in doubt about your ethnic heritage, it is better to have yourself checked.

$\mathcal{Y}$our Fourth Month

An ancient Oriental proverb tells us,
"To gain control,
one must first lose it."

Pregnancy epitomizes this.
You have lost control of life as you knew it before,
and you may be struggling to understand the meaning
of your new life.

Why did nature make pregnancy so difficult?
You might ask,
Am I bad for feeling so critical and
frustrated at times?
You might wonder,
Is it all worth it?

Until the moment you first hold your child to your heart,
you will continue to search for these answers.

When you hold your baby,
You will recognize how special and sacred
your journey has been.
And all of your questions will be answered.

Your pregnancy will have been
the smallest price to pay
for life's greatest gift.

YOUR BABY DURING THE FOURTH MONTH

- The length of your baby from the top of its head to the bottom of its buttocks will increase from 4 inches to 6 inches.
- Your tiny baby weighs 3 to 9 ounces.
- It has downy hair called "lanugo" over its head and body.
- It assumes more of an adult shape.
- Your baby looks like a small human being with a large head.
- It moves its arms and legs frequently and purposefully.
- All the joints in its limbs (elbows and knees) can move.
- Its heart chambers are completely formed.
- Tiny eyebrows and eyelashes have formed.
- Its fingers and toes have differentiated into their three bending joints.
- Its fingernails are well formed.
- Its external genitalia have developed, and you can tell if it is male or female.
- You can feel it move!

CHANGES YOU MAY NOTICE IN YOURSELF THIS MONTH

You may experience all of the changes from your prior months, plus the following:

- Your uterus will move from midway between your pubic bone and your navel all the way up to your navel.

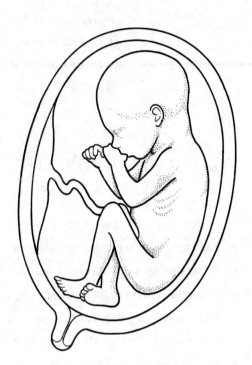

Your sixteenth week through your twentieth week is your fourth month of pregnancy. This is your baby at sixteen weeks.

- ◆ As your uterus is attached at its lower portion, the upper portion of your uterus may tilt slightly.

- ◆ Round ligaments from the sides of your pubic bone to the upper sides of your uterus may stretch and create a pulling sensation.

- ◆ Your vaginal discharge will increase.

- ◆ Gastritis and heartburn may increase.

- ◆ Your enlarged uterus may press on your sciatic nerve (located on the back wall of the pelvis) and cause shooting pains to radiate down the back of one or both of your legs.

- ◆ Varicose veins in your legs may enlarge and cause pain.

- ◆ More significant weight gain will begin.

- ◆ Sudden cramps may occur in the calf muscles of your legs.

UTERINE CHANGES

How large will my uterus be now?

Your sixteenth week is an important landmark. The top of your uterus will be midway between the top of your pubic bone and your navel. Your uterus will be up high enough for you to feel it—and for you to need new jeans. If you are in between your normal clothes and maternity clothes, a rubber band will help to hold your unbuttoned pants together.

I have a pulling sensation from the bottom part of my navel down to my pubic bone. Whenever I move, I feel it. Is this my uterus?

Most likely your urachus is pulling. Your urachus is a membrane that extends from your navel down to your pubic bone. This is a remnant from

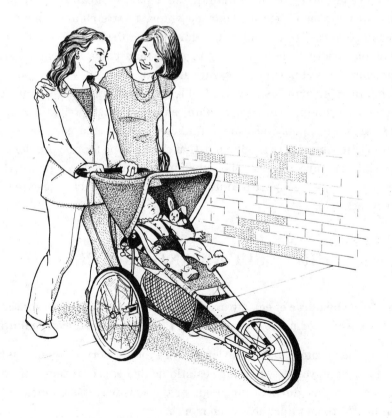

the days you were a fetus inside your mother. When you were a fetus, this extended from your bladder to your umbilical cord. As your abdominal wall is stretching during your pregnancy, your scarred and fibrotic urachus is pulling and will not give up without a fight. There is no danger from this. Eventually it will stretch out and will not harm your pregnancy.

My large uterus is putting a lot of pressure on my body. I find it difficult to move around and even to eat. Is this normal?

Yes, it is. Being pregnant is a profound, overwhelming, and humbling experience, more so than any of us would have imagined. As your uterus grows, loops of your intestines must be displaced from their usual locations and splayed to the right, the left, and the top of your uterus. Your intestines are attached to your body on the back wall of your abdomen by thin membranes, called "mesentery," which contain its blood supply. A woman's mesentery is longer than that of a man, so it can adapt to pregnancy. It is no small feat for your mesentery to stretch and your intestines to compress to the sides. In addition, the tissue and skin of your abdominal wall will be stretching to more than twice its original size. Your sensations of pain and pressure are justified.

In future pregnancies, you will feel less discomfort because your skin and your mesentery will stretch more easily. Although pregnant women try to act stoic, almost all women find carrying an enlarged uterus immensely difficult. There is not much that can be done for this problem because it is a natural physical phenomenon. You will need to cope with the pressure and just feel positive knowing that all of these changes are normal events.

URINE SUGAR AND PROTEIN

Why must the nurse check my urine sugar and protein every month? If my tests were normal last month, won't they be normal every month?

Even if your protein and sugar levels were totally normal when you became pregnant, you may develop gestational diabetes or toxemia of pregnancy at any time during your pregnancy. This is why it is important for your doctor to monitor these each month.

SUGAR

♦ Diabetes of pregnancy, called "gestational diabetes," may arise during the second half of pregnancy. If you develop this condition, there will be too much sugar in your blood, which will then spill out into your urine. This can be detected with a simple urine dipstick test.

♦ Decreasing sugars and calories in your diet may be all you need to do to return your sugar levels to normal.

PROTEIN LEVELS

♦ Toxemia of pregnancy may develop during the second half of pregnancy. If you start to develop toxemia, your body will not hold on to its protein, which will spill out into your urine.

♦ Simply resting can often control toxemia, but your doctor will have to monitor you and your baby very closely. Testing your urine for protein will help her gauge your health.

It is not uncommon for a pregnant woman to have small amounts of sugar, protein, or both in her urine. Do not panic if you have traces of either. Your doctor will consider many pieces of your individual health puzzle to form a complete picture. One test by itself is not cause for alarm.

THE VEGETARIAN WITH TWINS

I am carrying twins, and I am a strict vegan. Has the safety of a vegetarian diet been studied for women carrying twins?

Vegetarian nutrition in mothers of twins has been studied and has proven to be both adequate and healthy. Three percent of all pregnancies are twins, triplets, or a higher order of births. When women have assisted reproductive technologies performed to help them conceive, the rate of twin deliveries increases to 25 to 30 percent; triplets account for 5 percent of deliveries in this group of women. There are steps you can take to ensure your vegetarian diet provides adequate nutrition for your babies.

- Increase your total caloric intake so that you are consuming 300 more calories daily than you would if you were carrying a single pregnancy.

- Take iron supplements. Your body will need enough iron for yourself, two infants, and two placentas. Depending upon your initial blood count, you will probably need one or two 32-milligram elemental iron supplements daily. You should also have your doctor repetitively monitor your blood count for anemia.

- Increase your daily folic acid from 400 micrograms to 1 milligram.

- Maintain a healthy diet of fruits, vegetables, beans, grains, nuts, and tofu. You will not have a problem giving your babies all the vitamins they need.

IF YOU ARE STILL EATING MEAT OR FISH

I am in the process of becoming vegetarian, and I eat meat only once a week. What are the potential risks of adding some meat in my diet?

Since you are making a transition to a vegetarian diet, you already may have an idea of the health disadvantages of a meat-based diet. I'll discuss these here. Some are worse than others, but I hope this overview will help you decide how to shape your new vegetarian diet. Non-vegetarian potential problems include nitrites in meats, pesticides in meats, viral infections in meats, parasites in meats, cholesterol in meats, lack of fiber in meats, and weight gain from meats.

Nitrites

Nitrites are chemicals placed in certain meats when they are packaged to keep the muscle in the meat looking red. They are found in bacon and other cured meats such as ham, luncheon meats, bologna, frankfurters, meat pâté, and corned beef. Studies in humans and animals have shown that nitrites cause several kinds of cancer. Although there are no studies concerning nitrites and the development of cancer in pregnant women, I would suggest that you avoid these foods in pregnancy. It's best not to give your baby any chemicals that are potentially harmful to you.

Pesticides

Meat, chicken, and dairy products have more pesticides than any other food. Pesticides are originally sprayed on crops that animals eat. The animals store these pesticides in large quantities in their fat cells, where pesticides accumulate and remain for years. Meat and dairy products account for 60 to 85 percent of pesticides found in humans. You can wash pesticides off your lettuce, but you cannot remove them from the fat cells of your beef. If you are buying meat, try to choose products from organic or free-ranging farms.

Viral Infections

Mad cow disease (bovine spongiform encephalopathy) is a viral infection that spread in the meat supply of Europe, particularly in the United Kingdom, between 1995 and 1997. Over 160,000 cows contracted this disease because they were fed meat from infected sheep. At least twenty-five people in the United Kingdom and France contracted a similar human disorder, Creutzfeldt-Jacob disease, after eating beef infected with mad cow disease. This disease causes loss of coordination, jerking twitches, dementia, and eventually death. In the wake of this epidemic, the European Union now strictly regulates the feed given to animals. Still, before you purchase any beef, make sure you know where it comes from.

Parasites

There are three parasites found in undercooked pork that are a public health risk: trichinella, *Taenia solium,* and toxoplasmosis. Trichinella is a worm found in food sources—pork in 60 percent of the cases. It's usually found in sausage. *Taenia solium* is a pork tapeworm, often present in pigs in developing countries. With increased immigration, it has begun to surface in the United States more frequently. Toxoplasmosis is a parasite present in pork and can be passed to humans if the meat is not fully cooked. Eat pork products only if the meat is very well done.

Cholesterol

There is no cholesterol in any food that is not animal derived. The only foods containing cholesterol are meats, chicken, fish and shellfish, eggs, and dairy products. Studies have shown that vegetarians have mean blood cholesterol levels of 127 milligrams per deciliter, compared with mean cholesterol levels of 203 milligrams per deciliter in non-vegetarians. Thirty-five to 45 percent of the content of many types of meats is fat. These meats include steaks, ribs, pork chops, and ham. If you have high cholesterol, you can eat artichoke, avocado, beans, potatoes, and any other fruits or vegetables without raising your cholesterol.

Lack of Fiber

There is absolutely no fiber in any meat, chicken, fish, eggs, or dairy products. Pregnancy itself causes constipation. Evolution to a totally meat-free diet will help you increase your fiber intake and prevent this problem.

Higher Calories Contribute to Weight Gain

Vegetarians, on the average, weigh 10 percent less than their meat-eating peers. Studies show that when meat-eaters change to vegetarian diets, they lose an average of twelve to twenty-two pounds. If you are overweight or gaining too much weight and you want a healthy alternative, try switching to a diet rich in vegetables, fruits, grains, beans, and nuts.

I am trying to become vegetarian, but I eat fish. Should I avoid certain fish during pregnancy and nursing because of its mercury content?

People today have much higher levels of mercury in their bodies than their ancestors did. The Food and Drug Administration has advised pregnant and nursing women to exclude shark, swordfish, king mackerel, and tilefish from their diets. These fish contain high levels of methylmercury, a chemical that affects the developing nervous system of a fetus and young infant. The developing brain of an unborn child is very sensitive to mercury. A pregnant woman will have no signs of mercury toxicity, even though her fetus is being affected. Children exposed to mercury prior to birth have been shown to have an increased risk of developmental defects.

Mercury is present in various types of fish from both fresh and salt water. If you do eat fish, the FDA suggests you eat canned fish, smaller ocean fish, and fish that have been raised on farms. Larger fish like swordfish and shark have remarkably high mercury levels because they absorb mercury from the smaller fish they eat as well as from the seawater. If you eat tuna fish, it is best that you eat the canned type. Canned tuna fish contains much lower levels of methylmercury because the tuna used are smaller. Definitely, do not eat tuna in the form of steaks or any sushi because the fish used are larger and the levels of methylmercury within these larger tuna exceed the levels recommended by the FDA. Nevertheless, please do not eat canned tuna fish on a daily basis while pregnant or nursing. It is wise to rotate your fish sources so you are not eating only tuna.

Mercury contamination of many freshwater lakes has resulted in high levels of mercury in freshwater fish. The concentration of mercury is highest in catfish and other freshwater fish; large-size fish like swordfish, tuna, and sharks; and carnivorous, bottom-feeding fish.

The best way to check your mercury level is by hair testing. These levels have been shown to correlate with levels in your baby's umbilical cord. Studies of the hair of pregnant women have shown that levels as low as ten parts per million can affect fetal brain development.

If you want more information about fish and toxins, you can obtain it from the Environmental Protection Agency at www.epa.gov/ost/fish or the FDA at www.cfsan.fda.gov. Although fish is generally healthier for you than poultry or red meat, there are some medical disorders that you can develop from eating fish. These include toxoplasmosis, fish and shellfish poisoning, and worms.

Toxoplasmosis

In the United States, several thousand infants are born each year with congenital toxoplasmosis. Toxoplasmosis is a very serious illness if a mother contracts it either a year prior to becoming pregnant or during her pregnancy. If you are still eating fish, please eat it well-done and be sure the utensils you use are not the same ones that have been in contact with raw meat or fish. Toxoplasmosis can cause devastating brain damage in a newborn.

Fish and Shellfish Poisoning

Fish and shellfish receive toxins through the food chain from waterborne bacteria, viruses, and fungus. The toxin then moves up the food chain to humans. Fish and shellfish can tolerate high levels of toxins. These toxins cannot be detected by the appearance, smell, or color of the fish. When an unsuspecting woman eats fish or shellfish with a toxin, she may experience a variety of symptoms, depending on the specific toxin. The symptoms include diarrhea, gastroenteritis, paralysis, hives, and rashes. Numerous common fish and shellfish have been the agents in these poisonings, including tuna, bluefish, sardines, and mackerel. There are no specific studies concerning fish and shellfish poisoning in pregnancy. However, any type of infection you can avoid can only benefit your baby and yourself.

Fish Worms

There are many varieties of worms that women can contract by eating snails, crabs, and raw fish. When living in the human intestines, the worms will absorb all of the vitamin B_{12} that the mother has eaten. A mother will then be creating a vitamin B_{12} deficiency in her fetus. Cooking the contaminated fish and shellfish can kill many of these types of worms. If you are sitting at a sushi bar, do not permit the chef to cut your cooked vegetarian food with the same knife he used to cut raw fish.

WEIGHT WATCH

I already gained fourteen pounds during these first few months, and I am still hungry all the time. Have I lost the weight battle?

You have not lost the battle at all, and your rate of weight gain may suddenly decrease to a much less threatening level. Although much of the medical literature available suggests that you should not gain more than six pounds during your first three months of pregnancy, those are general guidelines and are definitely not applicable to every woman. Some women gain most of their weight initially, and some gain most at the end of pregnancy. Although only a small component of your weight gain up until this time has been for the growth of your uterus and baby, significant amounts may be attributed to changes in your breasts, as well as to fluid retention in your blood vessels and body tissues. Some weight, of course, may have gone to deposits in your fat tissues, but some of this was unavoidable, as most women gain four pounds of fat tissue by this time in their pregnancy anyway.

Try to evaluate your diet. If you have been craving foods like pickles, olives, salsa, spaghetti sauce, vinegar chips, or pickled beets and vegetables, you may be retaining large amounts of fluid. Although pickles and other heavily spiced foods may not be high in calories, they definitely are high in salt. By limiting your intake of these foods, you may notice a significant amount of fluid loss.

If you need to snack and nibble all the time to prevent nausea, please limit these snacks to raw vegetarian foods like crudités, apple wedges, sliced oranges, grapefruit, melon, bananas, rice cakes, dried fruits, and low-calorie protein bars (the high protein levels in the bars may actually help to suppress your appetite).

Please remember that each trimester of your pregnancy represents a total change in your appetite, nausea, organ growth, and fetal development. There is no reason to fear that this excessive weight gain will continue, and you will be doing the best you can for your baby if you focus on maintaining a healthy intake of nutrients, enriching your meals with fresh produce, and not worrying about your weight. It's hard to believe that extra weight is a positive thing, but this is absolutely true when it comes to pregnancy. Be good to yourself.

I travel frequently for my job. What should I look for when I eat in restaurants and hotels?

Foods in restaurants may be presalted or prespiced and may contain monosodium glutamate (MSG), which is a salt. Most chefs will be catering to individuals who do not have to worry about swelling, hypertension, or toxemia of pregnancy. It is simpler for you to ask that your meal be prepared without salt. Also, the chef may be concentrating all of his artistry in the meat portion of the menu, so don't be surprised if your vegetables come out boiled. These won't be very nutritious for you, since having been prepared this way, the vegetables will be depleted of all their B and C vitamins. Ask your server if you can have your vegetables steamed. If you snack on fresh fruits (such as grapes or apples) during the day, try to wash them to rinse off any pesticides before eating.

When you are not following your normal at-home routine, it's very easy to fall prey to convenience foods. Watch out especially for empty calories in the form of carbohydrates. If you are eating fried vegetables, try peeling off some of the batter. It has minimal nutritive value; all it does is fill you up and add calories. Salads may be prepared with large quantities of salad dressing, and similarly, your vegetables may be stir-fried in large amounts of oil. If your meal is very oily, just ask for an empty plate so you can take the food out of its oil bath and avoid consuming all that excess fat.

It can be difficult for you to get the nutrition you need if you are eating out all the time. Most restaurants try to accommodate vegetarians, but more often than not, you will feel protein deprived. Be prepared to discover that others, try as they may, may not understand how to prepare balanced vegetarian meals. To compensate for this, bring extra food rations with you on your trip, including protein bars, nut butters, and small boxes of high-protein cereal.

Should I eliminate Chinese food with MSG from my diet?

There has been much controversy surrounding MSG. MSG is a flavor enhancer that was originally extracted from molasses. Because some tests showed that MSG caused damage to the nerve cells of rats, it was banned from use in baby foods in 1969. It is not even possible to give a human being anywhere near the dose that was given to these rats. Medical studies in humans have shown that a baby can metabolize monosodium glutamate as well as you can and not have any side effects from it. No one has ever shown that MSG actually causes birth defects in humans.

Be that as it may, if you prefer, you can easily ask the staff in an Asian restaurant to eliminate MSG from your foods. If you had MSG before you knew you were pregnant, please do not worry at all. You can continue to eat your Chinese food, hopefully containing many stir-fried green, red, and yellow vegetables and tofu. During your pregnancy, if you start to retain fluids and swell, eliminate MSG with the same diligence with which you would eliminate salt.

> I always wondered why pregnant women were told not to eat foods containing MSG. There are two billion people in the Orient eating foods with MSG and reproducing quite satisfactorily.

NOTE ON NUTRITION: COPING WITH AN EATING DISORDER DURING PREGNANCY

I have had anorexia since high school. One of the reasons I first became vegetarian was to keep my weight down. How can I resolve my need to keep my weight down and still give adequate nutrition to my baby?

It will be very important that you find a nonjudgmental obstetrician or midwife with whom you can communicate. When you tell your doctor or nurse that you have anorexia, hopefully she will be accepting and informed about your condition. If she makes it seem insignificant or if she is judgmental, please find another individual who realizes you have a medical problem and will not treat you as though the problem is your fault.

When you go for your obstetrics visits, it might be better for you not to have your weight checked each time. Although your weight gain is important, it is your healthy diet that counts. Please ask your obstetrician if there are ways she can judge your health other than by taking your weight. Your doctor may just want to check you every three months if she believes your baby or you are not growing on schedule. It is also a good idea to record your food intake to make sure you are consuming sufficient quantities of starches and fats. You will need nuts, grains, breads, pastas, and oils in your diet to support your baby. Laxatives can be dangerous for your baby, and although they may help to eliminate calories, they also cause you to lose nutrients your baby needs. Of the many pregnant patients I have had with anorexia, not one has gained too much weight and not one has had trouble losing weight afterward. This is the one time you have to let go. Try to understand that this weight gain is a positive, natural, and healthy experience of pregnancy. Your baby and you will be happier for it.

If you are having difficulties letting yourself gain weight, seek counseling. There are many psychologists and psychiatrists who specialize in anorexia and will help you through each month of your pregnancy.

Anorexia and bulimia are lumped together as eating disorders; however, each has a different effect on a pregnancy. In anorexia, women and their babies lose the benefit of those nutrients they did not consume. In bulimia, women are losing not only those nutrients they took in, but also the many gastric chemicals and electrolytes that their body has mobilized to digest these foods. These electrolytes are very important to a baby's health.

Medical studies demonstrate that if you have anorexia or bulimia during your pregnancy, you have a higher risk of having a miscarriage, an infant with a low birth weight, obstetric complications, and postpartum depression. As a vegetarian, you are more likely to have a smaller baby than that of a meat-eating woman to begin with because your diet is lower in fats. If you compound being vegetarian with being anorexic and bulimic, your baby may be excessively small in both weight and length. It is not uncommon for anorexic women to resolve their condition during the pregnancy. However, it is easier to observe a change in your body image that makes you happy. Once you deliver, you may feel very unhappy with your body and experience a relapse. Try to be prepared for this and do your best to stay healthy and strong for your new baby.

AN OUNCE OF PREVENTION: SAFE, NATURAL HEALTH REMEDIES

Acupuncture

Acupuncture may be a great asset to help you cope better with nausea, food cravings, back pains, fatigue, and anxiety. I have sent women to acupuncturists who have been able to help them ovulate, conceive, cope with nausea and vomiting, and go into labor when they were overdue. As a society, we know so little about Eastern medicine, but that does not mean it has no validity and cannot be helpful to complement traditional Western treatments. There is nothing harmful about receiving acupuncture needles during your pregnancy. Receiving this treatment may help to decrease your need for other medications.

Chiropractic Treatments

Not only are they safe, chiropractic treatments may help you to cope with back discomfort for the duration of your pregnancy. While you are pregnant, your entire spinal cord will be shifting from a more vertical posture to one with your abdomen out and your shoulders back to counterbalance the weight of your growing abdomen. This postural change, along with an increased strain on your lumbar (lower back) disks and your sciatic nerves, contributes to many back problems during pregnancy. Chiropractic treatments will not hurt your baby, and they can help you feel better and decrease your need for pain medications.

Massage

Motion is the essence of health. If you can keep your circulation moving, your muscles invigorated, and your joints and ligaments limber, you will feel vibrant, alert, and refreshed throughout your pregnancy. When you are having a massage treatment, bring a pillow with you to keep yourself tilted, so that you are not lying flat on your back. When you are lying tilted on your abdomen, you can keep this pillow either under your abdomen or under your knee. The treatments will not only refresh your body, they will relax your mind, too.

Echinacea

There have been no studies showing any detrimental effects of echinacea during pregnancy. Echinacea is a Native American healing herb, but until recently it has been used more often in Europe than in our country. The Plains Indians used it on wounds and insect bites, as well as for colds, arthritis, and toothaches. The roots and leaves of this plant will help to stimulate your immune response, but your body metabolizes it quickly, so it must be taken several times a day to be effective. Use of the echinacea flower will not totally alleviate all cold symptoms by improving the immune response, but as an herbal remedy, it will help you to combat an infection more quickly. When your body cells are infected with a virus or bacteria, your body guides a substance into the surrounding cells to boost their immunity; echinacea has the same effect. If you are using ground echinacea leaves, you can take 1 teaspoon up to three times a day. If you are taking echinacea tablets, just follow the directions on the label.

Please confirm that the preparation you're using does not contain goldenseal—you should not take any form of this herb during your pregnancy. American Indians in the Northeast used this yellow root to fight skin wounds and sore throats. Although the roots of the goldenseal plant can stimulate your immune response and fight infection, they can also stimulate uterine contractions.

Vitamin C

Are there any specific types of vitamin C I should take to treat my cold? How much can I take without causing harm to my baby?

Your best choice of vitamin C is one that contains the complete C complex of bioflavonoids, hesperidin, and rutin. Rosehip also contains bioflavonoids and other enzymes that will help your body to digest the vitamin. Rosehip is actually formed in the bud of a rose and is the richest natural source of vitamin C. It is best that you not take the chewable form of the vitamin; vitamin C is ascorbic acid, and chewing it may erode the enamel on your teeth. You can safely take large doses of vitamin C— 500 to 1,000 milligrams three to four times a day—to fight your cold. Vitamin C is water-soluble and will be eliminated rapidly from your system, so a once-a-day dose will not be as effective. The higher your level of vitamin C, the more effective it will be at fighting your infection. It is best not to take very large doses of vitamin C *throughout* your pregnancy because high doses often cause mild anemia. Taking large doses while you are sick will help you; vitamin C fights many types of viral and bacterial infections and stimulates your general immune response. However, you do not want to increase your chances of becoming anemic, so reduce your vitamin C intake to normal once your cold is better.

CHAPTER 7

Your Fifth Month

Your pregnancy has not been easy.
But it never was supposed to be.

You may doubt yourself
and wonder, "Had I known . . . "
The truth is,
you would have done this again, at all costs.
You are having your baby in anticipation of the happiness
you know awaits you.

If you have given birth before,
you are doing it with reverence for this miracle of life.

Wherever you are on your journey,
your mind is enriched.

Pregnancy has imparted to you an increased respect for all life,
no matter how meek
no matter how tiny.

You will continue on your path as a vegetarian.
A path that extends the same compassion toward all of life
that has been shown to you.

YOUR BABY DURING THE FIFTH MONTH

- Your baby's length, from the top of its head to the end of its torso, grows from 6 inches to 9 inches.

- Its weight increases from 9 ounces to slightly over 1 pound.

- Its skin becomes thicker and less transparent.

- It develops a scant layer of fat under its skin.

- Its toenails start to grow.

- The nerve cells in its brain grow rapidly.

- Its scalp hair grows.

- It will swallow amniotic fluid.

- Its small intestine contracts and pushes material into its colon.

- Its pancreas starts to produce insulin.

- Its kidneys produce urine, which then becomes amniotic fluid.

- It can hear now—it hears your heartbeat, blood flow, and intestines moving.

- Its body will assume more adultlike proportions: its head, torso, and legs each make up a third of its total size.

CHANGES YOU MAY NOTICE IN YOURSELF THIS MONTH

You may still be experiencing all of the changes that have occurred within your prior months, plus the following:

- You may have pain in your lower back and hips.

- You may feel dizzy and faint while standing for prolonged times.

- You may feel nauseated and faint while lying on your back.

- You may feel sciatica, pains from your buttocks down to the backs of your legs.

- You may notice a sudden significant weight gain, well over five pounds this month.

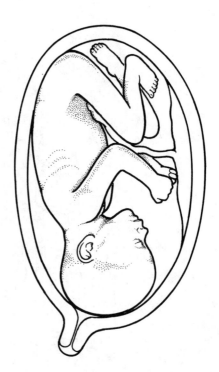

Your twentieth week through your twenty-fourth week is your fifth month of pregnancy. This is your baby at twenty weeks.

- ◆ Stretch marks on your abdomen and breasts may increase in width and number.
- ◆ You may have difficulty sleeping or experience insomnia.

MATERNITY CLOTHES

When will I need to buy maternity clothes?

Buying maternity clothes will give you a wonderful opportunity to create a new wardrobe for this special time in your life. However, you should try to keep this new wardrobe small because you may be going through two sets of wardrobes during these nine months. The first you'll buy when you're still small but can no longer fit into your old clothes. Then you'll need a second set when you are really large. Here's a way to gauge how large you will be at different phases of your pregnancy: At sixteen weeks, your uterus will be midway between your pubic bone and your navel; at twenty weeks, your uterus will be at your navel; at twenty-eight weeks,

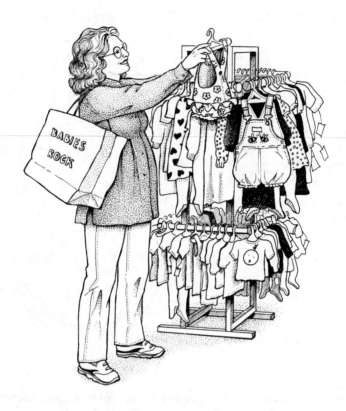

your uterus will be midway between your navel and your rib cage; and at thirty-six weeks, the top of your uterus will be under your rib cage. After your thirty-sixth week, your uterus will appear smaller as it drops into your pelvis.

What should you buy? That depends on your tastes, your job, your budget, and how comfortable you feel about your pregnant body. It will be more economical and practical if you buy tops that you can wear again. Although you will not be able to use your pants and skirts again, there's no reason you cannot use your tops. Keep in mind that you will be pregnant in two seasons and in many sizes. Some clothes you may barely have worn before it will be too cold or too warm to use them. Try wearing some of your husband's shirts, too. This will help him feel more a part of your pregnancy, and it will save you from spending too much on shopping. He will probably feel excited and happy to see you wearing his shirt to cover his baby.

NUTRITION AND ABDOMINAL HEALTH

I have had so many different abdominal pains during pregnancy. Which are related to my diet?

First, if you know the anatomy of your abdominal organs, you will be able to discern which organ is causing your pain. Then you will be better able to know how your diet may be related to the pains.

Gallbladder Stones and Inflammation

Gallbladder stones or inflammation cause pain under the right side of your rib cage, radiating to the right shoulder, usually after you eat. Gallbladder problems occur more commonly during pregnancy. The symptoms of either an inflamed gallbladder (cholecystitis) or stones in the

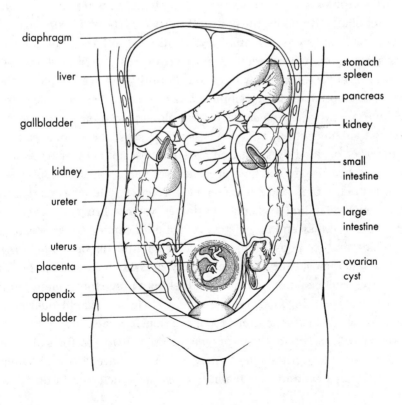

gallbladder (cholelithiasis) may be quite similar. Both conditions cause sudden sharp gripping pains under the right rib cage after meals. Medical students learn a common mnemonic for the type of person who usually develops gallstones—a fair, fertile female. This is because gallbladder disease is more common in Caucasians who are pregnant or have been pregnant. Your gallbladder is a saclike organ that contains bile, which is stored and then pushed through a tiny duct into your intestines to aid digestion when you eat fried, fatty, or raw foods. If you developed tiny stones in your gallbladder, these may block the duct and prevent bile from passing through. Typically, if a pregnant woman with gallbladder stones went to a sub shop and had a sandwich with cheese, onion, and oil or butter, within fifteen minutes after eating, she would experience a gripping right-sided pain. This pain occurs as the gallbladder cramps down to push out blocked bile. Pregnant women develop more stones because their bile is thicker and forms a kind of sludge that condenses into little stones.

If you have such pains after meals, you may feel better if you stand up and walk around. You may also feel like applying pressure on your right shoulder blade. Gradually, the pain will subside as the bile is able to ooze around your tiny stone. Eventually you will need to have your gallbladder removed. You will not want to let this pain continue through the rest of your life, but the surgeon will try to wait until you have completed the first three months of fetal development before scheduling the procedure.

While you are awaiting surgery, you will be placed on a very low fat diet. You should not eat fatty foods, such as eggs, cheese omelets, ice cream, or even salad dressing. You also had best not eat raw fruits and vegetables, because the cellulose of certain vegetables—such as apple peel, green pepper, onion, and cucumber peel—requires bile for digestion. If you eat such offending fruits and vegetables, you can bring on a gallbladder attack. You may end up existing on a diet of canned fruits, steamed vegetables, and ice pops. I had gallbladder pain during one of my pregnancies, and almost everything I ate as a vegetarian bothered me except Italian ices and ice pops. Not the ideal diet for a pregnant woman—but if you avoid all irritating foods for several days to let your gallbladder heal, you will be able to eat nutritional foods that much sooner.

The middle three months of pregnancy are considered the safest for gallbladder surgery. Although you may not wish to have your gallbladder removed, your pain and your inability to eat may dictate your decision.

All pregnant women are concerned, and rightly so, about anesthesia. But the anesthesiologist knows that you are pregnant and will use safe anesthetic medications, so you and your baby will be fine.

If you experience a gallbladder attack in your last trimester, your doctor may try to wait until after you deliver to remove your gallbladder. You will be placed on a rather limited fat-free and cellulose-free diet. Performing surgery now, when your uterus is so large and your gallbladder is squashed between your uterus and your liver, is a challenge for a surgeon. The surgery can be safely done, but not without difficulty.

After appendicitis, gallbladder surgery is the second most common nonobstetric reason women require surgery during pregnancy. Your gallbladder can be removed with either a small incision or through a scope. You will probably leave the hospital rather quickly, staying overnight just so the nurses can confirm that your baby is fine.

Gastritis

Gastritis causes a burning sensation in the midpart of the upper abdomen, directly under your breastbone. This sensation almost always occurs after eating and often after everything you eat. It is an irritation of your stomach lining. Years back, doctors believed it was caused by nervousness, but now they know there are many other causes, including bacteria that live in the stomach. Gastritis will feel like a burning or gnawing sensation in your middle-upper abdomen. You may feel it worse when your stomach is empty, when you drink caffeinated beverages, and when you eat spicy foods. You will probably be advised to eat a bland diet so as not to further irritate your stomach lining.

Your gastritis may be caused by an intestinal bacteria called *Helicobacter pylori*. A gastroenterologist will be able to diagnose it and treat you safely during your pregnancy with an antibiotic. Amoxicillin, which can be taken at any time during your pregnancy, and Flagyl, which can be taken after your first trimester, will help rid your stomach of this bacteria and give you much relief.

Although you may have always had mild gastritis, you may feel much worse during pregnancy because your body produces more gastric acids. These acids are actually eating your gastric lining, especially when you have no food in your system. That is why you feel worse when your stomach is empty. Conversely, some foods and beverages (such as spicy foods and coffee) will stimulate your body to produce even more gastric acid. That is why you may not want to eat frequently at an Indian or Thai restaurant while you are pregnant. You may feel best when you nibble small portions of steamed food that is mildly flavored. Your body will tell you which foods are safest.

Chamomile tea may have a calming effect on your gastric lining. If you are lacto-ovo-vegetarian, you may feel better eating ice cream, custard, or pudding. Although many people reach for antacids, you should try to alleviate your symptoms with natural foods rather than synthetic chemicals. Ice cream, ice pops, Italian ices, and other cold foods and beverages will actually decrease the penetration of the acid burn and help relieve your gnawing discomfort.

Kidney Stones

Kidney stones are caused by several factors, including diet, fluid intake, heredity, and the region where you live. The stones cause sudden gripping pains in the small of the back, often radiating around the side of the abdomen, and sometimes cause blood in the urine.

Kidney stones are very common—and very painful—but they will not affect your pregnancy. Stones form in the central part of the kidney and pass down through your ureter into your bladder. If a stone blocks the downward passage of urine, you will experience sudden gripping pains. The stone may also scratch and irritate the ureter on its way down, causing blood in your urine. The blood is actually a useful clue, because it confirms that you have a kidney stone.

For most people, the treatment for kidney stones is a natural one. It includes rest, pain medication to relax the spasms of their ureter, and large quantities of liquids to flush out the stone. Occasionally, a doctor must remove a stone, either by feeding a tiny basket up through the bladder into the ureter to pull it down or by lithotripsy, the use of an external laser beam to disrupt and break the stone. Lithotripsy cannot, however, be used in pregnant women.

Once you have kidney stones, you will need to modify your lifestyle. If you live in a region where your water contains a high mineral content, you may need to soften it to remove the minerals, because these can form stones. The Midwest region of the United States is an area where kidney stones are endemic owing to the high mineral content in the water. We lived in Chicago for two years, and the high mineral content in the water coated our cooking pots with minerals. Visualizing this mineral coating on pots helped me to envision the minerals that can build up in the urinary tract. Also, please don't drink mineral water, as you do not want to consume these extra minerals and risk developing more kidney stones. After you pass your stone, you will be advised to drink at least eight glasses of water every day, to dilute your urine and to prevent the formation of new stones.

Bladder Infection

I had a bladder infection that caused pain above my pubic bone and stinging when I emptied my bladder. Can I prevent this from recurring?

Many pregnant women develop bladder infections because their immune response is suppressed. This decrease in immune response is a protective mechanism so that women do not reject their own pregnancy.

Some signs indicating that you had a bladder infection were pain or irritation in the lower-middle portion of your abdomen, a need to empty your bladder frequently, pain at the end of urination, and burning within your urethra when the urine finally left. During pregnancy it will be best for women to take an antibiotic for bladder infections. The spasms and heat created from an infection in the bladder have been believed to cause premature labor because they irritate the adjacent uterus. There are many antibiotics that are safe to use during pregnancy.

Please drink large quantities of liquid to flush out the infection. Eating cranberry products will also provide relief because they prevent bacteria from adhering to the bladder wall. When the bacteria cannot adhere, you will void them. Cranberry products are not limited to juice; you can also eat fresh cranberry preserves and dried cranberries in a fruit/nut mixture to help treat your infection. You will not obtain the same relief with a mixed-juice drink, such as cranberry-apple or cranberry-pineapple juice. Pure cranberry juice works best. Within one day of taking antibiotics you should start to feel better. Please finish your entire course of antibiotics. Otherwise the antibiotic will destroy only the weaker bacteria; their resistant bacteria will take over and multiply and you will have a more difficult infection to deal with.

Appendicitis

I was admitted to the hospital last night because I may have appendicitis. Is it common to have appendicitis in pregnancy?

Your appendix is a tiny elongated structure in the right-lower region of your abdomen. It had a purpose in human beings centuries ago, but there is no known purpose for it now. The appendix can easily become inflamed, and if the inflammation causes the appendix to rupture, the situation will be more serious than having surgery.

Appendicitis is the most common reason pregnant women require surgery, aside from obstetric reasons. Appendicitis can occur at any time in a woman's pregnancy and can be somewhat more difficult for a physician to diagnose because the appendix has moved out of its typical location. As your uterus grows upward, your appendix will also be moved upward. In one study, out of almost forty-five thousand pregnant women, twenty-two, or 0.05 percent, had appendicitis. All of their children were delivered healthy, but several were born premature after their mother's appendix had ruptured in the later part of pregnancy. Although the appendix is part of the intestinal tract, no dietary changes could have prevented you from getting appendicitis.

Your doctor will check to see if you have pain in your lower abdomen, on an imaginary line between your navel and your right hipbone. If you locate the point two-thirds of the way from your navel toward your hipbone, that is McBurney's point, and that is where your appendix is normally located. During pregnancy, however, the appendix is pushed up each month of pregnancy to a higher level in your abdomen. If you develop pain on the right side of your abdomen, lose your appetite, have a slight fever, and have a high white blood cell count, your doctor will suspect that you have appendicitis. There is no reason to fear appendix surgery. The anesthesiologist will make sure that your baby is getting enough oxygen and that all of your medications are safe for your baby, and the nurses will make sure you do not have cramping after surgery.

ROUND LIGAMENT PAINS

I have started to feel pains on either side of my uterus, pulling from the sides of my uterus down to my pubic bone. Every time I rise from a sitting position, I feel this pulling sensation. Why is this happening?

You are describing round ligament pains. Your round ligaments extend from the side of your uterus down to your pubic bone. They help give your uterus support. Since they are strong supporting structures, they are tough and do not stretch easily. Your uterine muscles stretch much more easily than do your round ligaments. Eventually, the round ligaments will stretch adequately to support your growing uterus and your pain will resolve.

EYE HEALTH AND YOUR DIET

I am five months pregnant and my distance vision has changed. I know that this is common during pregnancy, but has my vegetarian diet contributed to this?

There are no dietary factors known to worsen vision during pregnancy. Two physical changes of your eyes have caused this shift in your ability to see distances. The curvature of your cornea, the surface of your eye, has changed its shape during your pregnancy, and the pressure of the fluid within your eye has decreased. Both of these changes often have an effect on refraction. These changes usually resolve after your pregnancy is completed, but your refraction may not return to its original level of acuity.

Actually, your vegetarian diet is healthier for your eyes both during pregnancy and throughout your life. Three vitamins—riboflavin, vitamin A, and vitamin D—are critical to good health for the eyes and are all present in large quantities in vegetarian diets. Riboflavin, one of the B vitamins, is commonly used to treat eye problems, visual refraction problems, and cataracts. You can obtain your riboflavin from vegetables as well as natural yeast.

Vitamin A, found in green leafy vegetables, yellow vegetables (such as carrots, sweet potatoes, and pumpkins), red cabbage, and fruits, is necessary for the production of a chemical that facilitates vision at night. When vitamin A is deficient, an individual will develop night blindness. Your vegetarian sources of vitamin A are abundant. However, it is important that you do not take an excessive amount of vitamin A, over 25,000 international units daily, in the form of supplements derived from animal sources. Vitamin A in vitamin tablets is frequently derived from animal sources, and excess quantities can cause birth defects. No vitamin A that you derive directly from plant sources causes birth defects.

Adequate vitamin D will decrease your chance of developing cataracts and other visual problems. Vitamin D is absorbed through your skin, and it will not be necessary for you to consume any animal products in order to obtain adequate amounts. Walking outdoors for fifteen minutes daily will be a perfect way to get all the vitamin D you need for a healthy life and a healthy pregnancy.

NOTE ON NUTRITION: CALCIUM AND VITAMIN D

I am a vegan, and I am concerned that I will not be able to consume enough calcium through my diet to have a healthy baby. Is my concern valid?

Being a vegan, you do not have to be concerned. You will be obtaining more than enough calcium from numerous vegetables and will be retaining more of the calcium you ingest within your body. There is a widespread misconception that because the calcium derived from vegetables is not absorbed as easily as is the calcium from dairy, you will become deficient in calcium. The reality is that even though you may absorb less calcium, you will retain more in your body and therefore have more to give your baby (see chapter 2).

In most individuals, calcium excess is not a health problem, though some people may deposit calcium in their muscles, bones, and soft tissues. In general, you should not take calcium supplements without a specific reason. Calcium deficiency can occur not only from low calcium in your diet, but also from high phosphorus in your diet. Phosphorus is present in carbonated drinks, meat, eggs, luncheon meats, and cheese spreads. The ideal diet should contain a ratio of phosphorus to calcium of one to one, but many Americans have a phosphorus-to-calcium ratio of four to one. These individuals may be losing most of the calcium that they take in and may actually deplete the calcium that has been stored in their bones.

I have heard that the calcium from vegetables is not absorbed as well as the calcium from dairy products. Is there anything I can do to increase my body's absorption of calcium?

Many factors influence your body's ability to absorb calcium. A healthy, balanced diet, with plenty of vitamin D, magnesium, and acid-rich foods like vitamin C, will increase your calcium absorption. Regular exercise is one of the best ways to increase calcium levels. Dairy products are the most obvious source of calcium-rich foods, so if you are a lacto-ovo-vegetarian, don't skimp on dairy. It is also good to know what foods inhibit calcium absorption. If your diet is high in fat, protein, phytic acid (found in whole grains), and oxalic acid (found in spinach, chard, beet greens, rhubarb, and cocoa), it will be more difficult for your body to retain calcium. That is why it is good for you to rotate the foods in your vegetarian diet: Foods have a variety of advantages and disadvantages. You may also decrease your absorption of calcium if the level of acid in your stomach is reduced from taking antacids.

One very positive fact for vegetarians to know is that although their absorption of calcium may be lower, they will retain more of the calcium they take in. Vegetarians do not lose the calcium in their body's waste products, as so often occurs in non-vegetarians and in individuals whose diets contain a lot of wheat, soda, alcohol, and tobacco.

Calcium Supplements

Which calcium supplements are the healthiest for me during pregnancy?

Calcium citrate is the most easily absorbed calcium supplement; you will actually get the most calcium per unit from one of these preparations than from any other calcium compound. Preparations containing calcium lactate and calcium carbonate, such as Tums, create an alkaline environment in your intestinal tract and actually slow down your calcium absorption. Dolomite and bone meal are two other forms of calcium supplements, but they are not as common—or as healthy—as calcium citrate. Dolomite may contain chemical impurities like heavy metals. Bone meal is made from ground-up cow's bones and may also contain chemical impurities. As a vegetarian, you'll find this supplement not very appealing.

Calcium supplements are effective if you are not able to get enough calcium from your diet. However, they are beneficial only to a point; your body will not absorb extra calcium once it has received maximum levels.

People tell me that my baby will have weak bones because I am a vegan and do not eat any dairy products. Is that true?

Most people assume that calcium is the primary element needed for bone development. The truth is, once a woman has a sufficient foundation of calcium in her diet, it is other elements and nutrients—namely, magnesium, phosphorus, potassium, and protein—that affect the bone density mass in her child. As a vegan, you will have no difficulty obtaining sufficient quantities of all these minerals and protein. And because your diet is so low in phosphorus, you will retain much higher levels of calcium in your system from your calcium-rich plant foods (see chapter 2).

If there is so much calcium in dairy products, why isn't dairy the best source of calcium?

When you eat dairy products, you are eating a food with both high levels of calcium and high levels of protein. Calcium is a positive ion, and therefore it is attracted to a negative ion. When you digest the protein derived from milk, it creates an acid residue. This acid residue is full of negative ions that bind with the positive ion from calcium, and both calcium and the protein acid residue are excreted together in your urine. When you eat dairy products, you may be losing much of the calcium you are taking in.

Are there other foods that create a high "acid residue" and pull calcium out of my body?

Yes. The five main products that cause your body to excrete calcium are meat, wheat, soda, alcohol, and tobacco. That is one reason osteoporosis is so common in our country, even though we have one of the highest per capita consumptions of calcium and protein. The tremendous acid residue created when Americans eat a hamburger on a roll and drink soda pulls the calcium out of their bodies faster than they can take it in. In numerous countries where people eat rice, vegetables, and water, they don't have a word for osteoporosis—that's how rare a condition it is. Vegetarians have half the rate of osteoporosis of our meat-eating counterparts because our diet enables us to retain more calcium.

Can I just take a blood test to know if my diet is low in calcium and if my body needs more calcium?

You cannot find out the actual amount of calcium in your bones from a blood test, unless your calcium level is extremely low. This is because your system tries to maintain a normal blood calcium level, even if it has to take calcium out of your bones to do this. Your blood level of calcium may be fine, but your bones and your baby's bones may be low in calcium. Under only a few circumstances will your blood calcium level be low. This is usually due to a metabolism problem, not to a low level of calcium in the diet. For example, if a woman develops toxemia of pregnancy and her doctor prescribes magnesium, the magnesium will bind with her calcium and lower her blood calcium level.

Since I have become pregnant, I have noticed my fingernails developing vertical ridges and becoming brittle. Do I need more calcium?

You may need more iron, calcium, and zinc. Most people believe that calcium is the only mineral needed for healthy nails, but iron and zinc are also very important. Brittle nails and vertically ridged nails are often a sign of iron-deficiency anemia. It will be best for your doctor or midwife to check your iron level. Also, please make sure you are taking a multivitamin with zinc.

Will I have symptoms that my calcium level is low?

Definitely. You may have any or all of the following: twitching, nerve sensitivity, brittle nails, insomnia, depression, numbness of your fingers and toes, and heart palpitations. In pregnancy, painful cramping of the calf muscles is a common symptom of calcium deficiency.

When this happens, you should break the cramp first. As soon as a cramp occurs and the sole of your foot tightens, get out of bed and flex your foot toward your knee to stretch your Achilles tendon. You will find it even more painful to do this, but it will break your cramp. Then place a heating pad or a heated thermal unit under your calf until all the tension is relieved. It is safe to sleep with a heating pad under and around your calf all night. To prevent future cramps, start eating foods high in calcium and foods that will help you absorb the calcium.

Do I need to eat dairy products to get vitamin D?

It is a common misconception that individuals must consume dairy products to obtain vitamin D. Dairy products may be fortified with vitamin D, meaning that vitamin D is added to them the way it is added to your vitamin pills, but most do not contain it naturally. Many vegetarian foods are also fortified with vitamin D, and nature has given us vitamin D in the form of sunlight; our bodies are able to manufacture their own vitamin D when exposed to the sun (see chapter 2).

Why do I need vitamin D for my baby to develop healthy bones?

If your body does not have sufficient vitamin D, it cannot absorb calcium. Regardless of how much calcium you ingest, your baby cannot use it without the help of magnesium and vitamin D. Vitamin D is very important for the growth and development of your fetus and for your own bones and tissues.

Will I be able to get enough vitamin D during my pregnancy even though I don't eat fish?

If you go into the sunlight for twenty to thirty minutes daily or get indirect sunlight in your home or office, you will have no problem at all getting enough vitamin D. If this is not possible, you can avail yourself of the numerous sources of vitamin D in both vitamin supplements and fortified foods.

AN OUNCE OF PREVENTION:
PREGNANCY AND OSTEOPOROSIS

I am very thin, and I know that thin women are more prone to osteo-porosis. Now that I am pregnant and vegetarian, will so much calcium go to my baby that I will be more likely to develop osteoporosis?

Whether or not you are vegetarian, you do not have to worry that pregnancy will place you at a higher risk for osteoporosis later in life. The calcium your baby and your placenta use during pregnancy will be restored naturally after you deliver by a regulation mechanism your body will put into action automatically. In addition, vegetarian women suffer less from osteoporosis than do non-vegetarian women.

A woman's requirement for calcium increases during pregnancy and breast-feeding to ensure adequate calcium for her baby—but she will be fine. Nursing women experience bone depletion that is transient, as their bone density returns to normal after nursing. Some women develop severe osteoporosis during pregnancy and sustain fractures while pregnant, but again, after delivery their bone density returns to normal.

Drinking milk and eating dairy do not prevent osteoporosis. Osteoporosis is a disease that results either from an increased excretion of calcium or from a deficient intake of calcium. The protein found in meat, fish, and chicken increases the loss of calcium through the urine and greatly contributes to the development of osteoporosis. When you eat vegetable sources of calcium—chick peas, dried fruits, sesame seeds, and soybeans—your body will absorb and retain consistently higher levels of calcium. Given this, it's not surprising that vegetarians have a lower rate of osteoporosis than non-vegetarians. Numerous medical studies have shown this to be true. One study in the *American Journal of Clinical Nutrition* showed that by the age of sixty-five, female meat-eaters had 35 percent bone loss, whereas female vegetarians had only 18 percent bone loss.

CHAPTER 8

Your Sixth Month

*You feel joy as you sense
the gentle life within you.
You sense when your baby is calm at rest
and strong at play.
You are already sharing one life.*

*Before you were pregnant, you may have thought
your baby and you would just share your bodies,
but by now, your bond has become much deeper than that.*

*The two of you will become one in spirit.
Hereafter, you will always be connected to
this life within you.*

*As your child grows, you will learn that although you
each have a unique self and purpose in life,
you will forever share
an inexplicable bond of strength with each other.*

*And while your child lives within you,
you will be teaching it peace and kindness and compassion
because you are a vegetarian.*

And it will carry that message
for the rest of its life.

YOUR BABY DURING THE SIXTH MONTH

- The length of your baby from the top of its head to the bottom of its buttocks will increase from 9 inches to 10 inches.

- Its total length from the top of its head to the tips of its toes will reach 15 inches.

- Its weight will increase from slightly over 1 pound to slightly over 2 pounds.

- Its skin will still appear wrinkled and quite thin.

- Your baby will develop a thin layer of fat under its skin.

- Its sucking reflex is strong.

- The retinas in its eyes develop distinct layers to receive light and to transmit images to the brain.

- The glands of its skin produce a cheesy vernix, which will spread over the surface of its body.

- Within its intestines the first stool, called "meconium," is forming.

CHANGES YOU MAY NOTICE IN YOURSELF THIS MONTH

You may still experience some or all of the changes you felt during your prior months, as well as the following:

- You may experience pressure under your diaphragm, making it difficult for you to eat large meals.

- You may have constipation, strained bowel movements, or hemorrhoids.

- Your ankles, hands, and wrists may swell.

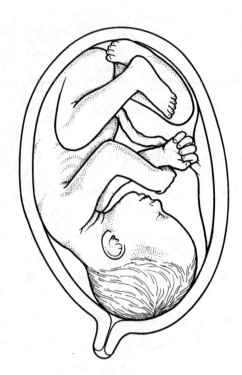

Your twenty-fourth week through your twenty-eighth week is your sixth month of pregnancy. This is your baby at twenty-four weeks.

- ◆ You may develop pain, swelling, and numbness of your hands and fingers, which are signs of carpal tunnel syndrome.
- ◆ When you exert yourself you may feel short of breath.
- ◆ You may have a tendency to feel faint when you are in a crowded room or when you stand.
- ◆ By the end of this month, your uterus will be 1 to 2 inches above your navel.

GESTATIONAL DIABETES

If there is no diabetes in my family, why must I be tested for it?

Having your blood sugar tested at around your twenty-eighth week of pregnancy is necessary because 2 to 3 percent of all women become diabetic during their pregnancies. Actually, diabetes is the most common medical complication that occurs in women during pregnancy. Of the women who develop gestational diabetes, 90 percent are not actually di-

abetic before they become pregnant. Diabetes of pregnancy usually resolves itself after delivery, but women who do become diabetic during
pregnancy are likely to become diabetic again, often within twenty years
after delivery.

What is gestational diabetes?

There are three types of diabetes: Type I, or insulin-dependent diabetes;
Type II, noninsulin-dependent diabetes; and gestational diabetes, which
develops during pregnancy. A small percentage of women who develop
gestational diabetes actually had Type I or II diabetes before they became pregnant but were unaware of it. If the diabetes persists after delivery, it was probably true diabetes all along, because gestational
diabetes usually resolves after delivery. If you are an older, heavy, or
sedentary woman, you will be more likely to develop gestational diabetes. Native American women are also more susceptible to developing
gestational diabetes.

How will I be tested for gestational diabetes?

You will be advised the month before you will be tested for gestational diabetes to drink or eat 50 grams of glucose one hour before your scheduled appointment. For this test, many doctors prefer to have their
patients drink Glucola, a medically designed liquid containing 50 grams
of glucose. Glucola is a caffeine-free noncarbonated high-glucose drink
that is, unfortunately, not very tasty. When you arrive for your office
visit, the receptionist will confirm the time that you ingested the glucose
so that she can check your blood sugar at the one-hour mark. If your
blood sugar level is over 130, you will need to have further testing, including a three-hour glucose tolerance test. A convenient alternative is
to drink either two 8-ounce glasses of orange juice or one can of Slice
soda. As long as you eat or drink 50 grams of glucose before the test, the
source is not important.

Why is a glucose test for diabetes performed so late in pregnancy?

The test is performed between the twenty-fourth and twenty-eighth weeks
of pregnancy because this is the period in which gestational diabetes

usually develops. Prior to this time, if a woman had diabetes but did not know it, her monthly urine glucose test would most likely have shown an elevated glucose level. Most women with Type I and Type II diabetes are well aware that they have this disorder before they become pregnant.

SLEEP AND DIET

Nightmares

I keep waking up at night with nightmares about my baby and myself. Is there anything I can do to prevent these?

The dreams of pregnant women have been studied for more than a hundred years. Most pregnant women dream about the safety of their unborn child. In fact, it is natural for your fears and worries to surface in your dreams. The frequency of your nightmares may increase as your delivery date draws near, as fear of the unknown is powerful. Just do your best to stay calm and happy; remember that you are taking good care of yourself and your baby.

Another possible cause of your bad dreams may be your diet. Try to remember what you ate at bedtime on the nights you have nightmares to see if there is a pattern of unpleasant dreams related to your food. If you do note a pattern, try to eliminate the offending foods. For example, watermelon often increases the frequency of nightmares in pregnant women.

Insomnia

I wake up several times each night. My sleep was never interrupted before. Why is this happening?

Sleep disturbances are so common during pregnancy that in one study, 88 percent of pregnant women reported an alteration in their sleep pattern. Whether you are experiencing difficulty falling asleep, having episodes of wakefulness during the night, or waking up permanently at four A.M. each morning, what you are experiencing is normal for pregnant women. Women frequently attribute their insomnia to things like heartburn, nausea, vomiting, backaches, hip pains, the need to urinate, and movement of their baby. These are certainly more than enough reasons to explain a significant loss of sleep during pregnancy. The only thing you can really do is accept that you will have nights like these—and plenty of them! When you wake up, try drinking a cup of warm milk. Warming the milk makes one of its amino acids, tryptophan, easier to digest. Tryptophan helps the body to relax. Do not take tryptophan capsules, however, because there is considerable controversy concerning their safety. If you still cannot go back to sleep, put on relaxing music, read a book, watch a movie, or knit or embroider an outfit for your baby. When I had insomnia, I used that time to do my craftwork in preparation for my babies' arrivals.

SALT INTAKE AND SWELLING

My legs are swollen; sometimes I have numbness and tingling in them. Is this dangerous?

The numbness and tingling is probably a result of swelling and fluid retention within your legs. In most women, swelling is normal in pregnancy, although sometimes it is a sign of a more serious problem. Ask your nurse to check your blood pressure, and your urine for toxemia. Once it is confirmed that you do not have a serious medical problem, you can try the following regimen.

To alleviate the swelling and numbness, keep your legs elevated whenever possible. It will be easier for the veins in your legs to bring the fluid from your body tissues back to your heart when your heart and legs are on the same level. Taking a warm bath also helps. The pressure of the bathwater on your leg veins will push fluids from your body tissues back to your veins. Your veins will then bring the fluid to your kidneys to filter the blood and eliminate excess fluids.

I have carpal tunnel syndrome, and each morning two fingers of my right hand are numb, painful, and swollen. Why did I develop this now?

Carpal tunnel syndrome affects 5 to 25 percent of all pregnant women. All people have a carpal ligament on the inner surface of their wrist, and nerves and blood vessels run under this ligament. During pregnancy, when you start to retain fluid and your body becomes swollen, the tissue under your carpal ligament often swells a great deal. This causes pressure and tension on the underlying nerves and blood vessels going to your hand and your fingers. The exact fingers that may be affected vary from person to person. In some women, one or two fingers are affected; in other women, all fingers of one hand are affected; and in still others, all fingers of both hands are affected. Both hands are affected in 50 to 75 percent of women with the disorder, and the right hand is affected more often than the left. Your fingers may or may not appear swollen, but they will invariably be uncomfortable and often quite painful. In 95 percent of these women, carpal tunnel syndrome resolves immediately after delivery. The other 5 percent of women usually experience a gradual resolution of the pain and swelling, but it can take up to two years.

What can I do to relieve the discomfort of carpal tunnel syndrome?

First, try to decrease the swelling in your entire body by eliminating foods containing salt. Do not use salt when you cook, and try to prepare most of your foods from scratch. Prepackaged food products like Rice-A-Roni, macaroni and cheese, and salad dressings all contain salt, as does any food you eat from a can. Canned foods frequently contain the preservative sodium benzoate. Sodium benzoate may not taste salty to your tongue, but its high sodium content will create salt in your body. It will be important for you to observe the sodium content on package labels. Soda, cheese, bread, cereal, and cake are often high in salt. Being a vegetarian and eating fresh produce should help you keep your sodium intake to a minimum.

How you position your arms and hands when you sleep may also influence how painful your carpal tunnel symptoms are. If you sleep with your hands over your head, near your pillow, your arm is high and your wrist is bent backward. This tightens the space between your carpal ligament and your wrist bone, compressing your carpal ligament. Reposition your arm alongside your body and bend your wrist so the pads of your fingers are closer to the inner surface of your wrist. This small change will give you immediate relief. You may also wish to purchase wrist supports to help keep your wrists in a flexed position. This will be particularly useful for you to use at night and at work. Ask your physician if she can write a prescription for the wrist splints, since insurance companies often cover the cost of this treatment.

My hands and fingers have become so swollen that I am afraid I will not be able to remove my rings. What can I do to decrease this swelling?

First, confirm with your doctor that you do not have a more serious problem, such as high blood pressure or toxemia of pregnancy, both of which would cause you to retain fluid. Your obstetrician will check your blood pressure and do a urinalysis to confirm that you are not developing either of these conditions. Try to stay in a cool place; you will retain less fluid in cool environments than in warm, humid ones. Simply increasing the air-conditioning in your home or at work may decrease the swelling. Again, do your best to limit your salt intake. By drinking plain water, you can pull salt out of your body tissues into your bloodstream and ease the swelling. Try not to drink mineral water, soda, or prepared juices, as these all contain salt.

Most important, you should remove your rings. Before your fingers become exceptionally swollen, place your hand in cool water to decrease the swelling and then apply an oily or a soapy solution. I have seen many women have their rings cut off in the emergency room. Although this can be a huge relief for the woman, it is quite destructive to the ring. If your ring is an heirloom, an engagement ring, or your wedding ring, it may never be the same again. When the emergency room physician cuts your ring, he may also need to rotate it or separate it from side to side so that it can slide off your swollen finger. It will be far better for you to remove your ring now, before medical removal becomes necessary.

THYROID DISEASE

I am hypothyroid, and my doctor has been checking my thyroid levels throughout my pregnancy. Does pregnancy significantly affect thyroid levels?

Yes, pregnancy has a significant effect on the function of the thyroid gland. That is because during pregnancy, the body produces high levels of estrogen, which then stimulates production of a protein that binds the thyroid hormone. This affects the functioning of the thyroid gland as well as the rest of the body. This binding also influences the results of your thyroid tests. That is why your doctor needs to check your thyroid levels often. You may need to adjust the amount of thyroid hormone you are taking, depending on how your levels have fluctuated during pregnancy.

I never had thyroid disease before my pregnancy, but when I had palpitations and went to the doctor, he discovered I was hyperthyroid. Will my thyroid function return to normal after I deliver?

Actually, your thyroid function will probably not return to normal after you deliver, but it may be easier to control. Many women develop thyroid disorders for the first time during or after pregnancy. The placenta produces hormones called "placental thyrotropins," which stimulate the thyroid gland to produce a large amount of thyroid hormone. When this occurs, women may experience a rapid heart rate, a visible enlargement of the thyroid gland, weight loss, and a slight bulging of the eyes. The treatment for hyperthyroidism is propylthiouracil; it is safe for use during pregnancy and is actually safer for a mother and her baby than if she were not treated at all. If placental hormones were the only cause of this problem, the condition would resolve after delivery. In some cases, women have begun to produce antibodies against their own thyroid gland. These antibodies continue to stimulate the thyroid gland to overproduce thyroid hormones long after the pregnancy is completed.

HEADACHES

Since I became pregnant, I have been experiencing frequent headaches. Can I do anything naturally to relieve them?

That depends upon the cause of your headaches. If you're having tension headaches, relaxation exercises and meditation may give you relief. If your headaches are caused by allergies, taking steps to remove the allergen from your environment and allergy desensitization may help. If you're suffering from migraines, there are some effective natural remedies you may want to try. Migraine headaches are common during the first three months of pregnancy and usually resolve after that time.

Try placing magnets on your head at the site of your headache. Using magnets for pain relief is very common in Eastern medicine. Magnets polarize the iron particles within your red blood cells, which may account for the success of this safe and effective treatment. The professional magnets from your pharmacy work well, as do standard refrigerator magnets. If the headache is at your temple region, place one magnet on either side of your temples and hold them for a minute or so, until your headache begins to fade. Occasionally, the pain of your headache may seem to migrate. Reapplying the magnets on your head wherever the pain has migrated will alleviate this. Within five minutes of magnet application, your headache will be gone. It will be wonderful if you treat your headaches with this simple physical modality instead of taking medication.

You may also wish to try massaging your head and neck. By massaging your tissues, you will increase circulation and help your body mobilize its natural self-healing powers. Similarly, if you stretch your neck and your upper arms, you may be able to decrease the intensity of your headache. If you find that you need pain medication, use plain Tylenol or its generic equivalent, acetaminophen. Tylenol has been used effectively during pregnancy for years with no negative side effects. Although numerous headache medications are available, none of them have withstood the test of time as long as Tylenol. If your headache does not resolve with these simple treatments, please discuss the problem with your physician.

GAS PAINS

This is my first pregnancy, and I became vegetarian only recently. I'm experiencing a lot of gas. Is this the result of my pregnancy or my vegetarian diet?

It is difficult to say if your gas pains are due to your dietary changes, your pregnancy, or a combination. Most vegetarians have adapted to vegetables, and they do not produce gas. Your body may still be adapting to this new diet. The main foods that create gas include legumes (beans and lentils) and the cruciferous vegetables (cabbage, Brussels sprouts, broccoli, and cauliflower).

In order to decrease your body's production of gas from eating legumes, soak your dried beans in water overnight. The volume of the water should be twice the volume of the beans. Discard this water in the morning. Your body produces gas as a reaction to the oligosaccharide covering of the beans, not from their inner contents. Soaking the beans and discarding the water will eliminate some of this covering. Try combining your beans with a grain, such as rice. This will also help to decrease gas production.

When you cook your vegetables, steam them well. The raw cellulose in plants triggers gas production, and steaming modifies the cellulose so your body will produce less gas. Some vegetables and fruits have a larger cellulose content that stimulates the body's production of gas. These include cabbage, broccoli, cauliflower, Brussels sprouts, onions, cucumber peel, and apple peel. Eating popcorn will help decrease gas production during pregnancy, as will strong chamomile tea made with two or three bags in each cup. Peppermint candy or tea will also relieve your gas, and cooking with seasonings like anise, caraway, coriander, fennel, and tur-

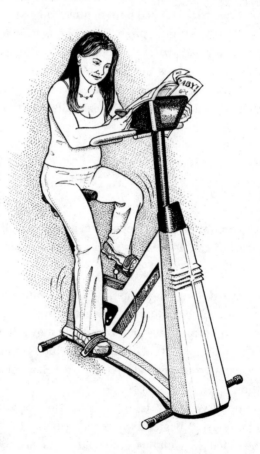

meric will provide some relief. You can also try using Beano tablets. Beano contains an enzyme that helps the body break down complex carbohydrates before they cause gas in the colon. Do not take activated charcoal tablets for gas. Although these tablets may help to relieve gas and symptoms of bloating, they have also been shown to cause cancer.

NOTE ON NUTRITION:
CONSTIPATION AND HEMORRHOIDS

Constipation

I eat a lot of fiber, but I still have severe constipation. Is this normal?

Yes, it is. During pregnancy, the body slows down the intestines so there is more time to absorb foods passing through the intestinal tract. Motilin is a hormonal peptide that normally functions to stimulate the bowel movement, but in pregnancy, your body decreases its production. Maintaining your vegetarian diet is the best way for you to combat constipation, but given these physiological changes, it can be difficult even for vegetarians to evacuate their bowels well. Every food that is recommended for constipation in pregnancy is vegetarian in nature. Humans have such a long intestinal tract that without fiber-rich vegetarian foods, the body requires three days for foods to digest fully. With fiber-rich foods, however, the body requires only eighteen hours. Fiber is particularly healthy because it removes toxins and bacteria with it as it is brushing along your intestinal tract.

To combat your constipation, eat fruits and vegetables, whole-grain cereal, rice, and bread. Drink at least eight glasses of water or other liquid daily, increase your exercise (this will speed up your intestinal transit time for foods), and increase your intake of vegetable oil or nut oil. Many pregnant women watch their weight and therefore limit their intake of oily foods. This decrease can contribute to constipation.

> *Think of your food as if it were going down a slide in an amusement park. If the slide is oily, there will be less friction and your food will go down much faster. Eating an oily Caesar or Greek salad may help your digestion regulate itself.*

Are over-the-counter products for constipation safe to take during pregnancy?

Many over-the-counter constipation products are safe and may be very helpful. These preparations include All-Fiber, Metamucil, Colace, Surfak, milk of magnesia, and Senokot. However, do not use Ex-Lax; natural products are more effective. Fiber products used for constipation, such as All-Fiber and Metamucil, are actually made from seeds. They give the intestinal contents bulk and fluid and help to move the contents along. Colace and Surfak will make the stool softer in consistency and help it to pass. They will not be absorbed into your body or into your baby's body. Milk of magnesia will soften the stool and stimulate your intestines. Senokot is natural (derived from tree bark) and is safe to take during pregnancy. It will stimulate intestinal movement. Choose one of these products and use it in moderation as an adjunct to your healthy vegetarian diet, not in place of it.

I have been so constipated that I developed hemorrhoids. Is this normal?

Yes. Women are likely to develop hemorrhoids during pregnancy for a number of different reasons. First, your enlarged uterus presses on the colon at the bottom of the pelvis, which prevents foods from passing easily. Second, your intestinal transit time is slower to provide more time for the body to absorb nutrients from your intestines. In doing so, the body reabsorbs water from the stools, making them harder and more difficult to pass. Third, all veins throughout the body dilate during pregnancy, including the veins around the anus. When pregnant women subject these dilated veins to the increased pelvic pressure of their large uterus as well as the increased pressure from constipation, it's no surprise they develop hemorrhoids.

Unfortunately, once you have developed hemorrhoids, they will probably recur later in your life. To alleviate your pain and swelling, you should eat fiber-rich foods like fruits and vegetables. Try eating more oily foods, too, like salad dressings and sautéed vegetables. These will relieve your constipation. And make sure you drink at least eight glasses of liquid daily. As a vegetarian, you will have no difficulty maintaining this optimum diet.

For hemorrhoid discomfort, it is safe to use topical preparations such as Anusol or Preparation H. Anusol contains zinc, which heals tissues. Preparation H contains yeast, which stimulates your own tissues to heal themselves. Preparations containing cortisone will heal your tissues and shrink your hemorrhoids. You will also be able to obtain relief by applying warm compresses, witch hazel pads, or Tucks pads. Tucks pads contain witch hazel, an astringent that helps shrink dilated veins and alleviate symptoms. If you find relief from your hemorrhoid problem before the end of your pregnancy, do not throw out your hemorrhoid medication. After you deliver your baby, your hemorrhoids may recur with a vengeance and you will want to have remedies at hand.

AN OUNCE OF PREVENTION:
ANEMIA AND IRON

What exactly is anemia?

Anemia is a common medical condition in which an individual's hemoglobin, the oxygen-carrying component of red blood cells, is deficient. Iron is a necessary component of hemoglobin, and that is why a deficiency in iron can create anemia. The primary function of iron is to form hemoglobin, which enables your red blood cells to carry oxygen. Almost 70 percent of all the iron in your body is in the hemoglobin of your red blood cells. Your liver, spleen, and bone marrow store the rest of your iron as a reservoir until your red blood cells require more.

There are several different reasons people may become anemic. Anemia may be caused by a hereditary abnormality of the red blood cells, a loss of iron from the body, a breakdown of red blood cells within the blood vessels, an inability of the intestines to absorb iron, a diet that prevents the absorption of iron, or insufficient iron in the diet. As long as you maintain a well-balanced and well-planned vegetarian diet, you should have no difficulty attaining adequate iron levels and preventing anemia.

Is it safe to take iron tablets? I worry about taking too many.

Unless you have a specific inability to tolerate iron, as an adult, you will not overdose on iron with two or three daily iron tablets that your obstetrician may have recommended for you. Some people are susceptible to iron toxicity. For example, if you have a genetic blood disorder called thalassemia, your red blood cells cannot store as much iron as the average individual's red blood cells. In this case, excess iron may accumulate in your liver and cause serious scarring. For most individuals, when iron toxicity does occur, it is usually caused by a huge amount of iron supplements, not from eating an iron-rich diet.

How will I know if I am anemic?

If you have iron-deficiency anemia, you may experience weakness, fatigue, shortness of breath, a rapid heart rate, and an increased susceptibility to infections. You may look pale, with pallor around your lips. The cornea of your eyes may appear pale; if you pull down your lower eyelid and look at the color of the blood within the blood vessels, you will see that these vessels are pale pink rather than their usual bright red color.

I am a strict vegetarian. Do you think I will have a greater chance of becoming anemic than will a non-vegetarian woman during pregnancy?

If you do not make wise and educated vegetarian food choices, you will be more likely to develop anemia. But the same can be said for any woman—vegetarian or not—who does not follow a balanced, nutrient-rich diet. With just a little planning and awareness, you will have no problem maintaining a normal blood count and preventing anemia with your vegetarian diet.

As a vegetarian, what can I do to make sure that I do not become anemic?

There are several things you can do to prevent yourself from becoming anemic, and you will understand these better by knowing how your body gets its iron from the foods you eat. The body absorbs only a small percentage of the iron we ingest. There are two types of iron in foods, heme iron and nonheme iron. Heme iron comes from animal muscle, and the body can absorb it easily. Nonheme iron is found in vegetation and egg yolk. This type of iron is a bit more difficult to absorb, but it is just as potent as heme iron.

Many factors affect your absorption of iron. Following a diet rich in vitamin C and citrus fruits and cooking with cast-iron cookware enable you to absorb more iron. However, if you have a low level of gastric acid, it will be more difficult for you to absorb iron. You may decrease your stomach acid if you take antacids regularly. Drinking milk and eating dairy products also reduces gastric acid levels. Additionally, certain chemicals in coffee and tea bind to iron, causing you to excrete it instead of storing it. Some vegetables like spinach, chard, and soy are high in iron but contain substances that decrease the body's ability to absorb iron.

As a vegetarian, you will need to remember that both dairy products and a few vegetables actually decrease your iron absorption, so that you should consume these at one meal and your other iron-rich vegetarian foods at another meal. Simple meal planning will help you avoid anemia.

How much iron will I need during my pregnancy?

When women are not pregnant, they need 15 milligrams of iron each day. That means they need 4,000 milligrams of iron over an average nine-month period. In pregnancy, that daily amount needs to double.

Over the course of your pregnancy, you will be giving 500 to 1,000 milligrams of iron to your baby. More than half of that amount will go to your baby during your last few months. You will increase your own blood volume by over 500 milliliters, will create 1,000 milliliters of blood for your placenta, and will lose an additional 1,000 milliliters of blood when your placenta separates (each milliliter of blood contains 1 milligram of iron). If you add these needs to your body's basic requirement of 4,000 milligrams of iron over nine months, you will need almost 8,000 milligrams of iron during your pregnancy. To be on the safe side, it is recommended that you take between 30 and 45 milligrams of iron each day.

I became anemic and was told to take iron supplements. Why can't my body keep up with its demand for iron?

It is a challenge for most women to obtain enough iron during pregnancy—vegetarian women are no exception. When your doctor checked your blood count for anemia at the beginning of your pregnancy, you learned that your blood count would inevitably decrease as your baby and placenta grew and used your iron. Supplemental iron is beneficial for pregnant women across the board. There is no shame in taking iron supplements; you will feel better through your entire pregnancy and after you deliver if you are not anemic.

Are there any side effects from taking iron?

Some iron supplements may cause intestinal upset, constipation, and blackening of the stool. These are most often caused by iron taken in the form of ferrous sulfate. The easiest forms of iron for an individual's intestinal tract are usually ferrous succinate, ferrous gluconate, and ferrous fumarate. These will cause less constipation and gastrointestinal upset. If you find it difficult to take some forms of iron, it is worthwhile to try different ones. We all have unique bodies, so it follows that some kinds of supplements will agree with you better than others.

I do not know how much iron is present in the vitamin pills I am taking. How much iron do I actually need?

Some vitamin supplement manufacturers describe iron as a compound and others describe it as elemental iron, so it can be difficult to figure out how much iron you are getting. Ferrous sulfate is the compound of iron and sulfate. One 325-milligram tablet of ferrous sulfate is 325 milligrams of the compound, but only 32 milligrams of elemental iron. Of that, you will probably absorb only 10 percent. Therefore, you will be obtaining only 3.2 milligrams of elemental iron daily from such a tablet. During your pregnancy, you need 30 to 60 milligrams of elemental iron daily. That is why your doctor will advise you to take two or three iron tablets daily in addition to an iron-rich prenatal tablet and your iron-rich vegetarian diet. If you take more than 60 milligrams of iron a day, many doctors recommend that you also take copper and zinc supplements to create a normal mineral balance in your body.

Has my vegetarian diet contributed to my developing iron-deficiency anemia?

It may have contributed to it, but iron deficiency is quite common during the last third of pregnancy: 55 percent of all pregnant women develop it by then. I cannot say whether or not your specific diet contributed to your anemia.

During your vegetarian pregnancy, strive to eat foods rich in vitamin C and take 250 milligrams of additional vitamin C with your supplemental iron tablet. Vitamin C is a reducing agent and will help your body convert ferric iron, the form iron takes in foods, to ferrous iron, which is the form your intestines will absorb into your body.

I have heard that the iron in a multivitamin is more difficult to absorb. Is that true?

Yes, this is particularly true because most pregnancy vitamins contain both iron and calcium, and calcium decreases an individual's absorption of iron. If your vitamin contains both calcium and iron, you may not be absorbing as much iron as you think you are. For the same reason, you may not absorb all of the iron if you are taking the vitamin with a calcium supplement, with milk, or with an antacid. You will absorb your iron tablets better if you take them with vitamin C and with juice. The acidity in these foods aids iron absorption.

CHAPTER 9

Your Seventh Month

Your pregnancy has touched your heart.
Being pregnant is all-encompassing for a woman.
It awakens your femininity
and moves you to exist on a new level,
a level of deep maternal satisfaction.

Women experience this sense of contentment and peace
many times during their pregnancies.
It is this awakening of the mother within you
that will bridge the gap between you and the dawning
of all new life.

As a mother
you are now in harmony with all of creation.
And a part of you will exist and perpetuate your spirit
for all time.

Can others sense this creative awakening within you?
Only a select few.
They are the few who have shared this same feeling
of connectedness.

This tiny life within you
has awakened you more fully

than you ever could have imagined
to the power and the possibility of life.

This tiny life,
will forever fill every hollow
of your mind and your heart.

YOUR BABY DURING THE SEVENTH MONTH

- Your baby's length from the top of the head to the end of the torso measures 10 to 11 inches.
- Its total length from the top of the head to the tips of the toes will increase from 15 to 17 inches.
- Its weight will increase from 2 pounds to 4 pounds.
- Your baby's eyebrows and eyelashes may become visible.
- Its eyelids will begin to open, and your baby will be able to differentiate light from dark.
- Its taste buds have developed.
- It will begin to deposit fat under its skin and to fill out its contours, so that your baby will begin to look plumper.
- Its brain is enlarging rapidly, and distinct folds are forming.
- Your baby can now grasp with its tiny hands.

CHANGES YOU MAY NOTICE IN YOURSELF DURING THIS MONTH

You may still experience some or all of the changes you felt during your prior months, as well as the following:

- Your uterus will enlarge and move closer to your diaphragm.
- You may experience shortness of breath with activity more often.
- Your feet and legs may become swollen often.

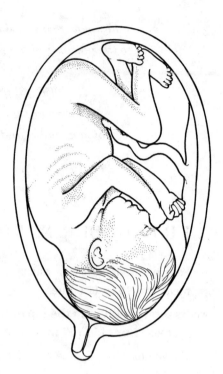

Your twenty-eighth week through your thirty-second week is your seventh month of pregnancy. This is your baby at twenty-eight weeks.

- You may experience more fatigue, especially after three P.M., and you need to rest more often.
- You will feel your baby move more often.
- You may feel Braxton-Hicks uterine contractions more often.

SHORTNESS OF BREATH

I have been feeling increasingly short of breath with each month of my pregnancy. My doctor says that my lungs are fine. Why is this happening?

It is common for women to have difficulty breathing as their pregnancy progresses. Your body gives preferential treatment to your baby, so a large percentage of your circulating blood volume goes directly to your placenta. If you try to visualize the numerous blood vessels supplying oxygen to your uterus and placenta, you will see that the more your baby

grows, the more oxygen it needs. It's only natural that your oxygen supply will be lower as you support this growing life inside you.

Another contributing factor is the pressure from your uterus on your
diaphragm and lungs as it continues to increase in size. The diaphragm
is a muscle, so it will stretch and push upward as your uterus expands.
During your pregnancy, it will elevate 1.6 to 2 inches and compress your
lungs. Your enlarged uterus also puts pressure on your inferior vena
cava. This is the main blood vessel bringing blood back from your lower
extremities to your heart. The major veins returning blood from each of
your legs join at the lower portion of your abdomen to form your inferior
vena cava. This large blood vessel then extends upward on the back part
of your abdominal wall to enter your heart. An enlarged uterus often
presses on the inferior vena cava and slows the return of blood back to
the heart.

Anemia in pregnancy is a common concern and may be another reason you're having difficulty breathing. In pregnancy, your body uses
much of its iron to create blood for your baby's body, your placenta, and
your uterus. Normally you would use this iron to form hemoglobin,
which carries oxygen throughout your body. Your hemoglobin count is
lower when you are anemic, which makes it more difficult for your red
blood cells to supply you with oxygen.

Your obstetrician or midwife will be checking your blood count often
to see if you are anemic. If you are significantly anemic, your doctor will
discuss how you might increase the iron content of your blood cells. In
chapter 2, you'll find specific information on how you can increase your
iron with a vegetarian diet. Please keep in mind that it takes 120 days, or
4 months, for a body to create a red blood cell. While you are waiting for
your body to form new red blood cells, try not to spend too much time in
warm, stuffy, poorly oxygenated areas, as these will further decrease
your supply of oxygen.

CHILDBIRTH CLASSES

Should I attend childbirth classes?

Childbirth classes will give you amazing insight into what it means to be
a mother. Your teachers will be nurses, childbirth educators, or mid-

wives who love the miracle of birth and will impart a sense of dignity and reverence to each aspect of your education. Although you may have read much about labor, there is no better way to prepare for it than by enacting labor during your class. Classes will not only share facts with you, they will also share emotions.

Childbirth classes empower you with the self-assurance and courage that you can gain only through learning. With this knowledge, you will be able to face from a position of strength all the challenges nature presents to you. You will learn how to cope with the intensity of labor, so you can maintain control and make choices wisely. You will learn why your labor proceeds as it does and why your health care team is making certain decisions, so that you will not feel vulnerable or intimidated. With this kind of understanding, all the pieces of your unique puzzle will fit together.

I do not want to experience pain; I plan to have an epidural as soon as I arrive at the delivery room. Do I still need classes?

Yes. Just because you want to go through labor without pain does not mean you should go through it without knowledge. Plus, something may happen while you are in labor that prevents you from receiving pain medication; it could be a problem with your own health or another emergency situation. It will be good for you to be prepared for this possibility. Childbirth classes will share with you much more than techniques about how to go through labor naturally. They will give you an overview of the entire delivery experience, including the process of labor, changes in your body, the effects of labor on your baby, what to expect from your health care team, and what you may be feeling during your own birth experience. The classes will teach you how to relax, how to breathe, how to position yourself, and how to move so you may better cope with your contractions, even though you may still wish to avail yourself of pain medication if and when you want. Please remember, this is your labor, and you can go through it any way you want. You do not have to meet anyone's standards other than your own.

> *When I had my first child, after twenty-one hours of back labor I had an epidural. With my third child, I delivered naturally after only four hours of labor. Anyone who brags that she went through labor naturally and thinks that you should too may not have gone through the twenty-one-hour*

labor I had or the twenty-one-hour labor you may have
had. Don't allow another woman's experience to influence
the choice that is right for you.

I would like to sign up for childbirth classes, but I do not know which
type is best for me. What is the difference between prepared child-
birth, Lamaze, and Bradley classes?

All types of childbirth classes will give you an overview of labor, vaginal
delivery, and cesarean section. They will help you to understand the basic stages of labor and how to best cope with the intensity of your experience. They will all impart a positive attitude and encourage you to see
your labor as the most exciting and rewarding period of your life. All
types of classes will try to alleviate any preconceived notions or fears
you may have had about giving birth.

Prepared Childbirth Classes

In a prepared childbirth class, you will learn about the physiology of
your labor and delivery; this will give you incredible knowledge and
strength. You will learn about the stages of labor and how delivery happens; how your baby will feel during labor; and what events during labor
will require a cesarean section. The classes will be factual and emotional,
but not opinionated. Your teacher will support you whether you want to
labor naturally or choose to have pain medication. She will supply the information you need to make choices. There is not just one way to deal
with the intensity of childbirth. The main objective of this type of class is
to provide the knowledge and practice you need to go into labor with as
little fear and anxiety as possible. You will also learn good ways to relax
and meditate, how to practice Lamaze breathing, and how to ask for help
during labor without losing your sense of dignity. Your teacher will respect your individual concerns about labor and encourage different
opinions about birthing sites, caregivers, and pain medications. Your
goal for this class should be to increase your knowledge and feel at peace
with your own labor.

One young patient of mine was so fearful of labor that she
could not relax at all; she shrieked for twenty hours and
ended up needing a cesarean section. It was only after her

delivery that I learned she never met her own mother. Her mother had died giving birth to her. This had been the most fearful moment of her life. She taught me never to judge the courage or fears of others, as we all have reasons for our choices.

Lamaze Classes

Lamaze classes are not just about breathing; they also cover relaxation techniques and movements, offer emotional support, and teach about massage. The classes will give you confidence in your own ability to give birth. This training will help you rely on yourself for strength instead of depending on others. Although the Lamaze philosophy concerning birth came to the United States from Russia, it has a distinctly Asian influence. It is a peaceful, calming, and introspective technique. During Lamaze classes, you will be taught the value of breathing, meditation, and concentration. Your partner will help you to keep focused by counting your breaths for you. By this transference of imagery, Lamaze will help you divert your conscious mind from the intensity of your labor to the peacefulness of your breathing.

I have delivered many women of Japanese descent. I have always admired their quiet inner strength and their ability to transport their minds to another place. I feel convinced that their relaxation contributes to their peaceful rapid labors. Lamaze training is quite similar to mind-body medicine, which Eastern medicine practitioners have been studying and developing for centuries.

Some women, unfortunately, become too rigid in their breathing patterns and try to adhere to a perfect technique. You should not lose sight of the purpose of the breathing: it is not a counting exercise; it is a relaxation technique, as is meditation. Lamaze has become the most popular type of childbirth in our country, for good reason. Lamaze cannot totally alleviate your pain, nor does it claim to. It can, however, help you cope remarkably well with the pain. Depending upon your pain threshold and the labor nature hands you, you will know if you need to receive pain medication. Even if you anticipate receiving pain medication during labor, you can use Lamaze techniques until that time. You may surprise yourself with your own inner strength. Nowadays, Lamaze instructors discuss all aspects of labor and birth, including narcotics, epidurals, spinals, and cesarean sections. There is not as much pressure placed on women to labor naturally as there had been just ten years ago.

> *When I had my children, I observed other women using Lamaze breathing techniques during labor, but I did not believe it worked. By the time I was halfway through labor, I began instinctively to concentrate on my breathing. It helped me so much to stay focused, to relax, and to refrain from "losing it" until I finally lost it.*

The Bradley Method

The Bradley method of childbirth is not as popular as Lamaze, but it has its own set of proponents. Your Bradley instructor will believe in nonintervention during labor, including the absence of all medications. Bradley instructors generally believe that women will do best if left alone during labor to handle their needs instinctively as they see fit and to breathe naturally. By that, they mean a woman does not need to focus on specific breathing techniques. They feel a woman should scream if she wants, thrash in the bed if she wants, and cry if she wants. This technique works well for those women who have a high pain threshold, are strongly motivated, and have relatively easy labors. If you know that you do not tolerate pain well, be honest with yourself. You do not want to feel disappointed if you cannot tolerate your labor pains and need to take pain medication. If you attempt to push yourself past the level of pain you can tolerate, you may only work yourself up into a frenzy without a plan of how to get a grip on yourself. The Bradley method will give you more freedom and a greater variety of methods to choose from while dealing with the pain of contractions, but it will not make the pains go away.

I have seen many women use the Bradley method, some with great success and some without. When a woman has a high tolerance for pain, this method can motivate her to succeed in her quest to have a natural birth. When a woman has a low tolerance for pain and a general fear of labor, this method may trigger a screaming, thrashing fit and only heighten her level of anxiety. Only you can be the judge, and labor may not be the best time for you to learn about your own pain tolerance.

You may do well with the Bradley method if you have an instructor who is a seasoned delivery room nurse and understands the complications that may arise during labor and the responsibilities of the delivery room team. If you are taught to distrust the team helping you, you will isolate yourself from their collective years of experience and wisdom. Remember that although birth is natural, nature never promised us birth without pain. In any labor, the goal is simply to have a healthy baby, not to test yourself.

Water Births

Water births are a relatively new phenomenon in our country. Dr. Michael Odent began his practice of birthing babies underwater in France. He would encourage women to rest in a warm bath to help them labor and, for some women, to help them give birth. His labor baths were two and a half feet deep, seven feet across, and wide enough for two people. Many of the women who used these baths felt that the calming effect and pressure of the water made their labors easier. Dr. Odent also noted in his patients what he called an "ejection response," meaning that when the women came out of the bath, they delivered their babies right away. He hypothesized that the sudden release of external water pressure they experienced when they came out of the water contributed to this response. It is difficult to know if his observation is medically valid; the speed, pain, and tolerance of each woman's labor is so unique that any change in a labor pattern is difficult to quantify.

Water births are now performed all over our country. An underwater birth may provide soothing pressure on your back, extra warmth, relief from sticky perspiration, and a strong sense of relaxation. While a woman is in the water, however, she will not be able to receive narcotic pain medications; since these affect motor skills, there is a risk she may fall and injure herself. She will also not be able to receive epidural anesthesia, as the catheter site might become infected in water. If you elect to have a water birth, you may need to rent the tub yourself if your hospital or birthing center does not have one. You will be able to rent one from a water birth agency. Discuss your wishes with your doctor or midwife, because your hospital may need to prepare a specific room for you to place your tub, inflow and outflow hoses, and other supplies. Your hospital may also need to check your local municipal water supply for a bacterial count. If your hospital already has a protocol concerning underwater births, it may not permit you to have a water birth if you have had an infection or a prior cesarean section, or any medical condition. That is why it is good to discuss this choice with your health care team.

You may wonder how your baby will be able to take its first breath underwater. Your baby will breathe when its chest expands after being tightly compressed within your uterus. Its chest will still be compressed while it is under the water, so it will not need to take its first breath until its placenta separates from your uterine wall or it is lifted out of the water.

Water and Births

Do you think it will be beneficial for me to shower or to sit in a bath during my labor?

As long as you feel the instinct to do so, yes, this can be helpful. If you just want to rest in bed or on a rocking chair, that is fine, too. There are many good reasons to use water during labor. Because we are accus-

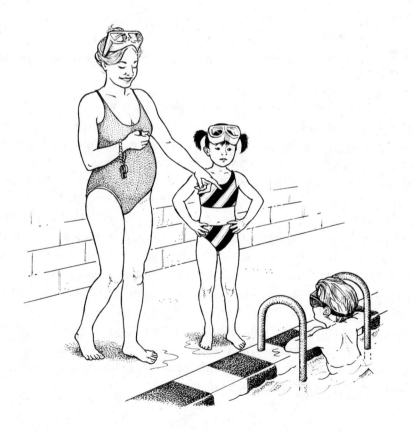

tomed to Western medicine, our concept of healing means using a chemical to change ourselves, like taking a medication. We are not as familiar with the healing power of physical modalities like water pressure, massage therapy, acupressure, acupuncture, and reiki. Just recall how relaxing and soothing it can feel whenever you place some painful part of your body in water. The use of water is not right or necessary for every woman, but it definitely will help some women.

Water can create counterpressure, and the pressure of water on your back may be as soothing as the healing pressure of a massage. During your labor, if you and your baby are doing fine and you have not had narcotics that may make you drowsy, you may be able to decrease the intensity of your pain by standing in a warm shower or sitting in a warm tub. Water will not eliminate all your pains, but it may help you to cope with them better. If you feel hot and sticky after hours of labor, you may be able to refresh yourself with a shower and have more energy to fuel the rest of your mission.

Leboyer Birth

What is the Leboyer method? Does this involve water for the baby or for myself?

Dr. Frederick Leboyer was a French obstetrician who considered the birth process from the perspective of the newborn. His was quite an innovative and compassionate approach. Dr. Leboyer recalled his own birth in a rebirthing experience and discovered it was very traumatic and laden with unnecessary shocks. His book, *Birth without Violence*, explored what a child's first impression of the world must be like. One of his most influential observations was how newborns react to light. He proposed that the delivery room should be dimly lit, because he felt it was too shocking for a child to arrive after nine months of total darkness into a world full of bright lights. During our adult lives, we often find ourselves sharing our most sensitive intimate moments in semidarkness. Dr. Leboyer believed that these moments of profound spiritual depth, including the moment of birth, require the kind of privacy and comfort that soft lighting provides. As a result of Dr. Leboyer's perceptive and compassionate insights, most birthing sites today allow you to lower the lights when you are ready to deliver.

Dr. Leboyer also believed that a newborn should be placed in a tub of body temperature water immediately after its birth to make the transition from its aquatic world less traumatic. This practice has not gained much acceptance in our culture. We generally believe that it is best for an infant to be held by its mother and father after birth. Parents cherish the opportunity to hold and caress their new baby, and we like to believe that the baby enjoys this new feeling, too.

Although we have not adopted all of Dr. Leboyer's childbirth philosophy, his insight into the newborn's first taste of life outside the womb has made a lasting impression on our beliefs about birth.

WEIGHT WATCH

I have gained twenty pounds! I don't know whether I should be happy or sad about this as I begin my last three months.

You should feel proud! So far, you have remained within a healthy, normal range of weight gain. You may gain anywhere between zero and fifteen pounds in your last trimester; the average gain in this period is eight to ten pounds. Of that, your baby will probably be gaining four more pounds, your uterus another pound, and your placenta almost another pound. In addition, you may be retaining significant amounts of fluid in your feet, legs, and fingers and (strangely enough) even around your nose during your last few weeks of pregnancy.

At this point, your levels of activity and exercise might be somewhat restricted owing to pressure from your uterus on your bladder, shortness of breath, and general fatigue. If your body is telling you that all you can do to maintain an active metabolic rate is to walk, then follow your instincts and do not push yourself. Please remember that you have the rest of your life to lose the weight, but only these nine months to create a healthy baby.

NOTE ON NUTRITION: VARICOSE VEINS AND YOUR VEGETARIAN DIET

Is there anything in my vegetarian diet I can do to strengthen my veins and prevent them from becoming varicose?

Your heredity, lifestyle, and diet are all contributing factors to varicose veins. Fortunately for you, many components of a healthy vegetarian diet may help you decrease your chances of developing varicose veins.

Fiber

As you know, fiber is essential to good digestion. A meat-based diet is low in fiber, causing elimination to be more difficult for a non-vegetarian. This kind of strain on the bowels increases intra-abdominal pressure and pushes down on the veins trying to return blood to the heart. Your high-fiber vegetarian diet decreases your need to strain to evacuate your colon and, therefore, will decrease your chances of developing or worsening your varicose veins.

Vitamin E

Oils derived from vegetables, seeds, and nuts are excellent sources of vitamin E, an essential nutrient for healing and strengthening body tissues. Because of its healing properties, vitamin E can be very helpful in preventing the development of varicose veins.

Vitamin P (Bioflavonoids)

Vitamin P strengthens capillaries and the collagen that binds capillary walls. It is usually found in the pulp (hence the *P*) of citrus fruits. It is also found in foods that contain vitamin C. Good sources of vitamin P are cherries, grapes, papayas, blackberries, green pepper, broccoli, and tomatoes. Vitamin P is not always found in vitamin C tablets, which is why it is important to eat natural fruits and vegetables. There is no vitamin P in any animal-based food, so vegetarians receive an excellent complement of this important vitamin.

AN OUNCE OF PREVENTION:
TOXEMIA OF PREGNANCY

My blood pressure is elevated, and my doctor is testing me for toxemia of pregnancy. What exactly is toxemia?

Although toxemia of pregnancy (also called "preeclampsia" and "pregnancy-induced hypertension") affects 6 to 8 percent of all pregnant women, no one knows what causes it. We do know quite a bit about the effects of toxemia, however; left untreated, it can harm a woman's organs, impact the growth and health of her baby, and lead to serious medical problems. Toxemia often runs in families, it occurs more often in a woman who has had hypertension, and it generally occurs more often during a first pregnancy. It usually develops after the twentieth week of pregnancy and is diagnosed when a woman presents with swelling, high blood pressure, and protein in her urine. As the disease progresses, it can damage the liver, the blood-clotting cells, and the kidneys.

What are the chances I will become toxemic?

Following is a list of specific factors that may increase your chances of developing toxemia.

- If this is your first pregnancy, your risk is increased three times.
- If you are over forty years of age, your risk is increased three times.
- If you are African American, your risk is increased one and a half times.
- If you have diabetes, your risk is increased two times.
- If you are having twins, your risk is increased four times.
- If toxemia of pregnancy runs in your family, your risk is increased five times.
- If you have high blood pressure, your risk is increased ten times.
- If you have chronic kidney disease, your risk is increased twenty times.

Toxemia can present at various times during a pregnancy. For most women, it occurs during the last trimester, but it can also occur any time before or after that. It may even occur when a woman is in labor or after she has delivered.

> *Toxemia has always been one of the mysteries of pregnancy. It usually resolves once a woman delivers her placenta, yet some women first develop it after they have finished delivering both their baby and their placenta.*

Symptoms of toxemia include high blood pressure, protein in the urine, fluid retention and swelling all over the body, fluid in the lungs, lower platelet count, changes in liver enzymes, visual changes of bright white spots, headaches, upper abdominal pains, and soreness on the right side of the abdomen (in the liver). If you develop toxemia, you may have only one or two of these symptoms or all of them. During toxemia, the uterine blood vessels that provide blood for the placenta may constrict and decrease its blood supply—causing babies to be smaller and experience distress during labor.

Toxemia of pregnancy runs in my family. Can a diet high in calcium help prevent toxemia in high-risk women such as myself?

There has been much medical debate over the effect calcium has in prevention of toxemia, but no one is sure if calcium helps at all. Taking high doses of calcium to prevent toxemia is a new theory, but according to a recent study by the National Institutes of Health of five thousand high-risk women, these higher doses of calcium did not prevent toxemia. Calcium is essential for your body to produce nitric oxide, a chemical that helps blood vessels relax. The blood vessels in women with toxemia spasm and constrict, which secondarily leads to an increase in blood pressure. The nitric acid that calcium causes to be produced may help to prevent this chain of events.

Prior to this study, however, other studies demonstrated fewer cases of toxemia when the high-risk women increased their calcium from the recommended daily dose of 1,000 milligrams to a dose of 2 grams. If you are a vegan, it will be best for you to make an effort to consume vegetables high in calcium and to consider calcium supplements (see chapter 2). For women who are at low risk for toxemia, calcium intake, whether high or low, does not seem to affect its incidence. Although the studies are conflicting, it cannot hurt to err on the side of caution. Without supplements, your calcium intake may be as low as 500 milligrams daily, so you will do well to consume a total of 2,000 milligrams of calcium daily, either from your diet, from calcium supplements, or from a combination.

Will my delivery be affected because I have toxemia of pregnancy?

Yes, it is very likely that toxemia will play a role in how your labor and delivery progress. Depending upon how far along you are, your doctor may induce your labor early; it is common for women with toxemia to experience serious problems as they approach their due dates. During your labor, your nurse will watch you very closely and repeatedly monitor your blood pressure, your urine output, and your reflexes. Your doctor or nurse may repetitively check your knee reflex to see if you are becoming twitchy, a sign that you may start to have a seizure. They will also test your blood and urine frequently to evaluate your blood-clotting parameters, your liver function, and your kidney function. In addition, during labor you may be given medications such as magnesium sulfate to prevent you from having a seizure. You may also not be allowed to have an epidural for pain relief. If your platelet count is too low, an epidural may cause bleeding around your spinal cord.

If it is critical for your health or your baby's survival that you be delivered immediately, and your labor is progressing slowly or not at all, your doctor may need to perform a cesarean section. Your blood may not be clotting well, so the doctor may use general anesthesia during the procedure. After your delivery or your cesarean section, you will most likely stay in the delivery room overnight so that your nurse can monitor your blood pressure, your urine output, and your reflexes.

What is the difference between toxemia of pregnancy and preeclampsia?

Toxemia of pregnancy is the general term for preeclampsia, pregnancy-induced hypertension, and eclampsia. In toxemic states, a woman may have high blood pressure, swelling all over her body, protein deposits in the urine, headaches, dizziness, vision changes, nausea, vomiting, stomach pains, and a decreased production of urine. In those cases where preeclampsia worsens and seizures occur, the condition is called eclampsia.

CHAPTER 10

*Y*our Eighth Month

*You are just one month away from holding your baby.
Your baby did not come to you by chance.
This is the baby destiny wished you to have.
You are part of the grand design
that has given this special child life.*

*You possess the instincts to protect your child,
and you will give it the courage
to be all it is meant to be in life.*

*You will teach your child to be honest, fair, and kind,
so that it will grow to respect itself and others.*

*You will share with your child your vision of kindness,
and your vegetarian principles,
so that it will revere and respect all living creatures.*

*As a mother,
you will enrich this baby's mind and soul.
You will shine a steady light upon its path
and inspire your child
to one day shine its own light.*

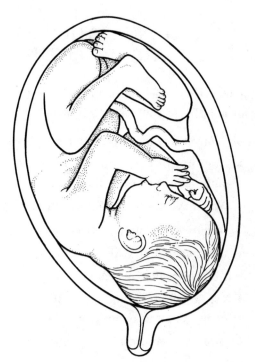

Your thirty-second week through your thirty-sixth week is your eighth month of pregnancy. This is your baby at thirty-two weeks.

YOUR BABY DURING THE EIGHTH MONTH

- ♦ Its length from the top of its head to the end of its buttocks is now 11 inches to 13 inches.
- ♦ Its full length from the top of its head to the end of its toes will increase from 17 to 19 inches.
- ♦ Its weight increases from 4 to 6 pounds.
- ♦ Its limbs become soft and plump.
- ♦ It may experience hiccups.
- ♦ Its fingernails have grown past its fingertips.
- ♦ Your baby's torso and limbs will be approaching newborn proportions.
- ♦ Your baby will begin to look more and more like a newborn.

CHANGES YOU MAY NOTICE IN YOURSELF THIS MONTH

You may still experience some or all of the changes you felt during your prior months, as well as the following:

- Your uterus now takes up most of your abdominal cavity.
- Your uterus will push your intestines to the sides of your abdomen and up toward your diaphragm.
- You may experience constipation frequently.
- You may feel vaginal pressure and swelling.
- You may notice varicose veins in your vulva.
- Your breasts may begin to secrete colostrum.
- While you are standing, active, or in a warm and stuffy environment, you may experience shortness of breath.
- You will feel pressure on your pubic bone, especially when sitting or walking.
- Your thighs may feel generally achy from the weight of your uterus.
- You will feel your baby move quite frequently.
- You may start to feel mild uterine cramps.

VULVA VARICOSITIES

I have huge, bluish red varicose veins on my labia, but none on my legs. My doctor says these are vulva varicosities. Will they go away after I deliver?

Yes, these large veins on your labia will disappear after your delivery. Numerous women develop extreme dilatation of the veins on either or both sides of their labia. These clusters of dilated veins can become so large that they become debilitating. They are unsightly to look at, may cause discomfort when you try to sit, and may make it impossible for you to have sexual relations. This condition is more common than you might think, but not surprisingly, most women do not discuss it openly.

Sometimes women have such large vulva varicosities that it looks as though the veins might rupture during delivery and cause excessive bleeding. Fortunately, that happens very rarely. The walls of these veins stretch just as the rest of the vulval tissues stretch, so in most cases women should not worry that these varicosities will rupture and bleed at delivery. Although varicose veins in your legs might not resolve completely after delivery, varicosities of the labia shrink and disappear totally.

BREAST CHANGES

My breasts have become much larger. They are sore, too, and are beginning to leak. Are these signs that I may deliver prematurely?

No, these are signs that your body is preparing for delivery normally, not prematurely. During your first six months of pregnancy, the ducts of your breasts grow. During the last three months, your tiny alveoli, the milk-producing glands at the ends of the ducts, are preparing. These alveoli become distended and start to fill with colostrum. Colostrum is the initial protein- and antibody-rich milk your body will produce. There is no normal amount of breast growth or discharge that occurs prior to delivery, so there is no need to worry that you will deliver prematurely. It is best not to squeeze your nipples to see if more colostrum will come, because that will cause more to come. The squeezing sends a reflex message back to your pituitary gland that you are ready to nurse; in response, your breast alveoli produce even more colostrum. If the discharge is a nuisance to you, simply purchase breast shields to prevent your clothes from getting wet.

The areolae of my breasts look much larger and darker in color. I know this does not happen to every woman. Should I be concerned?

We are all physiologically different and all have unique physical reactions to pregnancy. In many women, the pituitary, the master gland, produces more melanin-stimulating hormone than it does in other women. If your body is producing more of this hormone, you will develop a darker line down the middle of your abdomen (the linea nigra), darker pigment on the sides of your face, darker pigment on the inner surfaces of your thighs, and and darker pigment on the areola region of your breasts. This increase in pigment does not mean that you will deliver earlier or produce more or less milk. It is simply a normal change for some women. The pigment in your areolae may decrease somewhat after you deliver but probably will never be as light as before you were pregnant.

My breasts are so itchy now, what can I do?

The itchiness you are feeling is a result of your growing breast tissue. The same nerve fibers that carry the feeling of pain also carry itching and tickling sensations. You will not be able to alleviate the itching with oral medication, but you can treat it with cold compresses, topical Benadryl ointment, or solutions like Novocain and Lidocaine. Try not to scratch, because you might scratch enough to break the surface of your skin and develop an infection. Although cortisone is considered relatively safe for pregnant women to use for a serious dermatologic condition, you should not use it now, as it could penetrate your skin tissue. Consider wearing a bra made with finely weaved, smooth material. This may help by decreasing the surface irritation on your skin. If your breasts itch at night, keep this area cooler by using thinner blankets. Also, sleep on fine-weave bedsheets—with a 270 thread count or higher—to further decrease the surface irritation on your breasts.

Why do the veins in my breasts seem so much larger?

During pregnancy, collagen tissue in the walls of your blood vessels becomes softer; as this happens, the blood vessels dilate and stretch outward. At the same time, progesterone from your placenta decreases the tension in your blood vessel walls, so these same vessels dilate even further. Your blood vessels become so much wider that they become apparent on your breasts below the surface of the skin. After you deliver, these blood vessels will definitely return to their normal size.

Under both of my arms, the skin has become very swollen. Is this swollen breast tissue, swollen lymph nodes, or something else?

Although there are lymph nodes under your arms, what you are feeling now is swollen breast tissue. Every woman's breast tissue extends into the axillary region located under the arm. During pregnancy, it is not uncommon for the tissue to swell and cause some discomfort. There is not much you can do to alleviate this swelling, but you can take comfort in knowing that it is entirely normal. After you deliver and start to produce milk, the situation may become worse. The swelling may become tender and painful and prevent you from being able to put your arms down at your sides. If that happens, apply cold compresses to the breast tissue under your arms to decrease this milk production. The breast tissue on your chest wall will still continue to manufacture milk, but the axillary portion will not, so the pain and swelling here will ease up a bit.

I have inverted nipples. Will I be able to nurse my baby?

Many women have inverted nipples and are able to nurse, but you will not know until you try. It is a good idea to start preparing for nursing now. Meet with a lactation consultant or, if you prefer, a La Leche League representative; she will discuss the challenges you may face as well as the nursing methods that will be best for you. You may also want to purchase nipple shields, as they can help your baby to draw your nipple out while nursing. Try not to become discouraged before you start. You will never know if you can nurse successfully if you don't make an attempt.

I have silicone breast implants. Do you think it is all right for me to nurse?

Between one and two million women in our country have silicone breast implants. If you had a mammogram prior to becoming pregnant to confirm your implant had not ruptured, then it should be relatively safe for your baby to nurse. If you have not had a recent mammogram and now are not able to get one because of your pregnancy, you will have no way of knowing if silicone has leaked into your breast tissue. If there is a possibility that your implant has ruptured, it is best not to nurse. Studies have shown that a baby can ingest silicone from its mother's breast implants, especially if the implants have ruptured. As we do not know the future effects silicone might have on a baby who ingested it while nursing, there is reason for concern. Once you are nursing, you might ask your doctor to send a sample of your breast milk for microscopic analysis to check for particles of silicone.

I have saline implants in my breasts. Can I nurse with these implants?

For most women with saline implants, there is no medical reason not to nurse. How successful nursing is for these women often depends on the incision through which the implants were inserted. You probably will not experience any more difficulty, or pain, or be more likely to develop infections, while nursing if your doctor inserted your implants with an incision under your breasts or under your arm. If the implants were inserted through a small curved incision on the lower border of your areolae (the pigmented region around your nipples), you may experience difficulties. In this case, some of the ducts leading from the lower portion of your nipple to the glands in the lower portion of your breasts may have been cut. As a result, your glands will fill up with milk, but there will be no way for the milk to get to your nipple and to your baby. Having implants should not prevent you from trying to nurse, as numerous women with implants nurse without the slightest difficulty. Explain the details of your procedure with your doctor; she can help you determine whether or not nursing is a good option for you.

Will I be able to nurse if I had surgery to reduce the size of my breasts?

There is an excellent chance you will be able to nurse. Please discuss with your surgeon to confirm that during your operation he did not disrupt the ducts connecting your breast glands (the alveoli) to the final ducts that transport milk through your nipple.

NOTE ON NUTRITION: YOUR VEGETARIAN BABY'S SIZE

I have not gained much weight during my pregnancy; my doctor said that my baby might be small. Do you think this might be a result of my vegetarian diet?

Two basic factors contribute to your baby's size and weight at birth: the genetics of your husband and you, and your baby's environment during pregnancy. Your weight gain falls into the second category.

Weight gain is based purely on caloric intake; a non-vegetarian woman whose caloric intake is less than 1,500 calories daily will not have a significantly larger child than a woman who consumes the same number of calories on a vegetarian diet. Diet is not the only influence on a baby's weight; if you smoke cigarettes, your baby may weigh less than five pounds at birth. The average birth weight of an infant born to a smoker is one-half pound less than the weight of an infant born to a non-smoker. Your age also impacts your baby's growth. As an older mother, you will be more likely to have a smaller infant. Your baby's sex influences its size, too; female infants are generally four ounces lighter than male infants. Your medical and genetic history will also play a role in your baby's size and weight. If you have chronic kidney disease, hypertension, or severe anemia, you will more likely have a smaller newborn. If you previously had a small newborn, you are more likely to have another small one. Your own size relates to your baby, too; small women tend to have small babies. If you are carrying twins or triplets, they will most likely be smaller at birth than a single baby would have been. Identical twins (twins from the same egg) have a greater chance of being small than do fraternal twins (twins from two different eggs). That is because identical twins may be sharing all of their nutrition from the same placenta. The more babies you are carrying, the greater the chance they will be smaller. Alcohol and street drugs inhibit growth, so it is in your baby's best interest that you avoid these substances altogether.

How much influence does nutrition play in determining the size of my baby?

In a study of specific nutrients and their relation to the weight of newborns, vitamin C was the only nutrient that showed an impact on a baby's weight at birth. High levels of vitamin C increase a baby's weight by one to two ounces. As long as you're following a diet that provides a full complement of vitamins, minerals, and nutrients, your baby should have a healthy, normal birth weight.

In a study conducted in London, the newborns of vegetarian and of meat-eating individuals were compared. They show the following results:

	VEGETARIANS	Non-Vegetarians
BIRTH WEIGHTS	6.5 lb	7.2 lb
BODY LENGTH	20 cm	20.5 cm
APGAR SCORES	NO DIFFERENCE	
CONGENITAL DEFECTS	NO DIFFERENCE	

The newborns of vegetarian women were smaller, but otherwise their health was equal to that of non-vegetarian babies. The vegetarian children had the same amount of vitality at birth and no higher rate of abnormalities. It is difficult to evaluate how much of the size difference was due to environmental conditions and how much was due to diet.

I was not a vegetarian during my first pregnancy, but I am now. My first baby was too large to fit through my pelvic bones; she weighed nine pounds and three ounces. What are the chances this baby will be smaller because of my vegetarian diet?

The chances you will have a baby that is more in proportion to your pelvic cavity will actually be improved as a result of your maintaining a vegetarian diet. A vegetarian diet is not the total answer, however, because many factors go into creating the size of your baby, including your genetics, your husband's genetics, and your general health. Babies of vegetarian women are generally one-half pound smaller in weight than babies of non-vegetarian women. In your case, a baby one-half pound smaller may still not be small enough for you to deliver vaginally, because genetically you may be more likely to have large babies. A baby supported by a vegetarian diet will always weigh a little less than a non-vegetarian baby, no matter what your genetic profile is. When the size of a baby's head is not in proportion to its mother's pelvic bone, a cesarean section is usually necessary. In some women, the major problem is that they have a very small pelvis, but in the majority of situations, it is the baby's head that is too large.

Mothers born and raised in third world countries generally have nar-

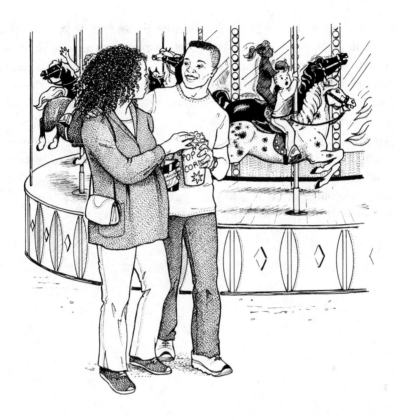

rower pelvic cavities; their babies are correspondingly smaller, and they are able to deliver their smaller babies without difficulty. When these same women move to our country and adopt our high-protein diet, they give birth to larger babies and have an increased need for cesarean sections.

AN OUNCE OF PREVENTION: COPING WITH NAUSEA

I am feeling nauseated again and do not want to eat anything. Is this normal?

During your last month of pregnancy, it is common to lose your appetite, be nauseated, feel that food is sticking like a lump in your esophagus, and feel full even after you have just a few bites of food. Part of your food aversion is due to the rapid decline in several of your pituitary gland's hormones as your body is getting ready to release your baby. Your loss of appetite is simply mechanical—as your uterus is placing so much pressure up and against your stomach and intestines, these will sense this outer pressure and resist your desire to eat (so as to avoid inner pressure).

Obviously, you will not be able to change these sensations and aversions, but you can work to balance them. Eat small meals of soft foods, do not lie down right after you have eaten, and keep yourself well hydrated. You may not be able to eat a salad, but you can certainly drink carrot juice, grapefruit juice, and vegetable soup.

CHAPTER 11

Your Ninth Month and Labor

Although each pregnancy lasts only nine months,
in your heart and your mind,
it may feel like a lifetime.
You have waited for the birth of your baby
and your dream of being a mother
to come true.

Yet you cannot understand why,
in spite of your excitement, your readiness, and your joy,
you are so fearful.
Although you feel happy, blessed, relieved, and prepared,
you are so very scared.

As a doctor,
and as a vegetarian,
I believe nature wishes us to deeply respect the sanctity of birth
and the experience of creation.

All women about to give birth have felt what you are now feeling.
Only women know what it is to create life,
and only women can understand intimately
the ecstasy of giving life.

Be patient with yourself.
Let yourself laugh or cry, smile or frown, sleep or run.

Your pregnancy may not have been easy,
and your labor may not be pleasant.
But without a doubt,
you will realize how every minute
of pregnancy and labor
has been worth waiting
a lifetime for.

YOUR BABY DURING THE NINTH MONTH

- ◆ Your baby's length from the top of its head to the bottom of its buttocks will increase from 13 inches to 15 inches.

- ◆ Its length from the top of its head to the tips of its toes will increase from 19 to 22 inches.

- ◆ Its weight will increase approximately from 6 to 8 pounds.

- ◆ Most babies will start to assume a head-down position by now.

- ◆ It will deposit more fat tissue under its skin, and it will have a softer look.

- ◆ Its kidneys are now fully mature and functional.

- ◆ Its lungs start to produce chemicals to help sustain its survival outside of your uterus.

- ◆ If your baby is a male, its testes will descend into its scrotum.

- ◆ Its proportions become more like adult proportions—its head and trunk make up 60 percent of its length, and its legs measure 40 percent of its length.

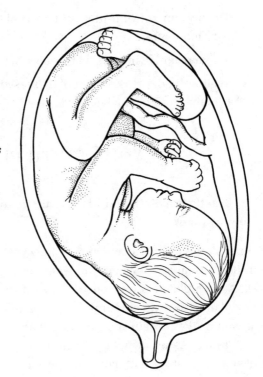

Your thirty-sixth week through your fortieth week is your ninth month of pregnancy. This is your baby at thirty-six weeks.

CHANGES YOU MAY NOTICE IN YOURSELF THIS MONTH

You may still experience some or all of the changes you felt during your prior months, as well as the following:

- ◆ Your uterus may begin to descend.
- ◆ You may feel less pressure on your diaphragm.
- ◆ Sometimes you may find it easier to breathe.
- ◆ The tissues of your vulva and lower extremities may become swollen.
- ◆ Your breasts may secrete a considerable amount of colostrum.
- ◆ Varicose veins in your legs may become worse, especially if you must stand for long periods of time.
- ◆ You may feel significant pressure on your pubic bone.

- The pressure of your uterus on your bladder may cause you to urinate more often.

- You may notice increasing mood swings.

- Feelings of depression and of increased emotional sensitivity may become more pervasive.

YOUR BIRTH PLAN

What exactly is a birth plan? Is it realistic to expect that my labor will follow my plan?

A birth plan is a general overview of how you wish to experience your labor. It is a template for how you want your labor to progress if all goes well. A birth plan lets your doctor know if you hope to deliver naturally, if you plan to have an epidural as soon as you enter the delivery room, if you would like to deliver in a particular position, and a multitude of other issues. As in all fields of medicine, your obstetrician or midwife will have a routine pattern in which she feels most comfortable. This does not mean she cannot change or does not want to change; it just means that unless you have specific requests, there is no reason for her to change. When a woman lets her physician know that she would like to follow another pattern during labor, more often than not, her physician will accommodate her. If you want to deliver squatting, with no medication, wearing your own clothes, with soft music playing in the background, there should be no problem in your doing so. As long as your wishes in no way jeopardize the health of either your baby or yourself, your doctor will be glad that you have shared your wishes with her.

Please consider the following choices when composing your birth plan:

- Is the availability of pain medication important to you?

- Is your freedom to move and walk around in labor an important factor?

- Is your labor or delivery position significant?

- How many people do you want to be with you during labor?

- Do you want close nursing/medical attention during your labor or only when it is necessary?

- ◆ Will you be able to bring personal items, including music, videos, or your own beverage, to labor with you?

- ◆ How long can your baby remain with you during your hospital stay?

If I were having a baby now, my only request would be that I have a quiet environment, with no "helpful" staff members yelling at me to push. I appreciate peacefulness. I would leave the rest up to what is meant to be.

Your birth plan cannot be a strict guideline; it is simply a wish list. It cannot formulate mandated roles for either your doctor or your nurse-midwife, because they must answer to a higher guideline. This is their ethical commitment, to deliver the healthiest child possible for you. Any unexpected changes or disappointments you encounter along the path to this goal are inevitable.

I hope that you will not be disappointed if your birth does not totally conform to your birth plan. It is not possible for us, as humans, to plan or control nature. No one can predict all of the events that might occur during labor. No one has knowledge or insight into how each baby, each placenta, or each uterus will react to that same experience of labor. As women, we all hope that our minds and our willpower will carry us through labor exactly as we wish, but we often forget that we must accept the realities of our bodies as much as we believe in the strength of our hope.

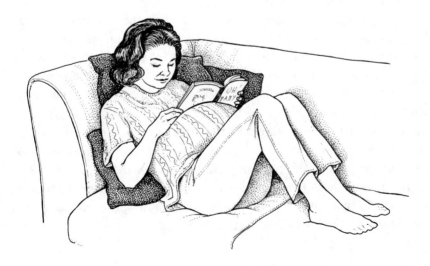

I always appreciated when women discussed their birthing plans, because they gave me a good sense of their thoughts and opinions about labor. Both they and I did our best to adhere to their plans, while still accepting the presence and power of nature in their childbirth.

> *During birth, you do not want to lose sight of the beauty of the forest by analyzing each tree. The plans of nature are usually far simpler to follow than are the plans of man.*

APGAR SCORES AND NEWBORN TESTS

Apgar Scores

What are Apgar scores?

The Apgar score was first devised in 1952 by pediatrician Dr. Virginia Apgar as way of evaluating a baby's health at birth. When a baby is born, the nurse or doctor will evaluate the baby at one minute after its birth and again at five minutes after its birth. The doctor or nurse will assess five aspects of the baby's appearance at birth: its heart rate, its breathing, its muscle tone, its reflexes, and its color. If a baby had a low Apgar score because of sudden fetal distress at birth, the medical team will continue to evaluate its Apgar score at ten minutes, fifteen minutes, and twenty minutes after its birth.

The higher a baby's Apgar score, the greater the indication that the baby was active and vigorous at its birth. Under optimum conditions, a baby should have a heart rate in the range of 120 to 160 beats per minute. It should begin to cry within its first few minutes of life, it should move its arms and legs, and it should flinch or withdraw its body and limbs when it is irritated. Its whole body will be either completely pink or mostly pink with bluish tinges at the ends of the fingers and toes. Although the top Apgar score is 10, this score is rarely assigned to a baby, because most babies are not completely pink at birth. The tips of the little fingers and toes of most babies are usually pale or blue at birth, even if the rest of their body is pink. The most common Apgar score given to a totally active, healthy baby at birth is 9.

YOUR BABY'S APGAR SCORE

For each of the five components below, your doctor will give your baby a 0, 1, or 2. These five scores added up make your baby's total Apgar score.

Component	SCORE		
	0	1	2
Heart rate	Absent	Less than 100 beats/min	More than 100 beats/min
Respiration	Absent	Weak cry and breathing	Good, strong cry
Muscle tone	Limp	Some flexion	Active motion
Reflexes	No response	Grimace	Cry or active withdrawal
Color	Blue or pink	Pink body with blue fingers	Completely pink

What do the results of an Apgar score really indicate about the health of my baby at birth and about its future health?

The Apgar cannot be used as an indication that a child will be a genius or will have learning difficulties. Many people mistakenly believe that there is a direct correlation between a newborn's Apgar score and its later intelligence quotient. This is not the case. The score cannot tell you if your child will read easily or have dyslexia, if your child will find learning easy or difficult, or if your child will have a normal attention span or will have an attention deficit disorder. The Apgar score is only an assessment of the condition of your baby at birth. And, most important for you as a vegetarian, there is no relationship between high/low Apgar scores and vegetarian/non-vegetarian diets.

The higher the Apgar score, the easier your baby's transition has been from life inside your uterus to life in our world. Most babies receive scores of 7, 8, or 9. The more important scores are actually a baby's five-minute and ten-minute scores, not the one-minute score.

Newborn Tests

Do I have control over what will be happening to my baby after it is delivered?

You will have a great deal of control of your baby's care after it is delivered; your greatest control will be in the pediatrician you choose. Although some treatments and some tests for newborns are federally mandated, others are left to the discretion of the pediatrician. This is why it will be good for you to either have a consultation with your pediatrician before your baby is born or for you to speak with other mothers who have used this physician so you can feel confident that you and your pediatrician are of like mind and spirit.

You need not agree with your pediatrician on all issues, but you should agree on some basic philosophical principles if you want to work together successfully to give the best health care to your baby. Each pediatrician has a list of his standing medical care protocol orders for the nursing staff to follow for all infants under his care. This does not mean that these requirements cannot be changed; they often are. They simply provide the nursing staff with a template for basic care. Please inform your pediatrician if you have special feelings or requests regarding your baby's care. If he does not agree with your views, it will be best for you to find another physician who does. As a vegetarian, you may have wishes that differ from those of the norm, so you and your baby's pediatrician will need to be in a mutually learning, growing, and respectful relationship with the welfare of your baby in mind at all times.

> *I did not believe in vaccinating my children until their first birthdays. I felt they would not have contact with tetanus, diphtheria, or other illnesses while they were infants, and I did not want them to receive vaccines when they weighed only six pounds. I found a supportive and understanding pediatrician, and we agreed to vaccinate the children when they were older and weighed twenty pounds. I appreciated the mutual respect my pediatrician and I shared.*

After you deliver and begin to raise your children, you will realize that the knowledge and expertise your pediatrician shares with you is one of the most important aspects in the care of your child. I hope that you will be able to find doctors with both skill and compassion as you begin your journey as a parent.

> *As a vegetarian mother who raised my children vegetarian, I was very blessed to have found an Indian pediatrician who respected my wish for our family to follow a diet that did not inflict harm upon animals, yet helped us to raise strong, healthy, bright children.*

What tests will be performed on my baby in the hospital?

Your baby will have numerous blood tests taken from its heel, its veins, and its placenta. Fortunately, several of the blood tests your baby will need can be taken directly from umbilical cord blood. The umbilical cord contains the same blood as that of your baby, which is why so many tests can be taken from it right after it is delivered. These tests will include a blood count for anemia, blood type, and Rh type. If you are Rh-negative, your baby's blood will also be tested for Rh blood antibodies. Other tests that your pediatrician may need to take from your baby include those for PKU, thyroid function, hepatitis, and oxygen content, as well as specific personal and genetic tests. Some of these may also be evaluated from umbilical cord blood.

I saw a nurse taking blood from a baby's heel. What was she doing?

The nurse may have been taking blood to test for phenylketonuria. PKU is a hereditary metabolic disorder that a child may develop if it receives a carrier gene from each of its parents. These parents probably do not know that they were carriers. If the disorder is detected and treated, the affected baby will suffer no adverse affects and will be able to live a normal life. Unfortunately, if this disease is not detected, it can lead to severe mental retardation. It is important for the nurse to check for this disease at birth, because the treatment to prevent serious outcomes includes the elimination of all milk and other dairy products from the infant's diet.

Is it necessary for the nurse to place eyedrops in a baby's eyes after birth?

The placement of antibiotic drops in the eyes of newborns is federally mandated to prevent specific infections transmitted during the birth process from scarring the eyes of some newborns. Many women carry vaginal infections like chlamydia and gonorrhea, which can infect their infants' eyes during birth. If chlamydia conjunctivitis is left untreated, this infection will cause much cell damage and scarring on the surface of an infant's eyes. If gonococcal conjunctivitis is left untreated, it will cause a pus-filled inflammation that can lead to blindness in the newborn. Erythromycin eyedrops or ointments are used to treat all infants after birth because it is effective against both chlamydia and gonococcal conjunctivitis.

Why does my infant need an injection of vitamin K at birth?

Vitamin K is essential for blood clotting. As adults, we do not obtain this necessary vitamin from our diets alone; we also obtain it indirectly from bacteria that live in the intestinal tract and produce it there. We live in a mutually beneficial relationship with these bacteria. This means that they need to live in our intestines for their survival, and we need the vitamin K that they manufacture for our survival. Newborns, however, do not receive vitamin K from their mother and have no bacteria in their intestinal tract; therefore they do not have vitamin K and may experience bleeding problems. To bridge this time gap from birth until an infant is able to manufacture its own vitamin K, all newborns are given an injection of this vitamin.

THE TRUTH ABOUT LABOR

What is labor?

Labor is a series of rhythmic uterine muscular contractions. These contractions work to open, or dilate, your cervix. Your uterus is like a container with a thick muscular wall. The hormones that trigger labor cause these uterine muscles to rotate and pull upward toward the top of the uterus. As a result, the top part of your uterus will become thicker, and the lower part will start to thin out. As the muscles move, each layer of muscle slides past the underlying one until the majority of your uterine muscle fibers are pulled at the top of your uterus. At this point, your cervix has become so thin that it will start to dilate. If you were to view your cervix from inside the vagina, its central area would look like the little eye opening of a kaleidoscope, rotating wider and wider in a circular fashion. All of these muscle fibers that have been encircling one another rotate in an increasingly wider circle as the cervix opens.

Is labor dirty and ugly?

Having been an obstetrician for most of my life, I find labor to be the most natural, pure, and earthy experience in a woman's life. Those who tell you that labor is dirty probably have not witnessed many births. Labor is as beautiful as any natural phenomenon. During your labor you will be in terrible pain, you will be sweating, bleeding, dripping amniotic fluid, or passing urine and feces as your baby's head is crowning. Despite all this, it is important to remember that beauty is in the eye of the beholder, and the beauty of birth is unsurpassed by any other beauty.

After you have completed the overwhelmingly powerful experience of labor and delivery of your baby, you will regain your composure. You will look down and see this brand-new cuddling life in your arms, this baby that fought just as hard as you have to find its way into the world. The lights in your room will be shining down on your baby, who does not yet recognize where she is or why she is here. She will begin to peep and whimper, and you and your husband will cry with joy and hold your precious baby.

Is this dirty? Labor represents the pure essence of creation and the purpose of our living. Please try to picture your labor and delivery as I have described it here, and you will see only beauty.

How will I know when my labor is starting?

This is the universal question. When your labor begins, your symptoms may be vague. And as with any natural event, their pattern will not be totally predictable. Your labor will start with one of two major events. Either your uterus will begin to contract or your water will break.

> *Think of your labor as a blizzard. Each blizzard starts with tiny snowflakes, a slowly approaching cloud, or a light, cool breeze. Just as each snowflake has its own pattern and each cloud its own shape, so too does each labor*

*follow its own predetermined path. As each storm pro-
gresses, the pattern unfolds in both intensity and duration. During your labor, you will have no doubt that you
have been placed in the middle of your own overwhelming
natural storm.*

If your labor begins with contractions, they may initially feel like a back-
ache or strong menstrual cramps. Your contractions will be far apart at
first, but gradually they will grow closer and closer together. Each suc-
cessive contraction will flow into the next, and you will have only a moment in between to prepare yourself. These contractions will also
become progressively stronger in intensity. If this is your first labor, your
contractions will precede delivery for an average of twelve hours. If this
is your second labor, your contractions may last anywhere between two
and ten hours.

There is a 25 percent chance that your membranes will rupture before
your labor begins. It is most common for the amniotic fluid sac to tear directly over your cervical opening; when this happens, you may leak a
large amount of fluid. If the leak is higher up, near the inner surface of
your uterine muscle, you may express only a few tiny drops. This is because the external pressure of the uterine muscle will create pressure
and block the flow of fluid. In this case, you may notice fluid leaking only
when you move in certain positions. This is why so many women are often uncertain if they are leaking amniotic fluid. When in doubt, please
call your doctor and tell all.

Most women relive their labors for the rest of their lives. These aren't
memories of pain or agony; those you will forget once you hold your newborn for the first time. Looking back on your labor, you will recall a profound sense of inner peace, much as artists must feel as they reflect on
their life's work.

Why must labor be so painful?

I have thought about this question on so many occasions, while watching
young women cry and thrash about in labor. I believe that the pain women
experience during labor must be a protective mechanism for us as humans, with its roots in the times of our earliest ancestors. Try to imagine
what birth was like for women at the start of human civilization. Thou-

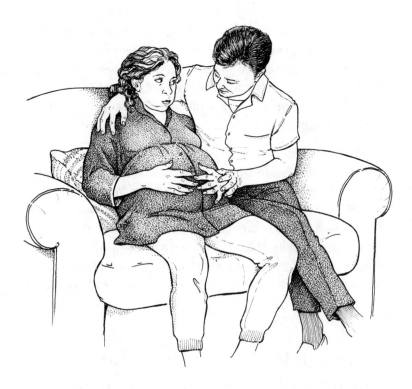

sands of years ago, humans lived in nomadic tribes. Women probably knew they were pregnant but had no idea when labor would begin. If the tribe had been traveling, labor pains would have forced women to leave the tribe. They would have sought refuge in a quiet place and would have started crying. Other women, usually the healers in the tribe, would have come to help them. Had they not heard the woman's cries, they and their babies might have perished. In those days, it would have been your pains and your cries that would have saved the lives of you and your baby. In this way, pain is a form of protection and self-preservation, set in place by the forces that created our species and intended for us to survive.

I do not tolerate pain well. What if I lose control and make a fool of myself?

Please do not worry about this. Losing control during labor is a normal response, and you will probably be acting just the way your doctor or nurse may have acted when they were in labor. No one in the maternity unit is judging you; you are not there to perform, you are there to have a baby. Almost all delivery room personnel are women who love the process of birth and are so excited for you to have your baby. There are no gold stars given to women who deliver naturally, who deliver quickly, or who deliver without crying. The only reward, and it is given equally to all participants of labor, is a beautiful baby. The entire birthing room staff knows that only you are feeling your pain, and none of them wish to judge it.

Many patients believe their obstetrician remembers how they screamed, cried, or kicked during their labor. As an obstetrician, I lived from emergency to emergency, trying to prevent complications from affecting a mother or a baby. I never judged women or focused on the small events. What I remember most vividly from each delivery is the look in a mother's eyes when she first sees her baby.

Standard Labor Procedures

Many years back, women were treated as though pregnancy and childbirth were an illness, so it was routine for them to be given enemas and have their pubic hair shaved when they arrived at the hospital. Nowadays, the only procedures that are standard are those that will ensure the safety of both mother and baby. These include checking blood pressure, heart rate, and temperature and taking blood and urine samples. Your doctor will monitor your uterine contractions and evaluate your cervix intermittently to gauge how much it has dilated. This will give you reassurance. As your labor is progressing, all the tests will not only reassure you, they will help you stay focused and strong as your delivery draws near.

It may not even be standard that you wear a hospital gown. If you want to wear your own clothes in labor, tell your doctor or midwife ahead of time; as long as these garments do not get in the way of caring for you or your baby, you should be able to wear them. Just remember that labor is not a clean, dry process, so don't plan on wearing your best outfit.

IVs

In general, women do not automatically need an IV just because they are in labor, but some physicians feel otherwise. Women have enough discomfort during labor and do not need the extra burden of an IV, but some doctors believe that laboring women should have an IV intact at all times in case of an emergency. Please discuss this issue with your obstetrician.

If you request narcotic pain medication, your nurse will probably need to start an IV line in a vein in your forearm or your hand. Sometimes women are given intramuscular injections, usually in the buttocks, for pain relief. The problem with intramuscular injections is that they take longer to act, are not quite as effective as intravenous pain medications, and do not leave the body quickly. This means that the baby will also have a residual narcotic within its system for a longer time.

If you plan to have an epidural for pain relief, you will be given an IV. Prior to receiving an epidural, you will need to receive IV fluids to reduce the possibility that the epidural will lower your blood pressure. An epidural relaxes your entire body, including your blood vessels. When your blood vessels relax, they dilate, and if they are low in fluids, their pressure will drop. IV fluids increase the fluid in your vessels and keep your blood pressure stable.

You may also need to have an IV line if you require a particular medication, specifically if you carry beta strep, have toxemia of pregnancy or diabetes, or experience any other medical or obstetric complications.

Fetal Heart Rate Monitors

There are two types of fetal heart rate monitors. The external monitor, located on a belt placed around your abdomen, is used most often. If your doctor cannot adequately observe your baby's heart well on an external monitor or if she is concerned about a potential problem with its heart rate pattern, she may use an internal monitor. To insert the internal monitor, she will pass a tiny catheter through your vagina with a coiled pin on the end and slide the coiled pin gently through the skin of your baby's scalp. This will not hurt your baby and will allow your doctor to monitor your baby's heart rate pattern continuously.

When your doctor checks your baby's heart rate pattern on the fetal monitor, she will be looking at the frequency of the beats, the variability or change in the beats, the reaction of the heart rate to contractions, and any decelerations in its heart rate. In general, the more variable your baby's heart rate appears, the better your baby is reacting to its labor. Variability is the squiggle in the heart rate line. Both the tiny squiggles and the long, broad up-and-down waves of the pattern indicate that your baby is reacting well to its environment and to its labor. As you observe your baby's heart rate, the monitor will print the number of beats per minute. A baby's normal heart rate generally ranges between 120 and 160 beats per minute. Its heart rate will also be printed as a horizontal line on a moving computer sheet. If your baby's heart rate pattern appears at a higher level on the monitor strip, that means its heart rate is rapid; if the pattern prints out lower, its rate is slower.

Your baby will always react to your contractions; it is considered normal and healthy if its heart rate goes up, goes down, or stays the same during contractions. What your doctor wants to see is your baby's long-term pattern. If its heart rate is going down repetitively and frequently after a contraction, she may be concerned. Heart rate decreases are common during labor, but as long as these decelerations are neither deep nor long, and do not occur after every contraction, they usually do not indicate a serious problem. If your baby has a very active heart rate pattern, this is a good sign, so don't panic if you see its heart rate moving all over the place. The nurse will be able to determine how each of the baby's heart rate changes correlates to your contractions and evaluate both your progress and your baby's readiness to deliver.

Sometimes during labor you may notice that the fetal monitor is not able to record your baby's heart rate continuously. If the baby's pattern is generally healthy, it is not necessary to record its heart every minute. In fact, it may be difficult to record continuously, because when your baby moves, its heart might not be in a position that allows the nurse to monitor it. Try not to worry about this; your nurse will know when she needs to start recording your baby again.

When you look at the fetal monitor strip, you will see two basic things: your baby's heart rate pattern and your uterine contraction pattern. As the monitors record these patterns, your nurse and your obstetrician will interpret them for you. Although you do not have the same level of experience and expertise in reading these monitor strips as your health care team has, that does not mean your input is not important, so feel free to ask them questions and share your impressions of what you see on the monitor.

On many occasions during my years as an obstetrician, observations from my patients and their husbands were both perceptive and helpful to me in delivering their babies.

Contraction Monitors

Your nurse will place a belt around your abdomen near the top of your uterus to monitor your contractions. When your uterine tone increases or decreases, the pressure reading on the monitor strip will also elevate or drop. Once an elevation on the monitor rounds the top of a rise, the peak of your contraction has passed. This external pressure monitor records the frequency of your contractions, not their strength. If this belt is applied tightly, your contractions will appear stronger. Also, if you are thin, there is less tissue between your uterus and the monitor, so your contractions will appear stronger. Conversely, if the monitor is applied loosely, or if you have more tissue between your uterus and the monitor, the contractions will appear weaker.

A contraction monitor correlates the intensity of one contraction with another, but it cannot provide an overall picture of how strong your contractions are. By observing your own contraction pattern, you will notice when they build in intensity and when they subside. Knowing this will help you prepare yourself psychologically for the onset of each one, and your husband will be better able to tell you when you have made it through the maximum phase of each contraction successfully. You will also be able to note the frequency of your contractions. When you are watching the monitor, count from the beginning of one contraction to the beginning of the next. When you experience at least one contraction every five minutes, you will know you have a healthy, normal labor pattern.

An internal contraction pressure monitor may also be used, but generally doctors and nurses prefer to feel a woman's abdomen to find out how intense her contractions are. If an internal monitor is necessary, your doctor will use a catheter to place one in your amniotic sac, where it can determine the intensity of your contractions more accurately.

Abdominal Palpation

When the pressure changes within your uterus, so will the feeling of firmness on the surface of your abdomen. The nurse will pat up and down on your abdomen prior to and during your contractions. First, she will feel the resting tone of your uterine muscle before a contraction begins. Then, as you are having a contraction, she will feel your uterus increase in firmness. When your uterus is not contracting, she will be able to press into your uterine muscle. Early in labor, your contractions will be mild in intensity and your uterus will feel as soft as your lips. When they build to moderate intensity, your uterus will become firmer and feel like the tip of your nose. Later in labor when your contractions are strong, your uterine muscles will feel as firm as the bone of your forehead.

RELAXATION

Labor is such a painful and emotional experience, I don't think I'll be able to relax. Will it really help if I can relax?

Yes, it will. It is so important to feel as relaxed as you can during labor. Because you are able to relax the muscles in your face, neck, shoulders, and limbs, your uterine muscles relax, too. Studies have shown that when people undergo medical or surgical procedures, those who are calm and positive fare better and have fewer complications. The benefits of relaxation techniques become most evident in the experience of labor. When a woman tenses her muscles, panics, or refuses to give in to the forces of nature at work in labor, she only frightens herself and prolongs the time she must spend delivering her baby. Each labor will follow the pattern it is destined to follow. Try to keep in mind that there is nothing to gain by worrying about what might happen or fearing pain before you feel it.

Yes, your labor will be intense, painful, long, and overwhelming. But it will also be miraculously productive, just the way it was meant to be.

> *There is an Oriental saying that the only tree left standing after a storm is the bamboo. The wind pulls up the rigid trees from their roots. The bamboo tree sways with the wind, so it can survive the storm.*

To become truly relaxed, you'll need to calm your mind, your body, and your environment. Meditation and visual imagery will help you picture yourself in a peaceful place, having successfully completed your labor, and holding your baby. To help you, bring something to use as a focal point during labor so you can take your mind off your contractions. This can be a photo, a picture, or a statuette that gives you peace and reassurance.

It may be beneficial if you ask your husband to learn some basic reiki techniques (the Japanese art of touch), so that he will be able to ease tension in your hands and feet. You can also try using metal Oriental balls (available in many Asian stores) to limber and relax the small muscles of your hands.

With respect to your labor environment, consider bringing scented essential oil into the delivery room. You can shake some of the oil on cotton balls and place them around your labor room or in a basin of water to let the aroma diffuse through the air. Lavender is an especially relaxing fragrance. Whatever personal, peaceful touch you can add to your environment will help you to relax and stay focused and encourage you to make this day into a fond and precious memory.

CESAREAN SECTIONS

I will be having a cesarean section. Should I support my vegetarian diet in any way to make sure I'm healthy for this surgery?

In general, most vegetarian women breeze through any surgery, and specifically cesareans, strong and healthy. There are several reasons for this success. One is that most of us have studied so much about nutrition that we have been living lives of optimum nutrition for years prior to the surgery and do not need to suddenly scramble to get our bodies in shape. Another reason is that a smaller percentage of vegetarians have cholesterol-related heart and blood vessel diseases, hypertension, diabetes, and obesity. All of these medical conditions contribute to poor tissue healing, so not having them contributes to good wound healing. A third reason is that, in general, vegetarians are more athletic, so their circulation is good, their muscles are strong, and their thoughts are positive.

You should have your blood count checked for anemia, because that is one of our challenges in pregnancy—but fortunately one you can easily correct with iron-rich foods and supplements. If you have a preexisting medical condition, such as cardiac disease or lung disease, your physician will let you know if you require any specific dietary supplements. In general, if you maintain a high intake of vegetarian protein and a high vitamin level, consume sufficient iron to prevent anemia, and exercise to keep your body strong, you will do wonderfully.

I am having a scheduled cesarean section. Will I feel as close a bond to my baby as a woman who delivers vaginally?

Yes, you will, without a doubt. You may feel drained, weak, and in more pain after your cesarean delivery, but as soon as you get to hold your baby, you will love it passionately. Remember that although most women deliver vaginally, most do not feel their delivery any more than you did because they have epidural anesthesia or pain medication that subdues or obliterates any sensation of delivering.

Having a cesarean section is as beautiful and spiritual an experience as having a vaginal delivery. Please try not to let public opinion convince you otherwise. After you have your cesarean delivery, if someone offers condolences, just reply that *you* are not sorry about it in the least. Feel overjoyed and blessed that you had the opportunity to create a new life. It is the creation of life that is beautiful, not the path that life chose for its arrival.

Your cesarean section will be a wonderfully exciting experience and certainly the most productive one of your life.

I had a cesarean section before, but now my doctor believes I should attempt to have a vaginal delivery. As a vegetarian, will I be strong enough to manage it?

Approximately 27 percent of all women who previously had a cesarean section attempt to have a vaginal delivery. These are a select group of women who do not have a recurring delivery problem, such as a small pelvis or a large baby, which is why their doctor encourages them to attempt vaginal birth. If you are within this group, vegetarian or not, the odds that you will be able to deliver vaginally will vary from 60 to 75 percent, depending upon the reason you initially needed your cesarean section. If your first cesarean section was for a totally nonrecurring problem, such as a prolapsed umbilical cord or a breech baby, your chances of having a successful vaginal birth after cesarean will be higher. If there are signs that the problem requiring your first cesarean section is recurring, your chances of success will be lower and your doctor will tell you so.

There is no reason to think that as a vegetarian you have a prior cesarean scar that has not healed as strongly as the scar of a non-vegetarian to withstand the contractions of an entire labor, and there is no reason to think you will not be able to push out your baby with as much muscle force as a non-vegetarian.

POSITIONS DURING LABOR

I do not want to be strapped down to a fetal monitor for my entire labor. Can I choose my positions?

Being in labor does not mean that you are ill. As long as all is well with your baby and you, there is no reason you should not move around or change your position. Your doctor will monitor you regularly to make sure everything is progressing normally. You may be in labor for hours; staying in bed may make your back pains worse and your labor seem longer and may actually make you feel ill. Before your labor, discuss your wishes with your doctor or midwife so that you can understand how each of you envisions your labor.

When you first arrive at the delivery room, your nurse or doctor will evaluate your baby on the fetal monitor for approximately thirty minutes. This procedure is necessary for the hospital staff to confirm that your baby is not experiencing fetal distress. In this case, your doctor will need to monitor you closely now. Studies have shown that this first evaluation of a baby in labor can accurately predict 50 percent of those babies who will end up needing a cesarean delivery for fetal distress. If the baby does show distress on admission, that may indicate it had distress at home when you were in early labor.

If your baby's monitor tracings appear fine, the nurse will let you walk around, sit in the rocking chair, take a shower, or do any number of things that will help you feel comfortable. Whether you decide to lie down, sit up, squat, or stand, she should have no difficulty monitoring you. If at any time, however, she needs you to lie in a specific position so she can accurately evaluate your baby's heart, please assist her as much as you can.

When I went on a tour of the delivery room with my childbirth class, I noticed that most women were lying down or reclining in bed. Why?

Lying down, or reclining with the head of the bed raised, is a popular and comfortable position for women during labor, mainly because the intensity and repetitiveness of labor contractions can be exhausting. Resting helps to regain your strength. If you think about the last time you had an intestinal virus, or about how drained you feel after a bout of cramps, you can imagine how totally exhausted a woman feels after hours of labor. If you choose to lie in bed, you will probably want to lie flat, slightly tilted to one side, with several pillows propping up your head.

Lying in bed will be necessary if you have an epidural or any pain medication. If you receive Demerol or another narcotic, you may feel sleepy and dizzy; your doctor will ask you to stay in bed for several hours until the medication wears off.

Women often achieve a measure of comfort while sitting up in bed with one or two pillows under their knees to support them. It will be good for you to bring two of your own pillows with you because hospital pillows may be uncomfortable. The hospital also may not have extra pillows for you to use.

Many women sit in a rocking chair during their labor because the repetitive rocking motion helps them to cope better with the intensity of their contractions. Under most circumstances, your nurse will be able to monitor both your baby's heart rate and your uterine contractions just fine when you labor in a rocking chair.

Is it safe for me to squat during my labor? I have been told it is a natural position for labor that will help me deliver more easily.

Squatting definitely has its place in labor, but it will not be easy for you to squat for long periods of time, even if you practice for months prior to your delivery. The norm in our country has been to treat childbirth like an illness, and for many years, lying in bed was the only accepted position for delivery. Nowadays, women listen to their natural instincts and are free to assume a number of positions during labor as long as they allow their doctors to evaluate their babies safely. When women try to squat, they often find it stressful on their thighs and their knee joints and difficult to balance on their feet, even when they try to squat for just an hour. Months of practicing squatting may help you, but since squatting is not a natural everyday stance for you, it will be hard to maintain this position through your entire labor.

During the pushing phase of your labor, squatting with support from your husband may be helpful, but it is not the panacea many people claim. Your husband will need to hold you during each contraction while you are on your haunches and then gently lay you down to recline between contractions. You may also use a birthing bar. With this bar, you can pull yourself up with each contraction and then recline back in bed to a sitting position until the next contraction.

Converting your bed to a sitting angle and slinging a full-length sheet over the middle of your birthing bar is another way to try squatting. With each contraction, bend your knees up in a squat, pull the sheet toward you, and bear down toward your vaginal area as you pull your torso up toward the sheet. I have often seen this technique help babies that appeared to be wedged in their mother's pelvis descend to the vaginal canal with great ease.

During my last labor, I did most of my pushing sitting on the toilet. Is this common?

Yes, sitting on the toilet is a very helpful position for many women during labor. In the bathroom, there is usually a wall rack to grip, a seat rim where you can place your legs, and an empty space below you so you do not restrict your baby's movement. Also, by sitting on the toilet, women can find the correct spot to bear down on when they are pushing, which helps to push the baby's head down quicker. If this is your second or third delivery, your doctor may be cautious about letting you sit on the toilet because this baby may deliver quickly; neither your doctor nor you will want your baby to have this kind of "water birth" in the cold toilet basin.

Can a birthing ball help me to cope better during my labor?

A birthing ball is a large, strong beach ball. It is two feet in diameter, made of firm plastic, contains air, and has a good bouncy spring to it. The rocking pressure of the spring is very comforting in labor, and since you are likely to move in various positions while using this ball, you will help your baby move closer to your pelvis.

When you use a birthing ball, you can place it against a wall and keep pressing into it to massage your back. You can also lean your abdomen into it and bend over on top of it. Instinctively, you will bob up and down, and this rocking motion will relax your muscles and help your baby descend. If your hospital does not have one, try purchasing a birthing ball from a maternity catalog. The ball will give you a soft surface to lean on, rock against, and apply pressure to your aching back and abdomen. The concept is so simple, it sound too good to be true, I know, but it does work and you may find it helps you immensely.

STAYING STRONG DURING LABOR

My friend says that as a vegetarian I will not have the muscle strength to push my baby out. Is there any truth to what she is saying?

Your friend apparently still believes in the widely accepted myth that consuming protein creates muscle mass. Protein does not create muscle; exercise does. When we consume foods high in protein, these foods do not create muscle, they create fat, which we use for energy. With exercise, that fat tissue is converted into muscle.

Just because you may consume less protein than your friend does not mean that your protein store is insufficient. The required amount of daily protein recommended in most reference charts is much higher than it needs to be for people to maintain good health. When the regulatory health boards determined the healthy range of protein levels, the highest level of protein within the range was selected, primarily because health officials believed that if some protein was good, more would be even better. With a healthy vegetarian diet, however, you will have no problem maintaining even this level. If you are in good physical and muscular form, if you have lived a healthy lifestyle, and if you have performed Kegel exercises (10 to 20 tightenings of your vagina several times a day to strengthen your vaginal muscles), you will have no problem pushing your baby out at delivery.

If I will not be allowed to eat solid foods during labor, how will I stay strong?

Fasting during labor is a time-honored tradition. In most birthing facilities, women are encouraged to drink clear liquids, chew ice chips, and suck on candies, but that is all. During labor, there is a natural delay in the time a woman's stomach ingests foods and when her stomach empties itself out. For example, if a woman ate a full meal at ten P.M. and then went into labor at midnight, the foods she had just eaten would remain in her stomach for a total of six to eight hours. Since it is common for women to experience nausea and vomiting during labor, whatever they had eaten for their evening meal they would likely revisit—and not nearly as happily—during their labor.

> *Many women suddenly vomit when they reach "transition," the point at which they move from the latent phase of labor to the active phase. Other women may vomit when they become fully dilated and their baby's head descends into their pelvic cavity. It will be best for you to eat light meals as you move close to your due date and avoid this kind of unpleasant moment.*

If you plan to have regional anesthesia, like an epidural or a spinal, it will take even longer for your stomach to digest foods, because these medications further delay your gastric emptying time. A full stomach can also pose a serious problem if you suddenly require a cesarean section. After having emergency general anesthesia, if your stomach is full, you may vomit violently when you wake up and risk breathing this into your lungs. This may result in a very serious and often life-threatening case of aspiration pneumonia.

There is no reason to believe that your health is at risk when you fast from solid foods during labor, so please do not worry that you are not eating. Chances are you will be so excited about your birth and focused on getting through your labor, you won't even be thinking about food.

AN OUNCE OF PREVENTION: WHEN PITOCIN IS NECESSARY

I would like my labor to be as natural as possible. Can you please discuss Pitocin and the circumtances under which my doctor may feel its use is warranted?

Pitocin is a synthetic form of one of the hormones our pituitary gland produces naturally to initiate labor. It functions to either bring on labor contractions or to increase the intensity of these contractions. It is administered at a very slow, steady rate, as a counted intravenous drip. The body begins to sense its effect within just three to five minutes. When given intravenously, it should reach its full effect within thirty minutes. If your doctor needs to give you Pitocin, she will start with the smallest dose in the IV drip and then gradually increase the quantity every half hour until your uterus is contracting adequately.

Pitocin will change the pattern of your uterine contractions in several ways. It will bring them closer together, it will make each contraction last longer, and it will increase the intensity of each contraction. You may need Pitocin to start your labor if you are overdue, if your doctor is concerned about your baby's heart rate pattern, if your membranes ruptured and labor did not start, if your baby has stopped moving regularly, if you had a prior stillborn infant, or if your baby is not growing well inside you. Pitocin is an effective means of increasing your contractions after you have started to labor naturally. When your labor loses intensity, your contractions are too weak to dilate your cervix; or if you have been in labor for a prolonged time with little progress, your doctor will want to give you Pitocin to make your labor more efficient. The exhaustion of a long labor can be counterproductive and torturous. Sometimes it is just simpler to get a jump start from Pitocin and progress during your labor at a normal rate.

Is the pain of a Pitocin-induced labor worse than that of natural labor?

Yes, the pains may feel stronger if you take Pitocin to induce your labor. If you were experiencing mild labor contractions and then received Pitocin to intensify the contractions, your labor will definitely feel worse, simply because the contractions are stronger. Even if you felt strong pains, it is easier to look up and see an IV bottle of Pitocin and hate that bottle, while it is harder to blame fate, God, your body, or nature for the pain. The pains of a Pitocin-induced labor may actually feel worse, because Pitocin-induced contractions do not begin as slowly and as gradually as do normal contractions. They strike suddenly, speed up quicker, and may not give a woman as much time to become accustomed to them. So even if they are not stronger in their total intensity, their pattern may be harder for you to tolerate.

During her first labor, a woman will usually push between a half hour and three hours. Some women have firmer pelvic tissues and others have larger babies, which makes the baby's descent more difficult and time-consuming. A doctor usually permits a woman to push as long as her baby is tolerating the labor well and she does not have fever, has the energy to push, and has the willpower to do so. If women have an epidural, they may need to push longer—from two hours to three hours—because they may not push with the same desperate intensity as they would were they feeling the pain.

If your baby's head is not perfectly aligned in your pelvis—if its head is tilted, for example, or facing your abdomen instead of your back—your pushing time may be longer. In both situations, your baby's head will need time to mold its shape and push through. The bones of a baby's head are not fused together into one large skull bone, as in an adult. When a baby maneuvers through the pelvis, its skull bones overlap and compress to fit through the pelvic outlet, which is often smaller than the size of the diameter of a baby's head. If you have delivered vaginally already, you may need to push for only one contraction. Oddly enough, some women who have delivered many children need to push for hours because their uterus may have lost its tone from having been stretched so many times.

Part III
Now That You Are a Mother

CHAPTER 12

Nursing as a Vegetarian

You are so excited to hold your baby close to you.
You long to feel the warmth of her flesh,
the groping of her tiny hands,
and the innocence of her eyes
as they peer searchingly
up into yours.

Yet you wonder, as do most new mothers,
if you will be able to nurse.
What if your breasts are too large, too small,
too sensitive,
or simply do not produce enough milk?

There is nothing to fear, as time will determine all.
Your baby and you will be on this special adventure together,
she learning to suck,
you learning to nurse.
Both of you learning to feel the emotions and needs of each other.

Whether you nurse for one day or one year,
whether you are her sole provider or provide along with formula,
whether you enjoy nursing or decide it is not your forte,

you will have experienced the joy, excitement, and enrichment
of nurturing
her new little life.

Please try to relax, accept, and enjoy your uncharted path
with your new little friend.

WHY BREAST-FEED?

I will be home from work with my baby for only four weeks after I deliver. Should I even attempt to breast-feed?

Even if you are able to breast-feed for only one week, the nutrients your infant will obtain will be truly beneficial. In 1971, only 25 percent of all women leaving the hospital after delivery started breast-feeding. By 1998, this had grown to 64 percent of women. The evidence continues to mount that breast milk supplies an infant with nutritional, immunologic, and developmental benefits that formula manufacturers have not been able to replicate. Although there are many practical obstacles that must be faced in the lives of many women, if it is at all possible, it would be best for you to attempt nursing your baby, even if only for a few fleeting days.

How will breast milk benefit my baby?

The American Academy of Pediatrics organized a work group to study the benefits of breast milk on infants. Their study included middle-class women from the United States, Canada, Europe, and other industrialized countries. They found strong evidence that breast-fed infants have lower rates of pneumonia and bronchitis, diarrhea, ear infections, infections in their blood, bacterial meningitis, and a type of intestinal disorder in premature infants called "necrotizing enterocolitis." Even when breast-fed infants did develop these disorders, they were much less severe in nature.

Other studies have shown that breast-fed infants have a lower inci-

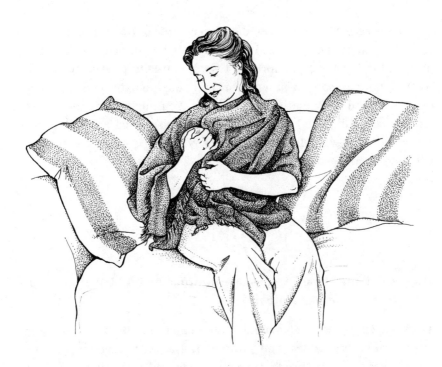

dence of allergies, digestive disorders, insulin-dependent diabetes, sudden infant death syndrome, ulcerative colitis, Crohn's disease, cancer of the lymph nodes, and a variety of other chronic disorders. Breast-fed babies have fewer illnesses in general and, as a result, fewer illness-related visits to both the doctor's office and the hospital.

PREPARING FOR NURSING

I plan to breast-feed my baby. What should I do to get ready?

You will need nursing pads and at least two nursing bras. Try to purchase pads without plastic backing so that air can circulate to your moist nipple region. Evaluate your nightclothes and tops so you won't need to lift up garments from your ankles to nurse. Loose-fitting garments that you can lift up from your waist or that unbutton in the front will be helpful. The best cream for your nipples, if they become sore, is your own milk applied over your nipple and areola. If you feel better with a backup cream, vitamin E cream or ointment will work well.

Also, please set up voice mail or make sure your answering machine is working so you will not need to stop nursing to answer your phone. To prepare for an emergency, locate a twenty-four-hour pharmacy or super-market that sells breast pumps, formula your pediatrician usually rec-ommends, and baby bottles with nipples. You might want to contact a lactation consultant, a La Leche League representative, or a relative who breast-fed. This way, should you have any breast-feeding questions, you will have someone to advise you.

BASIC NURSING GUIDELINES
FOR VEGETARIANS

What nutrients should I consume in order to fulfill the nutritional guidelines for nursing mothers?

The basic guidelines recommended for a balanced diet while nursing re-quires fruits, vegetables, and protein. The authoritative guidelines do not suggest that dairy products be included within your diet, nor do they suggest that protein be derived specifically from animal sources. To sus-tain and surpass nutritional requirements while nursing as a vegetarian, you will need to consume 1,000 milligrams of calcium, 65 grams of pro-tein, 5 micrograms of vitamin D, 700 milligrams of phosphorus, 1,300 mi-crograms of vitamin A, 2.6 micrograms of vitamin B_{12}, 320 milligrams of magnesium, 75 micrograms of selenium, and 19 milligrams of zinc daily. If your intake of any of these nutrients is slightly high or slightly low on a specific day, do not worry. Your food intake is not a direct pipeline to your baby, as most nutrients will be broken down, reprocessed within your body, and incorporated into your breast milk at a later date. It is your total nutritional health picture that is important, not your intake in a specific meal.

I cannot tolerate much dairy. Should I try to consume some and take Lactaid?

There is no need at all to consume dairy products and definitely no need to take another chemical. Nearly half the world's population is lactose in-tolerant, such that consumption of lactose (milk sugar) creates bloating, cramps, diarrhea, or a combination of these. If your body is telling you not to consume a specific food, listen to it.

More people are allergic, sensitive, or intolerant to milk than to any other food. An enormous number of children and adults develop eczema, skin rashes, and otitis media from forcing their bodies to consume lactose sugars, simply because they have been led to believe they need it. Your baby and you will be able to consume all the nutrients you both need from nondairy vegetarian foods, without taking a food that obviously is not right for you.

How many calories will I need daily while I'm nursing?

You will need between 2,200 and 2,700 calories each day to give your baby adequate nutrition and still maintain your own weight. Of that amount, 500 to 700 calories will be used specifically for breast-feeding needs. You may actually draw some of these calories from your own body fat. This is why some women lose the fat they gained during pregnancy and why many women who breast-feed lose weight faster than women who bottle-feed. Although the literature suggests that you need to increase your intake of liquids two to three glasses each day, your fluids will not affect the quality of your milk, just the quantity of it. It is your healthy diet that determines the adequacy of your milk.

As a vegetarian, will I have sufficient protein in my colostrum?

Yes. Your colostrum contains the same amount of protein as the colostrum of a woman consuming a high-protein meat-based diet. Studies have shown that even when women in third world countries are deficient in protein, this deficiency does not affect the protein content of their milk. Your own body will create the perfect amount of protein in your breast milk, regardless of the quantity within your system. It will also form the exact same quantities of carbohydrates and lactose as those formed in non-vegetarian women. Even severely protein- and calorie-deficient women in third world countries produce milk of the same quality; however, in those women, the volume may be decreased.

Actually, your body will create the correct quantity and quality of both colostrum and milk regardless of your age, ethnicity, number of prior pregnancies, or diet.

What nutrients are in breast milk, and how much milk will my body be creating?

Human milk contains over one hundred different constituents. These include proteins, fats, carbohydrates, and minerals. The minerals present in breast milk include sodium, potassium, chloride, calcium, iron, magnesium, copper, zinc, and phosphorus. Human milk contains all vitamins necessary for the total health of a baby, with the exception of vitamin K. Bacteria present in the intestines of humans manufacture vitamin K, and your newborn will eventually manufacture his own. Studies have shown that neither the total number of nutrients nor the relative amounts of the nutrients are appreciably different in the breast milk of vegetarian and non-vegetarian women.

You will produce 18 ounces of milk each day during your first week nursing. By the end of your third week, you will produce 27 ounces per day. Eventually, when your body has fully adapted to nursing, you will produce 60 ounces of milk daily.

I have been trying to nurse, but I'm having such a hard time. Why is something so natural so difficult?

Although nursing your baby is a very natural and earthy process, no one ever said it was easy, and it is not. Some women have been led to believe the word *natural* is synonymous with the word *easy*. This is not the case when it comes to pregnancy, labor, or nursing. Just as each of us must go through a learning curve to achieve many goals in life, so will you with nursing. To complicate the situation, your baby is learning, too. Eventually both of you will develop a pattern of timing, position, and techniques that are specific for the two of you. Even if you listen to advice from other women, your doctor, or your nurse, your baby and you will teach each other.

NURSING AS A VEGAN

I am vegan. Will my body be able to produce milk?

Without a doubt, your vegan diet contains every nutrient necessary to produce milk. The simplistic concept that women need to consume milk to produce milk has been disproved. For generations, women were encouraged to "drink plenty of milk," even if it gave them diarrhea and cramps and gave their babies gas. To produce milk, you need sufficient calories, liquids, and the following nutrients daily: 1,000 milligrams calcium, 65 grams protein, 5 micrograms vitamin D, 700 milligrams phosphorus, 1,300 micrograms vitamin A, 2.6 micrograms vitamin B_{12}, 320 milligrams magnesium, 75 micrograms selenium, and 19 milligrams zinc. The source of these nutrients need not be milk, as all are abundantly present in other foods. You do not need lactose sugar (milk sugar), nor do you need lactalbumin or milk casein (milk proteins).

Milk production is not under conscious control—your body has a hormonal reflex between your pituitary gland and your breast glands to stimulate lactation. This means that after you deliver your baby, your uterine hormones send a message to your brain that pregnancy is completed. This reflex is an integral part of your hormonal function as a woman and is not related to your dietary intake.

Will my protein intake be adequate for my baby?

You will produce sufficient milk if you increase your protein intake 15 grams above your base prepregnancy level. While you are breast-feeding, although you need to take in an additional 500 to 650 calories daily, your increased protein need is minimal.

Studies concerning protein needs are termed "nitrogen studies." Nitrogen is an important nutritional component derived from protein. When people eat protein-rich foods, their body breaks these down and stores them as amino acids containing nitrogen. When you need them, your body re-forms new proteins from the stored nitrogen in the amino acids. Nitrogen studies show that a minimal increase in your protein intake will ensure that a sufficient amount of protein is transferred to your baby.

YOUR BEST NUTRITIONAL SOURCES FOR NURSING

It will be so simple for you, as a vegan or vegetarian, to obtain more than all of the recommended nutrients for nursing from your diet.

Calcium

You need 1,000 milligrams of calcium daily and can obtain this from many sources, including ¼ cup sesame seeds (350 milligrams), 10 ounces frozen broccoli (159 milligrams), 1 cup bok choy (250 milligrams), 2 cups of green leafy vegetables (600 milligrams). Some examples of green leafy vegetables are collard, dandelion, kale, mustard, and turnip greens. If you are lacto-ovo-vegetarian, 1 cup of milk, yogurt, or pudding will supply you with 200 to 450 milligrams of calcium.

Protein

You will need 65 grams of protein daily. You can surpass this require-ment with ½ cup firm tofu (20 grams protein), ¼ cup cooked buckwheat kasha (64 grams protein), 2 potato knishes (16 grams protein), 1 cup lima beans (12 grams protein), 1 cup tempeh (18–30 grams protein), 1 cup blackbeans (15 grams protein), 1 cup granola cereal (10 grams pro-tein), 1 meat-substitute burger patty (10 to 20 grams protein). If you are lacto-ovo-vegetarian, try 1 cup plain low-fat yogurt (15 grams protein), 1 cup protein-fortified milk (10 grams protein), ½ cup ricotta cheese (14 grams protein), 1 cup cottage cheese (25 grams protein).

Vitamin D

In order to obtain the recommended 5 micrograms (equal to 200 IU) of vitamin D daily, you can drink 8 ounces soy milk (100 IU) and 8 ounces rice milk (100 IU), and eat 1 cup vitamin D–fortified cereal (40 IU), plus mushrooms and dark green leafy vegetables. If you consume dairy, you can have 1 cup homogenized milk (100 IU), 2 egg yolks (50 IU), and 1 pat of butter (2 IU) daily. As vitamin D is the sunshine vitamin, walking out-doors for fifteen minutes in sunlight daily (400 IU) or sitting near a sunny window will help you fulfill the nutritional needs for both your baby and yourself, even if you do not consume vitamin D–rich foods.

Phosphorus

Obtaining 700 milligrams of phosphorus will be easy. Phosphorus is present in seeds, nuts, grains, yeast, wheat germ, bran, and most fruits and vegetables. Some examples include 2 ounces tahini (416 milligrams),

½ cup bran cereal (294 milligrams), ½ cup baked beans (132 milligrams), ½ cup firm tofu (239 milligrams), ½ cup almonds (428 milligrams), ½ cup peanuts (280 milligrams), 1 cup of milk (232 milligrams).

Vitamin A

Yellow, orange, and red fruits and vegetables are abundant in vitamin A. Your recommended amount is 8,000 international units (or 1,300 micrograms) daily, and vegetarian sources include ½ cantaloupe (9,230 IU), 1 sweet potato (9,240 IU), 1 carrot (20,250 IU), 1 apricot (4,490 IU), 1 peach (1,330 IU), 1 tomato (2,170 IU), 1 cup of broccoli (4,000 IU). If you consume dairy products, you can have an 8-ounce glass of milk (500 IU), 1 tablespoon butter (430 IU), 1 ounce of cheddar cheese (300 IU), and 1 cup baked acorn squash (874 IU).

Vitamin B_{12}

While nursing, you need 2.6 micrograms of vitamin B_{12} daily. You can obtain this with 1 cup enriched cereal (2–6 micrograms), 4 ounces of tempeh (1–4 micrograms), and one 3-ounce veggie burger (3.5 micrograms). If you are a lacto-ovo-vegetarian, try 2 ounces of Brie cheese (1 microgram), 1 cup of Kellogg's Product 19 cereal (2 micrograms), 8 ounces of milk (1 microgram), and 1 ounce of cheddar cheese (0.3 microgram). One vegetarian vitamin B_{12} tablet daily will fulfill this vitamin's requirement.

Magnesium

The recommended dietary allowance of magnesium is 320 milligrams and can be obtained easily from 3 ounces of tofu (111 milligrams), ¼ cup brazil nuts (88 milligrams), ¼ cup almonds (96 milligrams), ¼ cup wheat germ (84 milligrams), 10 dates (58 milligrams), 5 dried figs (71 milligrams), 1 cup prune juice (26 milligrams), 1 ear of corn (58 milligrams). Lacto-ovo-vegetarians can have 8 ounces of milk (28 milligrams).

Selenium

Selenium is required in increased quantities while nursing—75 micrograms daily. This can be obtained from wheat germ, brewer's yeast, nuts, blackstrap molasses, barley, oats, mushrooms, and radishes.

Zinc

Finally, an average of 19 milligrams of zinc is recommended daily. Good sources are whole grains such as wheat, rye, and oats, plus gingerroot, mustard, chili pepper, and black pepper. Specific sources are 4 ounces of toasted sesame seeds (12 milligrams), 1 cup firm tofu (4 milligrams), ½ cup pecans (3 milligrams), 1 cup beans (2 milligrams), 10 brazil nuts (2 milligrams), 1 cup green peas (2 milligrams), 1 slice of whole-wheat pita bread (1 milligram).

INTRODUCING A BOTTLE

I will return to work when my baby is six weeks old and nurse him only in the mornings and evenings. How soon should I introduce bottle-feeding?

It will be best to give him a bottle two to three weeks before you plan your return to work. This might be difficult because he will still smell the odor of your skin and breast milk and may become so fussy that he will not accept the bottle at all. If this confusion occurs, ask your husband or mother to give him the bottle while you are in another room. This will be less distracting for him. Once he begins to accept the bottle, you can start alternating feedings, one with a bottle and the next with your breast. Within two or three weeks your baby should adapt to both means of sustenance.

I have never felt the instinct to breast-feed. I'd prefer to use bottles, but others are making me feel guilty. Is this the wrong choice?

This is your pregnancy, your birth, and your baby; you have a right to nourish this child in any way that will provide her with healthy nutrition. Bottle-feeding is well within the range of acceptable choices. Breast-feeding is wonderful for those who wish to do so, but it is not for everyone. Many people try to give pregnant women advice, but this advice should be offered in the spirit of sharing information, not with the intent to inspire guilt.

When I return to work, my baby-sitter will give my son my refrigerated breast milk. Are there any precautions she should follow?

When your baby-sitter removes your saved breast milk from the refrigerator, she can place the bottle in a small pot of warm water to take the chill out of it. As long as you have placed your milk in a clean container from a clean breast pump with clean hands, it will not be necessary for her to boil your milk. Boiling will actually remove some of the important vitamins. With time, your baby may become accustomed to drinking cold milk directly out of the refrigerator, just the way an adult does.

If your bottled breast milk has been out of the refrigerator, at room temperature or warmer, for over two hours, she should not place it back in the refrigerator for reuse. It will be safer if she discards that bottle of milk.

I plan to supplement with formula. Should I heat the formula so it will be the same temperature as my breast milk?

While you are nursing, your baby will probably prefer to drink formula at body temperature. Initially, take formula out of the refrigerator and place it in a small bowl of slightly warm water to take the chill out of it. Fairly soon, however, she may prefer her formula cool or even cold directly out of the refrigerator. This is similar to the way older children prefer cold milk rather than warm.

When I introduce a bottle to my breast-fed baby, are there any nipples I should use to prevent nipple confusion?

When you start to supplement your baby with formula, use small nipples that do not extend too far back into your baby's mouth. It will be slightly more difficult for your baby to obtain formula from these nipples and will create the more challenging situation—similar to what your baby experiences when he nurses from your breast. These smaller nipples can be obtained through Evenflo, Playtex, and Avent manufacturers.

My baby is four months old, and I will be going back to work. How will I know how much milk I should pump for her?

Your baby drinks between 2½ and 3 ounces of expressed milk for each pound of her body weight daily. If you plan to pump for a twenty-four-hour period and your baby weighs eight pounds, you need to pump between 20 and 24 ounces. If you are going to be away for eight hours, pump and store one-third of that, or 7 to 8 ounces.

CHOOSING A GOOD FORMULA

Which formula should I purchase?

Your pediatrician will determine the specific formula that is right for your baby. If you plan to bottle-feed, please contact your pediatrician prior to your giving birth so he can discuss his preferences with you and you can buy some prior to delivery. By being prepared, you will not need to run out after you deliver to purchase it. No one can determine which formula your baby will prefer, so don't buy a huge supply of any one kind. After your baby starts feeding and you observe how she reacts to the initial formula, your pediatrician and you will know whether or not to leave her on this brand or change to another. As your pediatrician has many years of experience observing babies' reactions to various formulas, he will know from your baby's reaction to one formula which brand might be best for her.

My baby does not want to drink any formula. Why?

Your baby may simply need time to get over his exhaustion from birth. Birth is a very traumatic experience, and he may not wish to exhaust himself by eating. He may be bruised and tired, and all he may need is rest. In addition, he has been consuming all the nutrition he needs directly through his umbilical cord, until the moment he was born. He may have a sufficient supply of nutrients for his first day or two of life. Some important clues to look for in assessing his need for nutrition: Is he fussy? Is he sleepy? Is he producing any urine? If he is producing urine, that is a positive sign that he is not dehydrated. Please inform your pediatrician as to how much liquid he has ingested and how much urine he is excreting, and she will let you know if you should be concerned.

POSITIONING YOUR BABY

What is the best way to hold my baby while breast-feeding?

Your baby might latch on and be more comfortable in one position than in another. You also may find you are more comfortable nursing your baby in certain positions. It is worthwhile to obtain breast-feeding books and attend a breast-feeding class to share information with other women. You can hold your baby in a typical cradle hold (both facing each other, with your baby's head resting in the crease of your elbow) when you start nursing. You may wish to lie down with your baby facing you, each of you lying on your side, with a rolled pillow behind him to prevent him from rolling back. You may then attempt to nurse your baby in a football hold (sitting up with your baby on his side, with his little head looking up at you and his little feet extending under your arm and toward your back). These are some of the positions that will help you at the start, but there are many that you and he will discover together.

> *You will probably start nursing your baby on your left breast, instinctively holding your baby in your left arm, close to your heart.*

IF YOU NEED HELP WITH NURSING

How can I get in touch with La Leche League?

The La Leche organization is composed of current and prior breast-feeding women who will assist you with breast-feeding problems. They will do their best to give you technical and emotional support if you are having nursing problems. The phone number is 1-800-La Leche. When you call this organization of experienced nursing volunteers, a member will help find a representative near your home who can help, guide, and motivate you. Your representative will be understanding of your individual situation and help you through your nursing problems.

What is a lactation consultant?

A lactation consultant is a professional who is educated and experienced in the process of breast-feeding. Often the consultant will be a registered nurse or other health care professional who has taken a rigorous course, attended special classes, and passed a certifying examination qualifying her to hold this title. She specializes in helping women through difficult nursing situations and will watch you nurse and give you suggestions as to how you can improve your technique. She will also give you little clues to help you avoid nursing problems. If you plan to nurse for a long time, she will be an invaluable asset to you. Most hospitals and birthing centers have lactation consultants who live in proximity to these sites and whose names and phone numbers will be made readily available to you. Your obstetrician, midwife, childbirth educator, or pediatrician will all know lactation consultants. If you have trouble reaching one, please e-mail ilca@erols.com for a consultant near your home.

NOTE ON NUTRITION: VEGETARIAN NUTRITION AND YOUR NEWBORN'S HEALTH

Could something in my vegetarian diet be causing my baby's fussiness?

Your baby's fussiness may be due to one of the components of your vegetarian diet, as some fruits and vegetables pass through breast milk to your baby and may be difficult for her to digest. In addition, your baby may simply be reacting to the acids within some of these fruits and vegetables, typically oranges, grapefruit, and tomatoes. The tomato category includes all tomato-based dishes, such as spaghetti sauces and pizza topping.

Some cruciferous vegetables—broccoli, cauliflower, Brussels sprouts, and cabbage—also cause fussiness and intestinal upset in babies. Other vegetarian foods that cause food sensitivity reactions in nursing newborns include beans, onions, turnips, and dried fruits such as prunes. In order to determine which food is affecting your baby, start an elimination diet one or two foods at a time to see if your baby's condition improves. Fortunately, there is such a variety of fruits and vegetables in a vegetarian's diet that even if you eliminate one group, you will have plenty of others to fulfill all vitamin and mineral requirements.

I eat large quantities of soy products. My pediatrician said that my son's gassiness might be related to a soy allergy. Can it be so?

Yes, it might be. More babies are allergic to dairy products than to soy; however, soy allergies do exist. Watch your diet carefully and eliminate tofu, tofu cheese substitutes, soybeans, textured soy protein, textured vegetarian meat substitutes, and even soy sauce. You may also need to stay away from Chinese restaurants for a while. The only way you can confirm that your son has a soy allergy is by eliminating these products and seeing if his condition improves. You can compensate for your decrease in vegetarian soy protein by increasing your intake of legumes, nuts, vegetables, and seeds.

Why is it that my baby becomes gassy and fussy when I eat some dairy products and not when I eat others?

Just as adults with lactose intolerance have varying degrees of sensitivity to various dairy products, so do babies. When you drink milk, your baby receives the full dose of lactose sugar that you receive. When you eat processed dairy products, such as a high-fat cheese, pudding, or even yogurt, your baby may not react at all.

If your baby reacts to all dairy products that you consume, then she may be reacting to caseins. Caseins are proteins present in all dairy products, cooked or not cooked, and high or low in fat content. Therefore your baby's reactions to these dairy products may be a clue as to whether she is reacting to lactose or casein.

I eliminated all dairy because the pediatrician said my baby's diarrhea was a reaction to this. He still has diarrhea. What can I do next?

A mother's ingestion of dairy can be one of the most irritating and allergy-producing irritants to her baby. Your baby may react to dairy products in a variety of ways, such as being fussy, gassy, or bloated or developing a skin rash. Evaluate your diet closely, since it may still contain milk components. For example, if you ingest a food with sodium caseinate, whey, solid milk products, or any product that begins with "lact," such as lactalbumin, that food contains dairy. Eliminate it from your diet. So many of these dairy-derived chemicals are present in processed foods that you will find life easier if you eat natural produce. Your baby will probably outgrow this dairy sensitivity by the time he is six months old. Meanwhile, avoid any prepared foods that may contain these dairy components.

My baby is colicky. Is my vegetarian diet making this worse?

It might be, but you can change that. The most likely cause of colic is iron in a mother's diet. If you take vitamins containing iron, please stop these and take a vitamin without iron. It may take four days to determine if your baby's condition improves after you eliminate iron. The next most common foods that produce colic are dairy products. You will be able to evaluate this as you eliminate milk, cheese, pudding, and ice cream from your diet. You will need patience, because it might take two weeks before you notice a change in your baby. The third most common cause of colic is soy products. This sensitivity might actually be a reaction to a mold that grows on soybeans. If you determine that soy is the causative agent, you will need to eliminate tofu, tempeh, and textured soy products.

Colic usually reaches a peak when a baby is six to eight weeks of age, then generally subsides by the time a baby reaches three to six months. Thank goodness it resolves naturally.

I sometimes eat fish. What are the dangers of fish to my nursing baby?

The Food and Drug Administration warns pregnant and nursing women to avoid shark, swordfish, mackerel, and tilefish. These all contain high levels of a form of methylmercury, a compound that affects a developing child's nervous system. These large fish prey on smaller fish and absorb mercury not only from the water in which they swim, but from the flesh of the smaller fish they consume. The FDA says you need not eliminate all fish from your diet, but you should definitely decrease your intake to a maximum of 12 ounces of cooked fish in any one week.

I eat tuna fish. Is it dangerous to eat tuna while nursing?

Controversy surrounds the question of the mercury levels of various types of tuna fish. The FDA has stated that small amounts of tuna are safe for pregnant and nursing women, yet the Center for Science and the Public Interest, a Washington-based consumer advocacy organization, states that tuna in sushi and tuna steaks contains levels of methylmercury that exceed acceptable FDA standards. Tuna in sushi and tuna steaks are derived from larger fish than those used for canned tuna and contain higher levels of methylmercury.

Although canned tuna contains lower levels of methylmercury, it is best that you not consume more than two cans of tuna in any one week.

If I do not go outdoors very often with my baby, should I supplement our diet with vitamin D?

Breast milk does not contain vitamin D, so all breast-feeding women, vegetarian or not, should seek to ensure that their breast-fed babies do not become deficient in this nutrient. There are only two sources of vitamin D: direct sunlight and direct dietary intake. Although few vegan foods contain vitamin D, many foods are supplemented with it. Formula and store-bought milk are supplemented with vitamin D, but obviously breast milk cannot be. There have been rare cases of vitamin D deficiencies in exclusively breast-fed infants of vegan mothers. These mothers had not maintained healthy vegetarian diets, followed healthy lifestyles, or taken the recommended supplements. These deficient children had been exclusively breast-fed for at least seven to nineteen months and actually required hospitalization for vitamin D deficiencies. Their mothers were darkly pigmented, obtained no sunlight, and did not fortify their infants' nutrition with vitamins.

If you are a darkly pigmented woman who does not venture outdoors, it will be beneficial and prudent for you to supplement your baby with vitamin D while nursing. In addition, please try to walk your baby outdoors for at least fifteen minutes each day. If you remain indoors, expose your baby and yourself to sunlight for part of the day.

HERBS AND MEDICATIONS
WHILE NURSING

I drink herbal tea. Might these dry my breast milk?

Suppression of lactation can occur with mint, ginger, barberry, or green tea. The term *herbal tea* is not specific to one category of herb or plant, as tea may be derived from a variety of leaves, fragrances, and spices. If you drink mint tea, ginger tea, barberry tea, or even green tea, you may notice a gradual decrease in your milk supply and will need to eliminate these from your diet.

Can certain herbs increase my milk supply?

Certain herbs increase milk production, but the effect is individual and varies from woman to woman. These include raspberry leaf, fennel, and fenugreek. Your health food store may carry a combination of these herbs in a product called Mother's Milk Tea. You can also purchase this in capsule form and may tolerate it better. Read the manufacturer's label on the capsule or tea container to determine how much you should take, as quantities of the herbs may vary from one manufacturer to another.

Which medications can I take for headaches?

It is always safest to avoid medications, and using magnets for your headaches (see page 242) might be a good alternative. If your headaches began while you were in the hospital and you had an epidural or spinal block, you may be suffering from spinal headaches. A spinal headache will usually exacerbate when you sit up and subside when you lie down. If this is your headache pattern, call your obstetrician; he will tell you to drink large quantities of fluid and lie down and may refer you to the anesthesiologist.

If yours is not a spinal headache, massage your head and neck at the site of your pain to stimulate circulation. If all else fails, start with Tylenol or Extra Strength Tylenol and evolve into using ibuprofen products such as Advil, Nuprin, or Motrin. It is wise to avoid aspirin products, as these pass to your baby and may increase the tendency for your baby to bleed.

I had a cesarean and I'm taking Demerol. Is it safe for me to nurse?

Yes. It is safe to take narcotics while nursing, but it's best if you can gradually decrease the narcotics you are taking. Your baby is receiving some of this medication while nursing, but these will not cause abnormalities or have long-term effects. She may, however, share some of your sleepiness and drowsiness from the Demerol, as it will be passed on in your breast milk. Hopefully you will not need to continue this medication more than a few days.

Will breast-feeding be effective as birth control?

There are some basic guidelines. You can use breast-feeding as a means of contraception only if you plan to totally, or almost totally, breast-feed your baby for the first six months of his life. It is 98 percent protective in preventing pregnancy during the first six months. You should not extend the interval between your feedings more than four hours during the day and more than six hours during the night. If you supplement your baby's feedings with formula, this should not exceed more than 5 to 10 percent of the total feedings from formula. For example, if more than one out of every ten of your baby's feedings is formula, this will decrease the chance that breast-feeding will be adequate contraception for you. As long as you adhere to this protocol, you should have a 98 percent chance of success in not becoming pregnant during these first six months.

Breast-feeding is not a substitute for traditional methods of birth control, even if you are not getting your period. When women breast-feed, they develop amenorrhea—meaning lack of menses. In general, women who do not have a menses do not ovulate. However, no one can predict when you will start to ovulate—and that will occur two weeks prior to your first menses. Therefore, you might conceive while breast-feeding, even if you have not had your first period yet.

> *I have had many of my nursing patients become pregnant,*
> *and they usually do not recognize that this has occurred*
> *for months.*

Some women begin their menstrual period two to three months after delivery, even if they are nursing. Once a woman resumes her period, she is ovulating. If you are such a woman, it is clearly best for you to use protection if you do not want to deliver two children within the same year.

Can I use birth control pills while nursing my baby?

There are some birth control pills that are considered safe to take while nursing, but they all contain hormones that you will pass on to your baby. Although you may have met many women who used birth control pills while nursing, no one can confirm that these are free of any effects. It is specifically important that you not use typical combined estrogen and progesterone birth control pills. Estrogen-containing oral contraceptives are not considered safe for a baby. The mini-pill is a birth control pill that contains progesterone and has no estrogen in it at all. You are permitted to take the "progesterone-only mini-pill" while you are nursing. This pill will not afford you the same degree of contraception as the standard combined estrogen and progesterone oral contraceptive, but it is considered safer while nursing. When women take these, they also experience more breakthrough bleeding, or spotting, during the month.

WEIGHT WATCH:
LOSING SAFELY WHILE YOUR BABY GAINS

My baby lost weight after birth. How can I be sure she is receiving enough colostrum?

Most babies lose weight during their first few days of life whether they are breast-fed or bottle-fed. Your colostrum is a clear to slightly yellow-tinged enriched solution that will supply your baby with all the nutrients she needs for her first three or four days of life. It is a very concentrated, well-balanced liquid packed with vitamins, antibodies, and other nutrients. Your baby needs only small amounts to be satiated—only an amount equal to a few spoonfuls during her first few days of life. Accordingly, she may wet her diaper only once on her first day of life, twice on her second, and three times on her third day. This is normal and healthy. By her second week of life, she will probably start to increase in weight and make up for her initial weight loss.

Can I safely lose weight yet supply healthy nutrition to my baby?

You will be able to give your baby excellent nutrition if you do not restrict your caloric intake too much. Your milk production will not decrease if you decrease your caloric intake gradually. For example, if you decrease your caloric intake by 100 calories each week, your milk supply should remain stable. If, however, you decrease your intake suddenly to only 1,500 to 1,800 calories daily, your milk supply will definitely decrease. You may not have to work as hard to lose weight while nursing as you would if you weren't. Just by your body's activity of producing milk, you will burn excess calories. That is why you may not need to start your diet immediately after delivery. Observe your weight fluctuation over these first two months, as you may be very impressed and satisfied by your own natural weight loss. The sites where you will lose the most weight while nursing will be your hips and thighs.

> *During times of famine, energy for nursing to newborns was obtained more easily from the fat of a woman's thighs than from any other site in her body. During those difficult times, women with heavier thighs kept their babies alive and sustained our species. Therefore, if you have heavy thighs, think of yourself as a natural survivor.*

CHAPTER 13

After You Deliver

For as long as you can remember,
you dreamed of having a child.
You dreamed of raising her, guiding her, teaching her,
and hugging her.
You will teach her to play, read, spell, and add.
To have values, be honest, and show respect.

Your baby was given to you for you to teach her,
but that is only a partial truth.
You will soon learn
that she was given to you
to teach you.

She will teach you to slow down, forgo selfish goals, find new needs,
and recognize the gifts you have been given.
She will teach you to be giving, caring, concerned,
and to share unconditional love.

Each of us learns so much from our children.
But only fate knows
which specific lessons you must learn,
as each of us is meant to learn different ones.

Your child knows what she must teach you,
so you will understand the purpose of your life.

ENERGY HIGHS AND LOWS

I am exhausted. How can I care for my baby when I can barely care for myself?

Pregnancy, labor, birth, and cesarean sections are exhausting. We have been led to believe that because pregnancy and birth are natural events, we will "spring" back to strength and health. In reality, pregnancy and birth are the most profound and significant events that occur in a lifetime. Women who have gone through these should be treated with respect, dignity, kindness, and compassion and given the help, pampering, and rest they deserve. Please do not try to be superwoman, as it will take

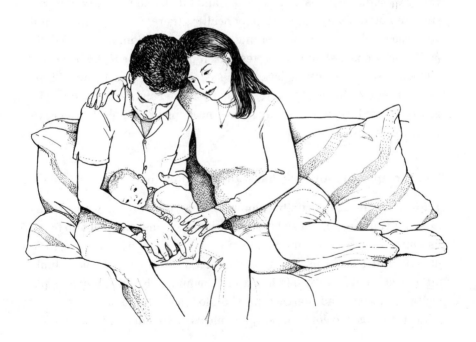

longer for you to regain your energy if you try to do too much now. This will be especially true if you have hemorrhoids, swollen legs, a bruised pelvis, burning when you urinate, difficulty with your bowel movements, swollen breasts, and total exhaustion. Pace yourself, and don't think about all you need to do. This way, you can prioritize and plan your life one week at a time.

Your baby's needs are few in number but great in time, frequency, and unpredictability. He will need to be fed, changed, held, rocked, and loved—very earthy needs. However, these will occur around the clock and quite frequently, and you will have to learn to squeeze in your other goals around your baby's needs. It will help if you localize your life with your baby, liquids, nourishment, rest area, and rest room all near one another. Your needs will be quite temporary, such as much sleep, daytime naps, liquids and nourishment, frequent access to a rest room and supplies to care for hemorrhoids, tears, or stitches. You may need help with doing the laundry and picking up pharmacy and supermarket supplies. After your baby's first four months, both your lives will be much easier.

Is my diet the cause of my exhaustion?

Every woman is exhausted after labor and birth, and if your doctor says you are nutritionally and medically healthy, there is no reason to think your vegetarian diet is contributing to your exhaustion. After you delivered, you probably had a blood test taken to determine if the blood you lost when your placenta separated caused you to become anemic. Please ask your doctor if your blood test results showed significant anemia, because if they did, you can easily follow the steps in chapter 2 to increase your iron levels.

Can I compensate for my exhaustion nutritionally?

You may be able to partially compensate nutritionally for your exhaustion, but your body has a right to feel exhausted, and you might do better listening to its wisdom and just take it easy. Your body is healing in its uterine lining, its bruised vaginal and rectal tissues, and its achy limbs after pushing. You probably lost a fair amount of blood when your placenta separated, had diarrhea in labor, lost body fluids in perspiration while laboring, and got your body chemicals out of balance vomiting. You may also be exhausted from having been pregnant for nine months, pushing for hours to deliver, and nursing your baby around the clock. The exhaustion might be an important clue telling you not to push yourself.

Nutritionally, please make sure you drink over eight glasses of water each day. Also, drink pineapple and papaya juices to increase the rate at which your tissues heal, eat vegetarian foods rich in vitamin C and zinc to support tissue healing, and eat foods high in magnesium to activate the enzymes your body uses to heal. Foods with iron will help to increase your blood count, especially if you lost a significant amount of blood. Minerals such as selenium, silica, and copper will also help your tissues heal faster so you will recover faster.

I have not had time to appreciate my baby; she is either fussing or crying or eating. Will I ever get back to my normal lifestyle?

The confusion will decrease a little each day as your baby adapts to this world and you adapt to your new life. When each of us first becomes a mother, it is a jolt to the status quo that we created in our lives over the prior twenty, thirty, or forty years. Your life is not confusing; it is just a new life. In your prior life, you were given assignments in your office, completed them, and they were done. In your new role as a mother, no task will ever be done, it will just be one of many waves rolling into another wave—all within a vast ocean of tasks that will continually present themselves. Being a mother is being at the mercy of nature; you will never be able to predict or control it.

If you try to accomplish all of the numerous things you did in your prior life, you will become stressed. At this time, your mission will be to put aside all other aspects of your life and concentrate on one little aspect, your baby. Try not to worry about all uncompleted tasks—they can all wait. Take pictures of your baby often, so when you feel overwhelmed, you will quietly and calmly look at these and reflect upon the blessings of your life.

TAKING OFF THE PREGNANCY POUNDS

I lost only twelve pounds after my delivery. How much weight do most women lose?

Most women lose between fifteen and twenty pounds by the time their baby is one week old. Your initial weight gain was due to the growth of your baby (seven and one-half pounds), body fat (seven pounds), tissue swelling (four pounds), blood vessel fluid (three pounds), enlarged uterus (two pounds), amniotic fluid (two pounds), placenta (one and one-half pounds), and breast swelling (one pound). All of these add up to more than a twenty-seven-pound weight gain.

After you deliver, you will lose only some of this weight immediately, obviously that related to your baby, placenta, and amniotic fluid. In addition, you may notice a sudden decrease in the amount of fluid you're retaining. The blood vessels on your hands may no longer appear swollen and distended. It may take you months to lose the fat tissue you accumulated, months for your uterus to fully shrink down, months for your breasts to return to their prior size, and weeks for all of your swelling to subside. Actually, some women gain weight after they deliver because they retain fluid temporarily for one to two weeks after delivery. Within two weeks after delivery, however, most women will have lost most of this fluid. Within four months after your delivery, you will probably have lost all the weight you are going to lose easily. By that time, you will need to face the reality that the rest of your weight loss will require exercise and diet control.

When I was pregnant, everyone told me to eat for my baby. Now I feel fat. I am so depressed. What can I do?

You are not alone, and you should not be hard on yourself. Over 90 percent of women feel the loss of their body image and loss of their self-esteem as a woman because of their body and weight changes after delivery. Every woman who delivers a baby has changed from her prior youthful shape to the shape of a mother. Please think about these changes objectively: your uterus stretched to create a new life and is still quite large, your abdominal muscles stretched to accommodate that uterus, you retained fluids in all your body tissues, and you gained weight as your body craved for you to carry and nurse a new life. You are no worse than any other woman—you are just a new mother.

With time, you will lose as much weight and regain as much of your prior shape as you want to work at. Please give yourself time and do not judge yourself harshly. When your baby reaches four weeks of age and you regain most of your strength, you will be able to reduce your caloric intake and begin a moderate exercise program. The values imposed on women, by placing them on a pedestal while they are pregnant and judging them harshly when they no longer look like a model, are unfair and unfortunate. Please do not let this get to you.

BODY CHANGES

My abdomen is still large, even though I delivered. Will it ever return to its normal size?

After delivery, a woman's uterus still remains the size of a four- to five-month pregnancy. The top of your uterus goes down, but only to the level of your navel, consistent with the height of a five-month pregnancy. Also, your abdominal muscles have been stretched over these past nine months and will not retract to their normal size and tone quickly. Please don't become discouraged if your abdomen is still large; most women are in the same situation as you.

It is not possible now to know if your abdomen will ever return to its prior size. The answer depends on how much your abdomen stretched, your abdominal tone before pregnancy, and the amount of exercise you will have the time and motivation to do now. You may never totally return to your previous size and shape, but you may come close.

My legs are more swollen after delivery than they were before. Why is this happening?

A large percentage of women have swelling in their legs after they deliver. This occurs often in women who had some swelling during pregnancy and whose fluid balance has not yet converted back to its normal state. If you are retaining much fluid, call your obstetrician. He will check your blood pressure and kidneys, because some women with these symptoms have developed toxemia of pregnancy after delivery. Once it has been confirmed that you are normal, you will not need to worry about your health. To lessen your swelling, decrease your salt intake, keep your legs elevated on a chair or a stool, wear support hose, and place them in a bath twice a day. When you sit in a bath, the pressure of the water on the external surfaces of your legs will push fluid from your body tissues back to your blood vessels and eventually out through your kidneys. All these techniques will help decrease your tissue swelling.

This was my third delivery, and my afterbirth pains are terrible! Why are they so strong?

Uterine cramps and contractions after delivery, known as afterbirth pains, increase in intensity after each subsequent pregnancy. However, they often peak during a third delivery and then remain at that level for all remaining deliveries. These afterbirth pains may reach very intense levels following both vaginal deliveries and cesarean sections. Because these pains are not that intense after first deliveries, many childbirth classes don't even mention them. Women learn the true meaning of afterbirth pains following their third baby. Fortunately, these pains usually subside three days after delivery. Until that time, place a heating pad over your abdomen or lower back to relieve some of your discomfort.

I delivered my baby three months ago and now have hair loss. Is my vegetarian diet contributing significantly to this?

Your vegetarian diet is not the primary cause of your hair loss after delivery, but it may be contributing to it. Hair loss occurs naturally after every delivery. As a vegetarian, you may have a diet that is lower in sulfur-containing amino acids than the diet of a meat-eater. Sulfur-containing amino acids—methionine, cystine, and cysteine—are all found in meats. Your hair contains and needs a constant supply of sulfur. To optimize the regrowth of your hair, you will need to consume dietary supplements or foods with sulfur-containing amino acids, plus biotin, inositol, choline, B and C vitamins, silicon, and omega-3 fatty acids.

Your hair will flourish if you consume a diet rich in cysteine, because this is the main amino acid constituent of your hair. As a vegetarian, you will find dietary sources of cysteine in red peppers, garlic, onions, broccoli, Brussels sprouts, yogurt, and egg yolks. If you do not consume a diet naturally rich in cysteine, a supplement of 1 gram of cysteine daily, taken between meals and with water or juice, will help you.

> *You will be able to distinguish some of the vegetarian foods that contain sulfur because of their characteristic odors. These foods include molasses, beans, and egg yolks, plus the odiferous vegetables—onions, garlic, cabbage, Brussels sprouts, and turnips.*

Biotin is a B vitamin, and it is the only vitamin that contains sulfur. It aids in the prevention of hair loss and balding. Please do not eat raw egg white, as this will deplete your body of its biotin supply. Vegetarian sources of biotin include brewer's yeast, unpolished rice, nuts, and cooked egg yolk. The quantities of biotin in vegetarian foods are somewhat limited, so you may want to supplement with 50 to 100 milligrams of biotin daily.

Inositol is a B vitamin that can also help prevent your hair from falling out. It is found in whole grains, citrus fruits (except lemon), cantaloupe, molasses, lima beans, and raisins. If you feel your diet is low in inositol, supplement it with 50 to 100 milligrams of inositol each day.

Silicon is a mineral that promotes healthy growth of hair, and vegetarians readily obtain it from plant fibers, including the hulls of wheat, oats, and rice, and from alfalfa, cucumbers, avocados, strawberries, lettuce, and a variety of other plants. You are most probably consuming enough silicon.

Omega-3 fatty acids are oils that help to promote growth and maintenance of healthy hair. As a vegetarian, you will not be obtaining omega-3 fatty acids from fish sources but will be able to obtain them from flaxseed oil capsules, 1,000 milligrams daily.

> *As a vegetarian, I feel my intake of cysteine, omega-3 fatty acids, and biotin is limited, so I supplement with these nutrients. If I am away from home several weeks and do not take these, my hair becomes thinner.*

NOTE ON NUTRITION:
VEGETARIANS AND TISSUE HEALING

Are there any vegetarian foods that will help my torn and bruised tissues heal?

Yes, and most of them contain papain. Papain is a compound that decreases tissue swelling and helps heal bruised tissues. It is present predominantly in pineapple and papaya. Years back, prescription medications were available that contained pineapple and papaya extract and were prescribed to promote tissue healing. I frequently recommended these extracts to soccer or basketball players, and their tissues healed with great rapidity—sometimes the bruises resolved overnight.

> *I had surgery several years ago and bought concentrated pineapple and papaya juice extracts, which I reconstituted at home. I drank these continuously and healed at an amazingly rapid rate.*

I pushed three hours and now have horrendous hemorrhoids. What can I do for these?

There are two components to dealing with your hemorrhoids: dietary and medical. The most critical factor is to not let yourself become constipated, and with your vegetarian diet, you will have a distinct advantage over other women. Eat large quantities of fruits, vegetables, and whole-grain breads and cereals. This roughage will keep your bowels moving quickly so the feces will not harden in your colon. Drink large amounts of liquid to keep your stool soft so you will not need to strain. Another important factor will be to consume a diet rich in oils to enable your foods to slide down faster. Vegetable oils are very healthy, not that fattening, and free from cholesterol—consider eating oily Caesar salads.

The medical treatment for your hemorrhoids includes methods to relieve pain and decrease tissue swelling. Tucks pads are witch hazel pads that shrink hemorrhoids and thereby decrease their pain. Effective topical hemorrhoid preparations include Anusol and Preparation H. Both creams reduce pain and help tissues to heal. Dermoplast spray numbs bruised vulval and hemorrhoidal tissues and will afford you great relief. After you go to the rest room, wipe the rectal area with moistened cotton balls so you do not irritate these tissues further. Last, sit in a warm sitz bath or bathtub, as this will greatly relieve your pain and heal your tissues.

I was anemic through my pregnancy, and then I lost blood during my delivery. What can I take besides iron tablets that will build up my blood count and not constipate me?

As a vegetarian, you have numerous dietary choices to help you restore your body's iron content. Eat an abundant quantity of dark green vegetables—the darker the green, the higher the iron. Therefore, eat the outer leaves of lettuce, the rabe of your broccoli, and dark green arugula in your salads. Next, use blackstrap molasses as your main source of sweetener on toast, over breakfast cereals, and in cakes or puddings. Molasses is an excellent source of iron and is not constipating. Limit your intake of dairy products, or just avoid them when you are eating your iron-rich foods, as they will decrease your absorption of iron. Last, sauté vegetables in a cast-iron skillet to consume iron from the particles precipitated from your pan. You will be surprised how quickly your iron increases without constipating supplements.

YES, YOUR BABY CAN BE A HEALTHY VEGETARIAN, TOO

My pediatrician has advised me that when I start to give my son food, he will need animal protein. Is this so?

Not at all. This particular pediatrician may not be familiar with the protein levels in many vegetarian foods. He also may not have thought about the low level of protein in human milk—5 percent—which has been able to sustain our entire species for centuries. Share some of your vegetarian information with your physician so the two of you will grow together—you may even want to lend him this book! If it is difficult for your pediatrician to reevaluate the nutritional concepts he has traditionally believed were true, it may be wise for you to seek health care for your baby from a provider who feels more comfortable with your vegetarian lifestyle.

RESUMING EXERCISE

I think I will feel better if I go back to the gym. How soon may I return?

Assuming that you do not have any maternity-related medical problems, such as persistent toxemia of pregnancy or hypertension, you should be able to resume exercising as soon as you feel the strength and motivation to do so. Although many health care providers state that women need to wait weeks, or even months, until they restart their exercise program, many of these providers have never been to a gym and do not recognize the physical and mental benefits of exercise. If you had a cesarean section, please wait until your physician has checked your incision several weeks after delivery. When you begin exercising, do not stress your abdominal wall. For example, use the stationary bike or the elliptical walker rather than abdominal exercisers. You should, however, be able to do arm exercises and use the weight machines, because no surgery or trauma affected the upper half of your body.

If you had a vaginal delivery, your choice of exercise will depend upon the type and extent of vulval trauma you experienced. If the bruising was minimal and you have no vaginal tears or lacerations, most exercises will be safe and beneficial just a few weeks after delivery. You will need to pace yourself, limit the level of intensity, and limit the duration of your workout. If you had an extensive episiotomy, you may want to do only stretching and arm exercises for several weeks, but at least you will be getting your body prepared for more strenuous exercise later.

Closing Thoughts

And so our journey together
through your pregnancy
has come to a close.

As vegetarians, and as mothers,
as seekers of truth, as humanitarians, and as caring,
compassionate women,
we are forever bonded.

We know that the place to look for truth
is not within present-day beliefs or in family traditions,
as these change with time.
Truth lies within the wisdom of our own hearts and minds.
These are the truths that will last forever.

As vegetarians,
we will have less cancer, less heart disease, and fewer infections.
Our bones and muscles will be stronger,
and we will survive longer.

Your commitment to a vegetarian lifestyle
truly blesses your baby and you
in body, mind, and spirit.

I wish peace, love, and blessings
for your new baby,
and thank you for letting me share
this important part of your journey
with you.

References

REFERENCES THROUGHOUT TEXT

American College of Obstetricians and Gynecologists. *Planning Your Pregnancy and Birth,* 3rd ed. Washington, D.C.: The American College of Obstetricians and Gynecologists, 2000.

As Your Baby Grows, *American Baby* vol. 8, no. 3, 1999.

Creasy, R., Resnick, R. *Maternal-Fetal Medicine,* 2nd ed. Philadelphia: W. B. Saunders, 1989.

Curtis, G. B. *Your Pregnancy Week by Week.* Edmonton, Canada: Fisher Books, 1997.

Danforth, D. *Obstetrics and Gynecology,* 4th ed. Philadelphia: Harper & Row, 1982.

Haas, E. S. *Staying Healthy with Nutrition.* Berkeley, Calif.: Celestial Arts, 1992.

Moore, K. L., Persaud, T. V. N. *The Developing Human,* 6th ed. Philadelphia: W. B. Saunders, 1998.

Nilsson, L. *A Child Is Born.* New York: Dell, 1990.

Prichard, J. A., MacDonald, P. C., Gant, W. F. *Williams Obstetrics,* 17th ed. East Norwalk, Conn.: Appleton-Century-Crofts, 1985.

Queenan, J. T., Queenan, C. N. *A New Life,* 2nd revised ed. Boston: Little, Brown, 1997.

Chapter 1: BEFORE YOU BECOME PREGNANT

Advanced Paternal Age: Risk to the Fetus. ACOG Committee Opinion 189 (Oct. 1997). American College of Obstetricians and Gynecologists, Washington, D.C.

Avery-Grant, A. *The Vegetarian Female.* New York: Avery Publishing, 1999.

Blackmore-Prince, C., Harlow, S. D., Gargiullo, P., Lee, M. A., Savitz, D. A. Chemical hair treatments and adverse pregnancy outcome among black women in central North Carolina. *American Journal of Epidemiology* 149 no. 8 (Apr. 1999): 712–6.

Borman, B., Cryer, C. The prevalence of anencephalus and spina bifida in New Zealand. *Journal of Paediatrics and Child Health* 29 no. 4 (Aug. 1993): 282–8.

Burnett, C., Goldenthal, E. I., Harris, S. B., et al. Teratology and percutaneous toxicology studies on hair dyes. *Journal of Toxicology and Environmental Health* 1 no. 6 (July 1976): 1027–40.

Burnett, C., Loehr, R., Corbett, J. Heritable translocation study on two hair dye formulations. *Fundamentals of Applied Toxicology* 1 no. 4 (July–Aug. 1981): 325–8.

Chambers, C. D., Johnson, K. A., Dick, L. M., Felix, R. J., Jones, K. L. Maternal fever and birth outcome: a prospective study. *Teratology* 58 no. 6 (Dec. 1998): 251–7.

Chatkupt, S., Skurnick, J. H., Jaggi, M., Mitruka, K., Koenigsberger, M. R., Johnson, W. G. Study of genetics, epidemiology, and vitamin usage in familial spina bifida in the United States in the 1990's. *Neurology* 44 (Jan. 1994): 65–70.

Ciacci, C., Cirillo, M., Auremma, G., Di Dato, G., Sabbatini, F., Mazzacca, G. Celiac disease and pregnancy outcome. *American Journal of Gastroenterology* 91 (Apr. 1996): 718–22.

Cnattingius, S., Nordstrom, M. L. Maternal smoking and feto-infant mortality: biological pathways and public health significance. *Acta Paediatrics* 85 (Dec. 1996): 1400–2.

Cox, T. M., Schofield, J. P. Gaucher's disease: clinical features and natural history. *Bailliers Clinical Haematology* 10 no. 4 (Dec. 1997): 657–89.

De Brandt, M., Palazzo, E., Belmatoug, N., et al. Outcome of pregnancies in lupus: experience at one center. *Annals of Medicine Interne* (Paris) 151 no. 2 (Mar. 2000): 87–92.

Delpixo, V. Epidemiological studies of work with video display terminals and adverse pregnancy outcomes (1984–1992). *American Journal of Industrial Medicine* 26 no. 4 (Oct. 1994): 465–80.

Diabetes and Pregnancy. ACOG Technical Bulletin 200 (Dec. 1994). American College of Obstetricians and Gynecologists, Washington, D.C.

Dlugosz, L., Vena, J., Byers, T., Stever, L., Bracken, M., Marshall, E. Congenital defects and electric bed heating in New York State: a register-based case-control study. *American Journal of Epidemiology* 135 no. 9 (May 1992): 1000–11.

Eliakim, R., Sherer, D. M. Celiac disease: fertility and pregnancy. *Gynecology and Obstetrics Investigation* 51 no. 1 (Jan. 2001): 3–7.

Eskenazi, B., Stapleton, A. L., Kharrazi, M., Chee, W. Y. Associations between maternal decaffeinated and caffeinated coffee consumption and fetal growth and gestational duration. *Epidemiology* 10 no. 3 (May 1999): 242–9.

Fernandes, O., Sabharwal, M., Smiley, T., Pastuszak, A., Koren, G., Einarson, T. Moderate to heavy caffeine consumption during pregnancy and relationship to spontaneous abortion and abnormal fetal growth: a meta-analysis. *Reproductive Toxicology* 12 no. 4 (July–Aug. 1998): 435–44.

Fonager, K., Sorenson, H. T., Olsen, J. Pregnancy outcome with Crohn's disease. *American Journal of Gastroenterology* 93 no. 12 (Dec. 1998): 2426–30.

Genetic Screening for Hemoglobinopathies. ACOG Committee Opinion 168 (Feb. 1996). American College of Obstetricians and Gynecologists, Washington, D.C.

Gershon, A. A., La Russa, P., Hardy, I., Steinberg, S., Silverstein, S. Varicella vaccine: the American experience. *Journal of Infectious Diseases* 166 suppl. 1 (Aug. 1992): S63–8.

Golderberg, R. L., Dolan-Mullen, P. Convincing pregnant patients to stop smoking. *Contemporary OB/GYN* (Nov. 2000): 35–44.

Goldsmith, J. R. Epidemiologic evidence relevant to radar (microwave) effects. *Environmental Health Perspectives* 105 suppl. 6 (Dec. 1997): 1579–87.

Guillonneau, M., Jacqz-Aigrain, E. Teratogenic effects of vitamin A and its derivatives. *Archives of Pediatrics* 4 (Sept. 1997): 867–74.

Hatch, E. E., Bracken, M. B. Effect of marijuana use in pregnancy on fetal growth. *American Journal of Epidemiology* 124 no. 6 (Dec. 1986): 986–93.

Hulse, G. K., Milne, E., English, D. R., Holman, C. D. Assessing the relationship between maternal cocaine use and abruptio placentae. *Addiction* 92 no. 1 (Nov. 1997): 1547–51.

Ida, A., Koyama, K. Ulcerative colitis and pregnancy. *Nippon Rinsho* 57 (Nov. 1999): 2603–7.

Immunization During Pregnancy. ACOG Technical Bulletin 160 (Oct. 1991). American College of Obstetricians and Gynecologists, Washington, D.C.

Jensh, R. P. Behavioral teratologic studies using microwave radiation: is there an increased risk from exposure to cellular phones and microwave ovens? *Reproductive Toxicology* 11 no. 4 (July–Aug. 1997): 601–11.

Kauppinen, K. Facts and fables about saunas. *Annals of the NY Academy of Sciences* 813 (Mar. 15, 1997): 654–62.

Kerem, B., Chiba-Falek, O., Kerem, E. Cystic fibrosis in Jews: frequency and mutation distribution. *Genetic Testing* 1 no. 1 (1997): 35–9.

Klebanoff, M. A., Levine, R. J., DerSimonian, R., Clemens, J. D., Wilkins, D. G. Maternal serum paraxanthine, a caffeine metabolite, and the risk of spontaneous abortion. *New England Journal of Medicine* 341 no. 22 (Nov. 1999): 1639–44.

Koren, G. Caffeine during pregnancy? In moderation. *Canadian Family Physician* 46 (Apr. 2000): 1569.

Little, B. B., Ghali, F. E., Snell, L. M., Knoll, K. A., Johnston, W., Gilstrap, L. C. Is hyperthermia teratogenic in the human? *American Journal of Perinatology* 8 no. 3 (May 1991): 185–9.

Locksmith, G. J., Duff, P. Preventing neural tube defects. *Obstetrics and Gynecology* 91 (June 1998): 1027–34.

McGowan, J. P., Shah, S. S. Management of HIV infection during pregnancy. *Current Opinions in Obstetrics and Gynecology* 12 no. 5 (Oct. 2000): 357–67.

Management of Herpes in Pregnancy. ACOG Practice Bulletin 8 (Oct. 1999). American College of Obstetricians and Gynecologists, Washington, D.C.

Marcus, M., McChesney, R., Golden, A., Landrigan, P. Video display terminals and miscarriages. *Journal of the American Medical Womens Association* 55 no. 2 (Spring 2000): 84–8, 105.

Martin, T. R., Bracken, M. B. Association of low birth weight with passive smoke exposure in pregnancy. *American Journal of Epidemiology* 124 no. 4 (Oct. 1986): 633–42.

Martinelli, P., Troncon, R., Paparo, F. Coeliac disease and pregnancy. *Gut* 46 (Mar. 2000): 332–5.

Maternal Serum Screening. ACOG Educational Bulletin 228 (Sept. 1996). American College of Obstetricians and Gynecologists, Washington, D.C.

Milunsky, A., Ulcickas, M., Rothman, K. J., Willett, W., Jick, S. S., Jick, H. Maternal heat exposure and neural tube defects. *Journal of the American Medical Association* 268 no. 7 (Aug. 19, 1992): 882–5.

Mindell, E. *Earl Mindell's Vitamin Bible for the 21st Century.* New York: Warner Books, 1999.

Morales, M., Berney, T., Jenny, A., Morel, P., Extermann, P. Crohn's disease as a risk factor for the outcome of pregnancy. *Hepatogastroenterology* 47 no. 36 (Nov.–Dec. 2000): 1595–8.

Muzaffar, F., Hussain, I., Haroon, T. S. Physiologic skin changes during pregnancy: a study of 140 cases. *International Journal of Dermatology* 37 (June 1998): 429–31.

Neiger, B. L. The re-emergence of thalidomide: results of a scientific conference. *Teratology* 62 no. 6 (Dec. 2000): 432–5.

Nevin, N. C., Johnston, W. P. A family study of spinida bifida and anencephalus in Belfast, Northern Ireland (1964–1968). *Journal of Medical Genetics* 17 no. 3 (June 1980): 203–11.

Nightingale, E. O., Schribanu, N., McCullough, D. C., Quinn, C. Observations on patients with neural-tube defects in a metropolitan hospital clinic: an epidemiological history. *Developmental Medicine and Child Neurology* 17 no. 5 (Oct. 1975): 574–9.

Norgard, B., Fonager, K., Sorenson, H. T. Birth outcome with celiac disease—nationwide study. *American Journal of Gastroenterology* 94 no. 2 (Sept. 1999): 2435–40.

Norgard, B., Fonager, K., Sorensen, H. T., Olsen, J. Birth outcome of women with ulcerative colitis: a nationwide Danish cohort study. *American Journal of Gastroenterology* 95 (Nov. 2000): 3165–70.

Novakov-Mikic, A., Vejnovic, T. Folic acid and prevention of neural tube defects. *Medianski Pregled* 52 (Nov.–Dec. 1999): 509–14.

Nybo Andersen, A. M., Wohlfahrt, J., Christens, P., Olsen, P., Melbye, M. Maternal age and fetal loss: population based register linkage study. *British Medical Journal* 320 no. 7251 (June 24, 2000): 1708–12.

Perinatal Viral and Parasitic Infections. ACOG Practice Bulletin 20 (Sept. 2000). American College of Obstetricians and Gynecologists, Washington, D.C.

Perinatal Viral and Parasitic Infections. ACOG Technical Bulletin 177 (Feb. 1993). American College of Obstetricians and Gynecologists, Washington, D.C.

Petersen, G. M., Rotter, J. I., Cantor, R. M., et al. The Tay-Sachs disease gene in North American Jewish populations: geographic variations and origin. *American Journal of Human Genetics* 35 no. 6 (Nov. 1983): 1258–69.

Physician's Desk Reference, 52nd ed. Montvale, N.J.: Thomson Healthcare, 1998, "Wellbutrin," p. 1120; "Zyban," p. 1139.

Planning Your Pregnancy and Birth, 3rd ed. Washington, D.C.: American College of Obstetricians and Gynecologists, 2000.

Preconceptional Care. ACOG Technical Bulletin 205 (May 1995). American College of Obstetricians and Gynecologists, Washington, D.C.

Psychosocial Risk Factors: Prenatal Screening and Intervention. ACOG Educational Bulletin 255 (Nov. 1999). American College of Obstetricians and Gynecologists, Washington, D.C.

Rasmussen, L. B., Anderson, N. L. Folate and neural tube defects. *Danish Medical Bulletin* 45 no. 2 (Apr. 1998): 213–7.

Recommendations for the Use of Folic Acid/Spina Bifida. Morbidity and Mortality Weekly Report 41 no. RR-14 (Sept. 11, 1992): 1–7.

Remington, S. R., Klein, J. O. *Infectious Diseases of the Fetus and Newborn Infant,* 3rd ed. Philadelphia: W. B. Saunders, 1990.

Robert, E. Intrauterine effects of electromagnetic fields (low frequency, mid-frequency RF, and microwave): review of epidemiologic studies. *Teratology* 59 (Apr. 1999): 292–8.

Scalera, A., Koren, G. Rationale for treating pregnant smokers with nicotine patches. *Canadian Family Physician* 44 (Aug. 1998): 1601–3.

Scheduled Cesarean Delivery and the Prevention of Vertical Transmission of HIV Infection. ACOG Committee Opinion 234 (May 2000). American College of Obstetricians and Gynecologists, Washington, D.C.

Schuchman, E. H., Miranda, S. R. Niemann-Pick disease: mutation update, genotype/phenotype correlations, and prospects for genetic testing. *Genetic Testing* 1 no. 1 (1997): 13–9.

Screening for Canavan Disease. ACOG Committee Opinion 212 (Nov. 1998). American College of Obstetricians and Gynecologists, Washington, D.C.

Screening for Tay-Sachs Disease. ACOG Committee Opinion 162 (Nov. 1995). American College of Obstetricians and Gynecologists, Washington, D.C.

Smith, D. W., Clarren, S. K., Harvey, M. A. Hyperthermia as a possible teratogenic agent. *Journal of Pediatrics* 92 (June 1987): 878–83.

Smoking and Women's Health. ACOG Educational Bulletin 240 (Sept. 1997). American College of Obstetricians and Gynecologists, Washington, D.C.

Substance Abuse in Pregnancy. ACOG Technical Bulletin 195 (July 1994). American College of Obstetricians and Gynecologists, Washington, D.C.

van Katwijk, C., Peeters, L. L. Clinical aspects of pregnancy after age 35 years: a review of the literature. *Human Reproductive Update* 4 no. 2 (Mar.–Apr. 1998): 185–94.

Wilson, P. D., Loffredo, C. A., Correa-Villasenor, A., Ferencz, C. Attributable fraction for cardiac malformations. *American Journal of Epidemiology* 148 no. 5 (Sept. 1998): 414–23.

Work place hazards. *Prolog Obstetrics,* 4th ed. Washington, D.C.: American College of Obstetricians and Gynecologists, 1998.

CHAPTER 2: VEGETARIAN NUTRITION DURING PREGNANCY

Avery-Grant, A. *The Vegetarian Female.* Garden City Park, N.Y.: Avery Publishing, 1999.

Bar-Sella, P., Rakover, Y., Ratner, D. Vitamin B_{12} and folate levels of long-term vegetarians. *Israel Journal of Medical Science* 26 (1990): 309–12.

Check it out! the food label, the pyramid, and you. *Home & Garden Bulletin* 266 (1994). U.S. Department of Agriculture, U.S. Department of Health and Human Services' Food and Drug Administration. U.S. Government Printing Office, Washington, D.C.

Dong, A., Scott, S. Serum vitamin B_{12}. *Annals of Nutrition and Metabolism* 26 (1982): 209–16.

Elliot, R. *Vegetarian Mother and Baby.* New York: Pantheon, 1986.

Graham, S. M. Long-term neurologic consequences of nutritional vitamin B_{12} deficiency in infants. *Journal of Pediatrics* 121 (Nov. 1992): 710–4.

Herbert, V. Vitamin B_{12}: plant sources. *American Journal of Clinical Nutrition* 48 (1988): 852–8.

Immerman, A. Vitamin B_{12} status on a vegetarian diet. *World Review of Nutritional Diet* 37: 38–54.

Klapper, M. *Pregnancy, Children and the Vegan Diet.* Umatilla, Fla.: Gentle World, 1987.

Kramer, M. S. Balanced protein/energy supplementation in pregnancy. *Cochrane Database Systems Review* 2 (2000): CD000032.

Kramer, M. S. High protein supplementation in pregnancy. *Cochrane Database Systems Review* 2 (2000): CD000105.

North, K., Golding, J. A maternal vegetarian diet in pregnancy is associated with hypospadias. The ALSPAC Study Team. Avon Longitudinal Study of Pregnancy and Childhood. *BJU International* (Jan. 2000): 107–13.

Sanders, T. A. The nutritional adequacy of plant-based diets. *Proceedings of the Nutrition Society* 58 no. 2 (May 1999): 265–9.

Young, V. R., Pellet, P. Plant proteins in relation to human protein and amino acid nutrition. *American Journal of Clinical Nutrition* 59 (5 suppl) (May 1994): 12035–125.

Chapter 3: YOUR MONTH OF CONCEPTION AND YOUR FIRST MONTH

Castleman, M. *The Healing Herbs.* Emmaus, Penn.: Rodale Press, 1991.

Dagher, S. M. Relationship of dietary intake to DDE resides in breast milk of nursing mothers in Beirut. *Food Additives and Contaminants* 16 (July 1999): 307–12.

Davis, J. R., Brownson, R. C., Garcia, R. Family pesticide use in the home, garden, orchard, and yard. *Archives of Environmental Contamination and Toxicology* 22 no. 3 (Apr. 1992): 260–6.

Dewailly, E., Ayotte, P. Inuit exposure to organochemicals. *Environmental Health Perspectives* 101 no. 7 (Dec. 1993): 618–20.

Hall, R. H. A new threat: organochemicals and food. *Nutrition and Health* 8 no. 1 (1992): 33–43.

Herrera, A. Persistent pesticides. *Bulletin of Environmental Contamination and Toxicology* 56 no. 2 (Feb. 1996): 173–7.

Longnecker, M. P., Rogan, W. J. Human health effects of DDT. *Annual Review of Public Health* 18 (1997): 211–4.

Newsome, W. H., Davies, D. J. Residues of polychlorinated biphenyls. *Food Additives and Contaminants* 15 no. 1 (Jan. 1998): 19–29.

Robbins, J. *Diet for a New America.* Tiburon, Calif.: H. J. Kramer, 1987, 342–6.

Schade, G. Organochlorine pesticides and polychlorinated biphenyls in human milk. *Science of the Total Environment* 215 nos. 1–2 (Apr. 1998): 31–9.

Chapter 4: YOUR SECOND MONTH

Al-Kanhal, M. A., Bani, I. A. Food habits during pregnancy. *International Journal of Vitamin Nutrition Research* 65 no. 3 (1995): 206–10.

Antimicrobial Therapy for Obstetric Patients. ACOG Educational Bulletin 245 (March 1998). American College of Obstetricians and Gynecologists, Washington, D.C.

Barnes, F. L. The effects of the early uterine environment on the subsequent development of the embryo and fetus. *Theriogenology* 53 no. 2 (Jan. 15, 2000): 649–58.

Flaxman, S. M., Sherman, P. W. Morning sickness: a mechanism for protecting. *Quarterly Review of Biology* 75 no. 2 (June 2000): 113–48.

Genital Human Papillomavirus Infections. ACOG Technical Bulletin 193 (June 1994). American College of Obstetricians and Gynecologists, Washington, D.C.

Hook, E. B. Dietary cravings and aversions during pregnancy. *American Journal of Clinical Nutrition* 8 (Aug. 1978): 1355–62.

Klebanoff, M. A., Koslowe, P. A., Kaslow, R. Epidemiology of vomiting in early pregnancy. *Obstetrics and Gynecology* 66 no. 5 (Nov. 1985): 612–6.

Symposium—Bacterial vaginosis in pregnancy. *Contemporary Obstetrics and Gynecology* 45 no. 12 (Dec. 2000): 37–51.

Vaginitis. ACOG Technical Bulletin 226 (July 1996). American College of Obstetricians and Gynecologists, Washington, D.C.

Zib, M., Lim, L., Walters, W. A. Symptoms during normal pregnancy. *Australian & New Zealand Journal of Obstetrics and Gynecology* 39 no. 4 (Nov. 1999): 401–10.

Chapter 5: YOUR THIRD MONTH

Avery, N. D., Stocking, K. D., Tranmer, J. E., Davies, G. A., Wolfe, L. A. Fetal responses to maternal strength conditioning exercises in late gestation. *Canadian Journal of Applied Physiology* 24 no. 4 (Aug. 1999): 362–76.

Clapp, J. F. III. The changing thermal response to endurance exercise during pregnancy. *American Journal of Obstetrics and Gynecology* 165 no. 6, pt. 1 (Dec. 1991): 1684–9.

Exercise During Pregnancy and the Postpartum Period. ACOG Technical Bulletin 189 (Feb. 1994). American College of Obstetricians and Gynecologists, Washington, D.C.

Garcia-Closas, R., Garcia-Closas, M., Serra-Majem, L. A cross-sectional study of dental caries. *American Journal of Clinical Nutrition* 66 no. 5 (Nov. 1997): 1257–63.

Grindefjord, M., Dahllof, G., Nilsson, B., Modeer, T. Stepwise prediction of dental caries in children up to 3.5 years of age. *Caries Research* 30 no. 4 (1996): 256–66.

Hanada, N. Current understanding of the cause of dental caries. *Japanese Journal of Infectious Diseases* 53 no. 1 (Feb. 2000): 1–5.

Jones, R. L., Botti, J. J., Anderson, W. M., Bennett, N. L. Thermoregulation during aerobic exercise in pregnancy. *Obstetrics and Gynecology* 65 (Mar. 1985): 340–5.

Klebanoff, M. A., Schiono, P. H., Carey, J. C. The effect of physical activity during pregnancy on preterm delivery and birth weight. *American Journal of Obstetrics and Gynecology* 163 no 5, pt. 1 (Nov. 1990): 1450–6.

Lotgering, F. K., Spinnewijn, W. E., Struijk, P. C., Bloomsma, F., Wallenburg, H. C. Respiratory and metabolic responses to endurance cycle exercise in pregnant and postpartum women. *International Journal of Sports Medicine* 19 no. 3 (Apr. 1998): 193–8.

McMurray, R. G., Katz, V. L. Thermoregulation in pregnancy. Implications for exercise. *Sports Medicine* 10 no. 3 (Sept. 1990): 146–58.

McMurray, R. G., Katz, V. L., Meyer-Goodwin, W. E., Cefalo, R. C. Thermo-regulation of pregnant women during aerobic exercise on land and in water. *American Journal of Perinatology* 10 no. 2 (Mar. 1993): 178–82.

MacPhail, A., Davies, G. A., Victory, R., Wolfe, L. A. Maximal exercise testing in late gestation: fetal responses. *Obstetrics and Gynecology* 96 no. 4 (Oct. 2000): 565–70.

Manders, M. A., Sonders, G. J., Mulder, E. J., Visser, G. H. The effects of maternal exercise on fetal heart rate and movement patterns. *Early Human Development* 48 no. 3 (May 1997): 237–47.

Marquez-Sterling, S., Perry, A. C., Kaplan, T. A., Halberstein, R. A., Signorile, J. F. Physical and psychological changes with vigorous exercise in sedentary primigravidae. *Medicine and Science in Sports and Exercise* 32 (Jan. 2000): 58–62.

Milgrom, P., Riedy, C. A., Weinstein, P., Tanner, A. C., Manibusan, L., Bruss, J. Dental caries and its relationship to bacterial infection, hypoplasia, diet, and oral hygiene in 6- to 36-month-old children. *Community Dental and Oral Epidemiology* 28 no. 4 (Aug. 2000): 295–306.

Planning Your Pregnancy and Birth, 3rd ed. Washington, D.C.: American College of Obstetricians and Gynecologists, 2000.

Riemann, M. K., Kanstrup Hansen, I. L. Effects on the foetus of exercise in pregnancy. *Scandinavian Journal of Medicine & Science in Sports* 10 no. 1 (Feb. 2000): 12–9.

Vinitketkumnuen, U., Chewonarin, T., Kongtawelert, P., Lertjanyarak, A., Peerakhom, S., Wild, C. P. Aflatoxin exposure is higher in vegetarians than in nonvegetarians in Thailand. *Natural Toxins* 5 no. 4 (1997): 168–71.

Whitaker, T. B., Springer, J., Defize, P. R., deKoe, W. J., Coker, R. Evaluation of sampling plans used in the United States, United Kingdom, and the Netherlands to test raw shelled peanuts for aflatoxin. *Journal of Association of Annals of Chemistry* 78 no. 4 (July–Aug. 1995): 1010–8.

Wolfe, L. A., Mottola, M. F. Aerobic exercise in pregnancy: an update. *Canadian Journal of Applied Physiology* 18 no. 2 (June 1993): 119–47.

Wood, G. E. Aflatoxins in domestic and imported feeds. *Journal of Association of Annals of Chemistry* 72 no. 4 (July–Aug. 1989): 543–8.

Chapter 6: YOUR FOURTH MONTH

Andre, J., Boudou, A., Ribeyre, F., Bernhard, M. Comparative study of mercury accumulation in dolphins (*Stenella coeruleoalba*) from French Atlantic and Mediterranean coasts. *Science of the Total Environment* 104 no. 3 (May 15, 1991): 191–209.

Blais, M. A., Becker, A. E., Burwell, R. A., et al. Pregnancy: outcome and impact on symptomatology in a cohort of eating-disordered women. *International Journal of Eating Disorders* 27 no. 2 (Mar. 2000): 140–9.

Brown, P. The risk of bovine spongiform encephalopathy ("mad cow disease") to human health. *Journal of the American Medical Association* 278 no. 12 (Sept. 1997): 1008–11.

Burket, R. C., Hodgin, J. D. Factors predicting reluctance to seek treatment in patients with eating disorders. *Southern Medical Journal* 86 no. 5 (May 1993): 529–32.

Campbell, T. C. Diet, lifestyle, coronary disease. *American Journal of Cardiology* 82 no. 10B (Nov. 26, 1998): 18T–21T.

Conti, J., Abraham, S., Taylor, A. Eating behavior and pregnancy outcome. *Journal of Psychosomatic Research* 44 (Mar.–Apr. 1998): 465–77.

Curk, A. Bovine spongiform encephalopathy crisis in Europe and its impact on beef consumption in Slovenia. *Review of Science Technology* 18 no. 30 (Dec. 1999): 758–63.

Dalgard, C., Grandjean, P., Jorgensen, P. J., Weihe, P. Mercury in the umbilical cord: Implications for risk assessment for Minamata disease. *Environmental Health Perspectives* 102 nos. 6–7 (June 1994): 548–50.

Despommier, D. D., Gwadz, R. W., Hotez, P. J. *Parasitic Diseases*, 3rd ed. New York: Springer-Verlag, 1995.

Fairburn, C. G., Stein, A., Jones, R. Eating habits and eating disorders during pregnancy. *Psychosomatic Medicine* 54 no. 6 (Nov.–Dec. 1992): 665–72.

Franko, D. L., Spurrell, E. B. Detection and management of eating disorders during pregnancy. *Obstetrics and Gynecology* 95 pt. 1 (June 2000): 942–6.

Gamble, H. R. Parasites associated with pork and pork products. *Review of Science Technology* 16 no. 2 (Aug. 1997): 496–506.

Garcia, H. H., Del Brutto, O. H. Taenia solium cysticerosis. *Infectious Disease Clinics of North America* 14 no. 1 (Mar. 2000): 97–119.

Grandjean, P., Weihe, P., Needham, L. L., et al. Relation of a seafood diet to mercury, selenium, arsenic, and polychlorinated biphenyl and other organochlorine concentrations in human milk. *Environmental Research* 71 no. 1 (Oct. 1995): 29–38.

Grandjean, P., Weihe, P., White, R. F., et al. Cognitive deficit in 7-year-old children with prenatal exposure to methylmercury. *Neurotoxicology and Teratology* 19 no. 6 (Nov.–Dec. 1997): 417–28.

Groschup, M. H. Bovine spongiform encephalopathy in ruminants and the new variant of Creutzfeldt-Jakob disease in humans. *Deutsche Tierarztliche Wochenschrifte* 106 (Aug. 1999): 329–31.

Harrison, L. J. Poisonous marine morsels. *Journal of the Florida Medical Association* 78 no. 4 (Apr. 1991): 219–21.

Hillerton, J. E. Bovine spongiform encephalopathy: current status and possible impacts. *Journal of Dairy Science* 8 (Nov. 1998): 3042–8.

Josephson, J. Cows for fear: is BSE a threat to human health? *Environmental Health Perspectives* 106 no. 3 (Mar. 1998): A134–8.

Kannan, K., Smith, R. G. Jr., Lee, R. F., et al. Distribution of total methyl mercury in water, sediment, and fish from south Florida estuaries. *Archives of Environment Contamination and Toxicology* 34 no. 2 (Feb. 1998): 109–18.

Koli, A. K., Williams, W. R., McClary, E. B., Wright, E. L., Burrell, T. M. Mercury levels in freshwater fish of the state of South Carolina. *Bulletin of Environmental Contamination Toxicology* 17 no. 1 (Jan. 1997): 82–9.

Lipp, E. K., Rose, J. B. The role of seafood in foodborne diseases in the United States of America. *Review of Science and Technology* 16 no. 2 (Aug. 1997): 620–4.

Mabs, D. Occurence and sequestration of toxins in food chains. *Toxicology* 36 (Nov. 1998): 1519–22.

Meat eaters gain weight. *Good Medicine* 6 no. 4 (1997): 4.

Meyers, G. J., Davidson, P. W. Does methylmercury have a role in causing developmental disabilities in children? *Environmental Health Perspectives* 108 suppl. 3 (June 2000): 413–20.

Mines, D., Stahmer, S., Shepherd, S. M. Poisonings: food, fish, shellfish. *Emergency Medicine Clinics of North America* 15 no. 1 (Feb. 1997): 157–77.

Morehead, A., Grunenwald, P. E., Dietz, V. J., Schantz, P. M. Trichinellosis in the United States, 1991–1996: declining but not gone. *American Journal of Tropical Medicine and Hygiene* 60 (Jan. 1999): 66–9.

Morgan, J. F., Lacey, J. H., Sedgwick, P. M. Impact of pregnancy on bulimia nervosa. *British Journal of Psychiatry* 174 (Feb. 1999): 135–40.

Oskarsson, A., Lagerkvist, B. J., Ohlin, B., Lundberg, K. Mercury levels in hair of pregnant women in polluted area in Sweden. *Science of the Total Environment* 151 no. 4 (July 4, 1994): 29–35.

Pennington, J., Bowes, A., Church, H. *Bowes & Church's Food Values of Portions Commonly Used,* 14th ed. New York: HarperCollins, 1984.

Pilgrim, W., Poissant, L., Trip, L. The northeast states and eastern Canadian provinces mercury study: a framework for action; summary of the Canadian chapter. *Science of the Total Environment* 261 nos. 1–3 (Oct. 16, 2000): 177–84.

Stack, P. S. Trichinosis. Still a public health threat. *Postgraduate Medicine* 97 (June 1995): 137–9, 143–4.

Stegink, L. D., Pritkin, R. M., Reynolds, W. A., Filer, L. J. Jr., Boaz, D. P., Brummel, M. C. Placental transfer of glutamate and its metabolites in the primate. *American Journal of Obstetrics and Gynecology* 122 no. 1 (May 1975): 70–8.

Steuerwald, U., Weile, P., Jorgensen, P. J., et al. Maternal seafood diet, methylmercury exposure, and neonatal neurologic function. *Journal of Pediatrics* 136 no. 5 (May 2000): 599–605.

Tan, L., Williams, M. A., Khan, M. K., Champion, H. C., Nielson, N. H. Risk of transmission of bovine spongiform encephalopathy to humans in the United States: report of the Council of Scientific Affairs. American Medical Association. *Journal of the American Medical Association* 281 no. 24 (June 23–30, 1999): 2330–9.

Taylor, D. M., Woodgate, S. L. Bovine spongiform encephalopathy: the causal role of ruminant-derived protein in cattle diets. *Review of Science Technology* 16 no. 1 (Apr. 1997): 187–98.

Todd, E. C. Seafood associated diseases and control in Canada. *Review of Science and Technology* 16 no. 2 (Aug. 1997): 661–72.

Tosteson, T. R. The diversity of origins of toxins in ciguatera fish poisoning. *Puerto Rican Health Science Journal* 14 no. 2 (June 1995): 117–29.

Toth, L., Karesu, S., Feledi, J., Kreutzberg, G. W. Neurotoxicity of monosodium-L-glutamate in pregnant and fetal rats. *ACTA Neuropathologica* (Berlin) 75 no. 1 (1987): 16–22.

Trevino, S. Fish and shellfish poisoning. *Clinical Laboratory Science* 11 no. 5 (Sept.–Oct. 1998): 309–14.

Walker, R. The significance of excursions above ADI. Case study: monosodium glutamate. *Regulatory Toxicology and Pharmacology* 30 no. 2, pt. 2 (Oct. 1999): S119–21.

Waugh, E., Bulik, C. M. Offspring of women with eating disorders. *International Journal of Eating Disorders* 25 no. 2 (Mar. 1999): 123–33.

Chapter 7: YOUR FIFTH MONTH

Ferrero, M., Ducons, J. A., Sicilia, B., Santolaria, S., Sierra, E., Gomollon, F. Factors affecting the variation in antibiotic resistance of *Helicobacter pylori* over a 3-year period. *International Journal of Antimicrobial Agents* 16 no. 3 (Nov. 2000): 245–8.

Gompel, A., Truc, J. B. Role of calcium at different ages. *Presse Medicale* (Paris) 22 no. 18 (May 22, 1993): 864–9.

Jones, G., Riley, M. D., Dwyer, T. Maternal diet during pregnancy is associated with bone mineral density in children: a longitudinal study. *European Journal of Clinical Nutrition* 54 no. 10 (Oct. 2000): 749–56.

Phillips, A. J., Ostlere, S. J. Pregnancy-associated osteoporosis. *Osteoporosis International* 11 no. 5 (2000): 449–54.

Power, M. L., Heaney, R. P. Role of calcium in health and disease. *American Journal of Obstetrics and Gynecology* 181 no. 6 (Dec. 1999): 1560–9.

Serenius, F., Elidrissy, A. T., Dandona, P. Vitamin D nutrition in pregnant women at term and in newly born babies in Saudi Arabia. *Journal of Clinical Pathology* 37 no. 4 (Apr. 1984): 444–7.

Topping, J., Black, A. J. Osteoporosis in pregnancy. *Professional Care of Mother and Child* 8 no. 6 (1998): 147–50.

Warren, J. R. Gastric pathology associated with *Helicobacter pylori*. *Gastroenterology Clinics of North America* 29 no. 3 (Sept. 2000): 705–51.

Chapter 8: YOUR SIXTH MONTH

Diabetes and Pregnancy. ACOG Technical Bulletin 200 (Dec. 1994). American College of Obstetricians and Gynecologists, Washington, D.C.

Suzuki, S., Dennerstein, L., Greenwood, K. M., Armstrong, S. M., Satohisa, E. Sleeping patterns during pregnancy in Japanese women. *Journal of Psychosomatic Obstetrics and Gynaecology* 15 no. 1 (Mar. 1994): 19–26.

Thyroid Disease in Pregnancy. ACOG Technical Bulletin 181 (June 1993). American College of Obstetricians and Gynecologists, Washington, D.C.

Chapter 9: YOUR SEVENTH MONTH

Burkitt, D. P. Varicose veins: facts and fantasy. *Archives of Surgery* 111 no. 12 (Dec. 1976): 1327–32.

Cornu-Thenard, A., Boivin, P. Importance of familial factor in varicose disease. *Journal of Dermatology and Surgical Oncology* 20 no. 5 (May 1994): 318–26.

Creasy, R. K., Resnick, R. Biologic adaptation to pregnancy. *Maternal-Fetal Medicine,* 3rd ed. Philadelphia: W. B. Saunders, 1989.

Di Cintio, E., Parazzini, F., Rosa, C., Chatenoud, L., Benizi, G. The epidemiology of gestational trophoblastic disease. *General and Diagnostic Pathology* 143 nos. 2–3 (Nov. 1997): 103–8.

Hypertension in Pregnancy. ACOG Technical Bulletin 219 (Jan. 1996). American College of Obstetricians and Gynecologists, Washington, D.C.

Lopez-Jaramillo, P. Calcium, nitric oxide, and preeclampsia. *Seminars in Perinatology* 24 no. 1 (Feb. 2000): 33–6.

Lopez-Jaramillo, P., Teran, E., Moncada, S. Calcium supplementation prevents pregnancy-induced hypertension by increasing the production of vascular nitric oxide. *Medical Hypothesis* 45 no. 1 (July 1995): 68–72.

Management of Gestational Trophoblastic Disease. ACOG Technical Bulletin 178 (March 1993). American College of Obstetricians and Gynecologists, Washington, D.C.

Martin, P. M. High frequency of hydatidiform mole in native Alaskans. *International Journal of Gynaecology and Obstetrics* 15 no. 5 (1978): 395–6.

Melet, J. J. Western diet: risk for varices. *Phlebologie* 34 no. 2 (Apr.–June 1981): 235–43.

Melet, J. J. The importance of nutrition among the risk factors in varicose veins. *Phlebologie* 34 no. 3 (July–Sept. 1981): 469–88.

Palmer, J. R. Advances in the epidemiology of gestational trophoblastic disease. *Journal of Reproductive Medicine* 39 no. 3 (Mar. 1994): 155–62.

Chapter 10: YOUR EIGHTH MONTH

Abitbol, M. M., Taylor-Randall, U. B., Barton, P. T., Thompson, E. Effect of modern obstetrics on mothers from the Third-World countries. *Journal of Maternal and Fetal Medicine* 6 no. 5 (Sept.–Oct. 1997): 276–80.

Bridges, A. J., Vasey, F. B. Silicone breast implants. History, safety, and potential complications. *Archives of Internal Medicine* 153 no. 23 (Dec. 1993): 2638–44.

Brzozowski, D., Niessen, M., Evans, H. B., Hurst, L. N. Breast-feeding after inferior pedicle reduction mammoplasty. *Plastic and Reconstructive Surgery* 105 no. 2 (Feb. 2000): 530.

Grant, S., Edelman, D. A. Pregnancy, lactation and the use of silicone breast implants. *Advances in Contraception* 10 no. 3 (Sept. 1994): 187–93.

Harris, L., Morris, S. F., Friedberg, A. Is breast-feeding possible after re-duction mammoplasty? *Plastic and Reconstructive Surgery* 89 no. 5 (May 1992): 836–9.

Marshall, D. R., Callan, P. P., Nicholson, W. Breastfeeding after reduction mammoplasty. *British Journal of Plastic Surgery* 47 no. 3 (Apr. 1994): 167–9.

Mathews, F., Yudkin, P., Neil, A. Influence of maternal nutrition on out-come of pregnancy. *British Medical Journal* 319 no. 7206 (Aug. 7, 1999): 339–43.

Reddy, S., Sanders, T. A. B., Obeid, O. Influence of maternal diet. *European Journal of Clinical Nutrition* 48 (1994): 358–68.

Chapter 11: YOUR NINTH MONTH AND LABOR

Buggy, D., Hughes, N., Gardiner, J. Posterior column sensory impair-ment during ambulatory extradural analgesia in labour. *British Jour-nal of Anaesthesiology* 73 no. 4 (Oct. 1994): 540–2.

Collis, R. E., Harding, S. A., Morgan, B. M. Effect of maternal ambulation on labour with low-dose combined spinal-epidural analgesia. *Anesthesia* 54 no. 6 (June 1999): 535–9.

Dystocia and the Augmentation of Labor. ACOG Technical Bulletin 218 (Dec. 1995). American College of Obstetricians and Gynecologists, Washington, D.C.

Fernandez-Guisasola, J., Garcia del Valle, S., Gomez-Arnau, J. I. Com-bined subarachnoid-epidural technique for obstetric analgesia. *Revista Espagnola de Anestesiologia y Reanimacion* 47 no. 5 (May 2000): 207–15.

Fetal Heart Rate Monitoring: Monitoring, Interpretation, and Man-agement. ACOG Technical Bulletin 207 (July 1995). American College of Obstetricians and Gynecologists, Washington, D.C.

Harper, B. *Gentle Birth Choices.* Rochester, Vt.: Healing Arts Press, 1994.

Induction of Labor. ACOG Practice Bulletin 10 (Nov. 1999). American College of Obstetricians and Gynecologists, Washington, D.C.

Nikodem, V. C. Immersion in water in pregnancy, labor and birth. *Cochrane Database Systems Review* 2 (2000): CD000111.

Obstetrical Analgesia and Anesthesia. ACOG Technical Bulletin 225 (July 1996). American College of Obstetricians and Gynecologists, Washington, D.C.

Operative Vaginal Delivery. ACOG Practice Bulletin 17 (June 2000). American College of Obstetricians and Gynecologists, Washington, D.C.

Prolog Obstetrics, 4th ed. Washington, D.C.: American College of Obstetricians and Gynecologists, 1998.

Rate of Vaginal Births After Cesarean Delivery. ACOG Committee Opinion 179 (Nov. 1996). American College of Obstetricians and Gynecologists, Washington, D.C.

Schauble, P. G., Werner, W. E., Rai, S. H., Martin, A. Childbirth preparation through hypnosis: the hypnoreflexogenous protocol. *American Journal of Clinical Hypnosis* 40 no. 4 (Apr. 1998): 273–83.

Shennan, A., Cooke, V., Lloyd-Jones, F., Morgan, B., de Sweit, M. Blood pressure changes during labour and whilst ambulating with combined spinal epidural analgesia. *British Journal of Obstetrics and Gynaecology* 102 no. 3 (Mar. 1995): 192–7.

Sleutel, M., Golden, S. S. Fasting in labor: relic or requirement. *Journal of Obstetric, Gynecologic, and Neonatal Nursing* 28 no. 5 (Sept.–Oct. 1999): 507–12.

Use and Abuse of the Apgar Score. ACOG Committee Opinion 174 (July 1996). American College of Obstetricians and Gynecologists, Washington, D.C.

Vaginal Birth After Previous Cesarean Delivery. ACOG Practice Bulletin 5 (July 1999). American College of Obstetricians and Gynecologists, Washington, D.C.

Vaginal Birth After Previous Vaginal Delivery. ACOG Practice Bulletin 5 (July 1999). American College of Obstetricians and Gynecologists, Washington, D.C.

Chapter 12: NURSING AS A VEGETARIAN

Breastfeeding: Maternal and Infant Aspects. ACOG Educational Bulletin 258 (July 2000). American College of Obstetricians and Gynecologists, Washington, D.C.

Martin, C. *The Nursing Mother's Problem Solver.* New York: Simon & Schuster, 2000.

Melton, L. J. III, Bryant, S. C. Influence of breast feeding on bone mass. *Osteoporosis International* 3 no. 2 (Mar. 1993): 76–83.

Zemlickis, D., Lishner, M., Degendorfer, P., et al. Maternal and fetal outcome after breast cancer in pregnancy. *American Journal of Obstetrics and Gynecology* 166 (1992): 781–7.

Index